STEWART HOCKENBERRY

Gateway to Memory

Issues in Clinical and Cognitive Neuropsychology
Jordan Grafman, series editor

Patient-Based Approaches to Cognitive Neuroscience, edited by Martha J. Farah
and Todd E. Feinberg, 1999

*Gateway to Memory: An Introduction to Neural Network Modeling of the
Hippocampus and Learning,* Mark A. Gluck and Catherine E. Myers, 2001

Gateway to Memory

An Introduction to Neural Network Modeling of the
Hippocampus and Learning

Mark A. Gluck and Catherine E. Myers

A Bradford Book
The MIT Press
Cambridge, Massachusetts
London, England

This book was set in Palatino by Interactive Composition Corporation

Printed and bound in the United States of America.

Library of Congress Cataloging-in-Publication Data

Gluck, Mark A.
    Gateway to memory : an introduction to neural network modeling of the
hippocampus and learning / Mark A. Gluck and Catherine E. Myers.
        p.   cm.
    "A Bradford book."
    ISBN 0-262-07211-4
    1. Hippocampus (Brain)—Computer simulation. 2. Neural networks
(Neurobiology). 3. Memory—Computer simulation. I. Myers, Catherine.
II. Title.
QP383.25 .G58 2000
612.8′2′0113—dc21   00-058681

To Herman R. Gluck,
   mentor and muse.
          —M.A.G.

To Harriet F. Kihlstrom,
   for everything, especially the scones.
                    —C.E.M.

Contents

Preface

Have computational models really advanced our understanding of the neural bases of learning and memory? If so, is it possible to learn about them without delving into the mathematical details? These two questions, asked over and over again by many colleagues, have inspired us to write this book.

Some of these colleagues were experimental psychologists who wished to understand how behavioral theories could be informed by neuroscience; others were neuroscientists seeking to bridge the conceptual gap from studies of individual neurons to behaviors of whole organisms. Clinical neurologists and neuropsychologists have also asked us whether neural network models might provide them with clinically useful insights into disorders of learning and memory. Unfortunately, many of these people found that their initial interest in modeling was thwarted by the mathematical details found in most papers and textbooks on computational neuroscience. Unable to follow the mathematics, these aspiring readers were left with the options of either accepting the author's conclusions on blind faith or ignoring them altogether.

Mathematics has long had the ability to inspire apprehension and awe among those not trained in its formalisms. A story is often told about the eighteenth century mathematician Léonard Euler, who was summoned to the court of Catherine the Great, the Czarina of Russia. She commissioned him to debate the French philosopher Diderot, who had offended her by questioning the existence of God and encouraging the spread of atheism in her court.

Appearing before the assembled courtiers, the two men faced off. Euler went first and announced that he had a mathematical proof of the existence of God. Advancing toward Diderot, Euler gravely explained:

"Monsieur, $(a + b^n)/n = x$, hence God exists!"

Of course, this claim was nonsensical, but Diderot—who understood no mathematics—could not make any response or rebuttal, and Euler won the argument by default. Soon after, Diderot left the royal court and returned to his native France.

Although mathematicians sometimes tell this anecdote to poke fun at the uninitiated, there is another more serious side to this tale. Euler won the debate not because his claims were valid, but simply because he couched his argument in mathematical jargon too esoteric for Diderot to understand. Over two hundred years later, researchers who develop computational models of brain and behavior still sometimes use the same ploy: masking their descriptions in complex mathematical equations that only other mathematicians can easily evaluate. This leaves the reader who lacks such training with two equally unpalatable options: either accept the modelers' (often grandiose) claims at face value or else—like Diderot—simply walk away.

However, we think there is a middle ground. It should be possible to communicate the fundamentals of connectionist modeling to a broader scientific community, by focusing on the underlying principles rather than the mathematical nuts and bolts. Like electrophysiology or neuroimaging, computational modeling is a tool for neuroscience and, while the methodological details are important, it is possible to appreciate the utility—and limitations—of these techniques without absorbing all the technical details. To this end, we have tried to describe the computational models in this book at an intuitive rather than a technical level, using illustrations and examples rather than equations. We have assumed no prior knowledge of computational modeling or mathematics on the part of the reader. For those who wish to delve more deeply into the formal details of the models, we have provided supplemental (but optional) MathBoxes, which appear throughout the text, as well as appendices that contain further implementation details for the model simulations.

We have two groups of readers in mind for this book: those with a specific interest in learning and memory and those who want to understand a sample case study illustrating how computational models have been integrated into an experimental program of research. To this broad readership, we have aimed to convey an intuitive understanding and appreciation of the promise, as well as the limits, of neural network models. If at the same time we excite a few of our readers to go on to become modelers themselves or to incorporate computational modeling into their own research programs through collaboration with modelers, all the better.

We believe that good models are born amidst a wealth of experimental studies and justify their existence by inspiring further empirical research. We had this in mind when we chose the word "modeling" rather than "models" in our subtitle: The emphasis here is on the process of modeling within the broader program of learning and memory research, rather than on the fine details of the models themselves. In contrast to the individual journal papers in which many of these modeling results were first reported, we have sought to convey a larger and more integrative picture here. This book tells the story of how models are built on prior experimental data and theoretical insights and then evolve toward a more comprehensive and coherent interpretation of a wide body of neurobiological and behavioral data.

We wrote this book in two parts. Part I (chapters 1 through 5) provides a tutorial introduction to selected topics in neuroscience, the psychology of learning and memory, and the theory of neural network models—all at the level of an advanced undergraduate textbook. We expect that some of this will be too elementary for many readers and therefore can be skipped, while other chapters will provide background material essential for understanding the second half of the book. Together, these early chapters are designed to level the playing field so that the book is accessible to anyone in the behavioral and neural sciences.

Part II, the core of the book, presents our current understanding of how the hippocampus cooperates with these other brain structures to support learning and memory in both animals and humans. In trying to answer the question, "What does the hippocampus do?" researchers have been forced to look beyond the hippocampus to seek a better understanding of the hippocampus's many partners in learning and memory, including the entorhinal cortex, the basal forebrain, the cerebellum, and the primary sensory and motor cortices.

Our emphasis throughout this book is on the function of brain structures as they give rise to behavior, rather than the molecular or neuronal details. Reflecting this functional approach to brain modeling, many of the models that we describe have their roots in psychological theories and research. We believe that appreciating these psychological roots is of more than just historical curiosity; rather, understanding how modern neural networks relate to well-studied models of learning in psychology provides us with an invaluable aid in understanding current efforts to develop models of the brain mechanisms of learning and memory.

In addition to covering our own theories and models in part II of the book, we review several related computational models, along with other qualitative and experimental studies of the neurobiology of learning and memory. In covering a range of models from a variety of researchers, we have tried to convey how it is possible for different models to capture different aspects of anatomy and physiology and different kinds of behaviors. In many cases, these models complement each other, the assumptions of one model being derived from the implications of another.

Given the wide range of academic disciplines covered in this book, many terms are used that may be unfamiliar to readers. The most important of these are printed in boldface when they first appear in the text and are accompanied there by a brief definition. These terms and definitions are then repeated at the end of the book in a glossary for easy reference.

Mark A. Gluck
Catherine E. Myers

Acknowledgments

We are indebted to many people who helped make this book, and our research, possible.

For their helpful comments and advice on select chapters of the first draft of the book, we are grateful to many friends and colleagues, including Gordon Bower, Gyorgy Buzsáki, Helena Edelson, Howard Eichenbaum, Jordan Grafman, Michael Hasselmo, Chip Levy, Somporn Onloar, Nestor Schmajuk, Larry Squire, Paula Tallal, Richard Thompson, and David Touretzky.

Special thanks to Herman Gluck, who read and commented on each chapter in many early drafts and who often served as a model reader through long discussions on how to present this material in a manner accessible to the nonspecialist.

Many students and postdoctoral fellows in our lab at Rutgers-Newark contributed to the research reported here and read and commented on early drafts of the book. For these efforts, we are indebted to M. Todd Allen, Danielle Carlin, Judith Creso, Brandon Ermita, Eduardo Mercado, Itzel Orduna, Bas Rokers, Geoff Schnirman, Daphna Shohamy, Adriaan Tijselling, and Stacey Warren. Several Rutgers-Newark undergraduates contributed throughout the years to our research and to pulling this book together; these include Christopher Bellotti, George Chatzopoulos, Arthur Fontanilla, Omar Haneef, Adrianna Herrera, Valerie Hutchison, Alexander Izaguirre, Priya Khanna, Timothy Laskis, Vivek Masand, Omar Nabulsi, Yahiara Padilla, Bettie Parker, Anand Pathuri, Teresa Realpe, Janet Schultz, Souty Shafik, Omar Toor, and many others. And keeping all the people and material organized and flowing smoothly would not have been possible without the efforts of Connie Sadaka. The laboratories, resources, and environment within which we conducted all of our own research reported here, as well as wrote this book, would not have been possible without the support of Ian Creese and Paula Tallal (Co-directors of the Center for Molecular and Behavioral Neuroscience, Rutgers-Newark) and Stephen José Hanson (Chair of Psychology, Rutgers-Newark).

We are indebted to the agencies, foundations, and organizations that provided financial support for our research and the writing of this book: the Alzheimer's Association, the Healthcare Foundation of New Jersey (especially Ellen Kramer), Hoechst-Celanese Corporation, Johnson & Johnson Corporation, the James S. McDonnell Foundation, the Pew Charitable Trusts, the National Institute of Mental Health, the National Institute on Aging, the National Science Foundation, the Office of Naval Research (especially Joel Davis, for fifteen years of continuous support), and Rutgers University (especially Associate Provost Harvey Feder).

Our editor at MIT Press, Michael Rutter—along with Sara Meirowitz—showed valiant persistence, unflagging energy, and deep enthusiasm throughout the project. We are grateful to them, to Peggy Gordon, and to the rest of the production, graphics, and marketing staff at MIT Press for seeing this book through to the final finished product.

Mark A. Gluck
Catherine E. Myers

I Fundamentals

1 Introduction

1.1 COMPUTATIONAL MODELS AS TOOLS

At some point in our childhood, many of us played with model planes made of balsa wood or cardboard. Such models often have flat wings and a twisted rubber band connected to a small propeller; when the plane is launched into the air, the tension on the rubber band is released, driving the propeller to spin, and the plane soars through the air for a few minutes of flight. A future scientist playing with such a toy could learn many general principles of aviation; for example, in both the toy plane and a Boeing 747, stored energy is converted to rotary motion, which provides the forward speed to create lift and keep the plane in the air.

Aerodynamic engineers use other types of airplane models. In the early days of aviation, new planes were developed by using wooden models of airplane shapes, which were placed in wind tunnels to test how the air flowed across the wings and body. Nowadays, much of the design and testing is done with computer models rather than wooden miniatures in wind tunnels. Nevertheless, these computer-generated models accomplish the same task: They extract and simplify the essence of the plane's shape and predict how this shape will interact with wind flow.

Unlike the toy airplane, the engineer's aerodynamic model has no source of propulsion and cannot fly on its own. This does not mean that the toy airplane is a better model of a real airplane. Rather, each model focuses on a different aspect of a real airplane, capturing some properties of airplane flight. *The value of these models is intrinsically tied to the needs of the user; each captures a different design principle of real planes.*

A model is a simplified version of some complex object or phenomenon. The model may be physical (like the engineer's wind tunnel) or virtual (like the computer simulation). In either case, it is intended to capture some of the properties of the object being modeled while disregarding others that, for the time being, are thought to be nonessential for the task at hand. Models are especially useful for testing the predictive and explanatory value of abstract theories. Thus, in the above examples, theories of propulsion and lift can be tested with the toy plane, while theories of aerodynamic flow and turbulence can be tested with the engineer's wind tunnel model or the computer simulation of that wind tunnel.

Of course, these are not the only models that could be used to test principles of aviation; many different models could be constructed to test the same ideas. The superficial convergence of a model and the world does not prove that the model is correct, only that it is plausible.

We believe that models should be evaluated primarily in accord with how useful they are for discovering and expressing important regularities and principles in the world. Like a hammer, a model is a tool that is useful for some tasks. However, no single tool in a carpenter's kit is the most correct; similarly no single model of the brain, or of a specific brain region, is the most correct. Rather, different models work together to answer different questions.

In evaluating a model's usefulness, it is important to keep in mind that the utility of a model depends not only on how faithful it is to the real object, but also on how many irrelevant details it eliminates. For example, neither the rubber-band toy nor the aerodynamic model incorporates passenger seating or cockpit radar, even though both features are critical to a real airplane. These additions would not improve the toy plane's ability to fly, nor would they add to the engineers' study of wind resistance. Adding such details would be a waste of time and resources and would distract the user from the core properties being studied.

The ideals of simplicity and utility also apply to brain models. Some basic aspects of brain function are best understood by looking at simple models that embody one or two general principles without attempting to capture all the boggling complexity of the entire brain. By eliminating all details except the essential properties being studied, these models allow researchers to investigate one or two features at a time. *By simplifying and isolating core principles of brain design, models help us to understand which aspects of brain anatomy, circuitry, and neural function are responsible for particular types of behaviors.* In this way, models are especially important tools for building conceptual bridges between neuroscience and psychological studies of behavior.

The brain models presented in this book are all simulated within computers, as are the aerodynamic models used by modern airplane designers. Chapters 3 through 5 will explain in more detail how such computer simulations of neural network models are created and applied.

Most of the research described in this book proceeds as follows. A body of behavioral and neurobiological data is defined, fundamental principles and regularities are identified, and then a model is developed and implemented as a computer simulation of the relevant brain circuits and their putative functions. Often, these brain models include several components, each of which corresponds to a functionally different region of the brain. For example, there might be one model component that corresponds to the cerebral cortex, one for the subcortical areas of the brain, and so forth. By observing how these components interact in the model, we may learn something about how the corresponding brain regions interact to process information in the normal brain.

Once we are confident that a model captures observed learning and memory behaviors and reflects the anatomy of an intact brain, we can then ask what happens when one or more model brain regions are removed or damaged. We would hope that the remaining parts of the model behave like a human or animal with analogous brain damage. If the behaviors of the brain-damaged model match the behaviors of animals or people with similar damage, this is evidence that the model is on the right track. This is the approach taken by many of the models presented in this book.

The usefulness of the models as tools for furthering research comes from novel predictions that the models make. For example, the model might predict that a particular form of brain damage will alter learning and memory in a particular way. These predictions are especially useful if the predictions are surprising or somehow unexpected given past behaviors or data. If the predictions are correct, this strengthens one's confidence in the model; if the predictions are incorrect, this leads to revisions in the model.

However, even a model of relatively simple behaviors can quickly become so complex that it seems an advanced degree in mathematics is required just to understand it. When theories and models are comprehensible only to other modelers, they lose their ability to function as effective tools for guiding empirical research. Rather, *it should be possible for most psychologists and neuroscientists to understand the intuitive ideas behind a computational model without getting mired in the details.*

In this book we have tried to summarize—at a conceptual level—neural network modeling of hippocampal function with little or no reference to the underlying math.

1.2 GOALS AND STRUCTURE OF THIS BOOK

The goal of the first five chapters—constituting part I—is to level the playing field so that the rest of the book is accessible to anyone in the behavioral and neural sciences, including clinical practitioners such as neuropsychologists, psychiatrists, and neurologists.

Some of the material in part I is likely to be too elementary for many readers. For example, we expect that many neuroscientists and their graduate students will be able to skip chapter 2 ("The Hippocampus in Learning and Memory") because that material is covered in most neuroscience graduate programs (and some psychology programs). In contrast, chapters 3 through 5 cover material that is likely to be too rudimentary for computer scientists, engineers, and others with a strong background in the formal basis of neural network models. These readers may wish to skip from chapter 2 to chapter 6, the beginning of part II.

As a caveat, we note that the tutorial material in part I does not conform to the standard organization and scope found in most textbooks. Rather, we have given the material our own spin, emphasizing the themes and issues that we believe are most essential to appreciating the models and research presented in the second half of the book.

For example, our coverage of the hippocampus and memory in chapter 2 focuses not on the more traditionally recognized hippocampal-dependent behaviors—such as the recall of past episodes or explicit facts—but rather on simpler behaviors, especially classical Pavlovian conditioning, that have formed the basis for a great deal of computational modeling.

To better understand the methods of information-processing theories of brain function, chapters 3 through 5 provide an introduction to the fundamentals of neural network modeling. Again, this tutorial is nonstandard in that it emphasizes the historical roots of neural network theories within psychological theories of learning and the relevance of these issues to modern studies of the hippocampus and learning behaviors.

Chapter 3 serves as an introduction to simple neural network models. It focuses on learning rules used for the formation of associations and the relevance of these rules to understanding the neural circuits necessary for classical conditioning. For continuity with the rest of the book, these networks will be illustrated through their application to classical conditioning. In this chapter, we introduce an early forerunner of modern neural network theories: the Rescorla-Wagner model of classical conditioning, which is in many ways a "model" model. It has stood for nearly thirty years as an example of how it is possible to take a set of complex behaviors, pare away all but the essence, and express the underlying mechanism as an intuitively tractable idea. Moreover, it now appears that the Rescorla-Wagner model may be more than just a psychological description of learning; it may also capture important properties of the kinds of learning that occur outside the hippocampus, especially in the cerebellum.

Chapter 4 introduces a fundamental problem that is common to the fields of psychology, neuroscience, and neural networks: How are events in the outside world transformed into their neural representations, that is, the corresponding physical changes and processes within the brain? Researchers from each discipline have grappled for years with the problem of representation, and each group has added important novel insights to our understanding of this problem.

Chapter 5 considers how animals and people learn from just the mere exposure to stimuli and what kinds of neural networks can capture this type of learning. It introduces a class of neural network architectures, called autoassociators, which have often been used to describe the functional significance of the very specialized circuitry found in the hippocampus. Interestingly, it is exactly this kind of learning from mere exposure that seems to be especially sensitive to hippocampal-region damage in animals. In addition, an autoassociator is capable of storing arbitrary memories and later retrieving them when given partial cues—exactly the sort of memory ability that is lost in amnesic patients with hippocampal-region damage.

This completes part I.

Part II of the book gets into the details of modeling hippocampal function in learning. Chapters 6 through 10 share a common format and organization. Each introduces a different behavioral or neurobiological phenomenon, reviews one or more computational models of these phenomena, relates these models to qualitative (noncomputational) theories of learning and the brain, and then closes with a discussion of the implications of these models for understanding human memory and its clinical disorders.

Chapter 6 builds on the discussions in chapters 4 and 5 of representation and mere-exposure learning and describes how these issues have motivated two different models of the interaction between the hippocampus and cortex during associative learning. These hippocampal models are compared to several qualitative noncomputational theories of the interaction between the hippocampus and cortex. The chapter shows how modeling of animal conditioning has led to new insights into why brain-damaged amnesic patients can sometimes learn associations faster than normal control subjects.

Chapter 7 focuses on the role of the hippocampus and medial temporal lobes in the processing of background stimuli such as the constant sounds, noises, and odors that are present in an experimental laboratory. Indeed, several early influential theories of the hippocampus argued that its chief function was in processing this kind of contextual information.

To more fully understand what the hippocampal region is doing, it is necessary to have some understanding of its inputs—and hence what the sensory cortices are doing to information from the eyes, ears, and other sense organs before they pass this information on to the hippocampus. Chapter 8

shows how certain types of network models can be related to cortical architecture and physiology. It presents a specific model that combines a cortical
module with a hippocampal-region module and explores how these brain
systems might interact. Finally, chapter 8 presents an example of how research into cortical representation has led to a real-world application to help
children who are language-learning-impaired.

Chapter 9 continues the discussion of cortical representation by focusing
on one particular region of cortex: the entorhinal cortex. The entorhinal
cortex is physically contiguous to the hippocampus and is considered part of
the hippocampal region as that term is used in this book. This chapter
reviews three different computational models of the entorhinal cortex and its
interaction with other brain regions. It then discusses the implications of
theories of entorhinal (and hippocampal) function for understanding and
diagnosing the earliest stages of Alzheimer's disease, which is characterized by cell degeneration and physical shrinkage in the entorhinal cortex and
hippocampus.

An emerging theme from these studies and models is that the hippocampal region does not operate in isolation; rather, to understand the hippocampus, one must understand how it interacts and cooperates with the
functioning of other brain regions. Accordingly, chapter 10 considers additional brain regions that provide chemical messengers that alter the functioning of hippocampal-region neurons. This chapter first provides a brief
review of neurotransmission and neuromodulation, with particular attention
to acetylcholine and how it affects memory. Next, the chapter discusses computational models that suggest that acetylcholine released from the medial
septum into hippocampus is integral in mediating hippocampal function
and a model that addresses the effects of changes in acetylcholine levels on
learning and memory.

The final chapter, chapter 11, reviews several key themes that recur
throughout the book. They are:

1. Hippocampal function can best be understood in terms of how the
hippocampus interacts and cooperates with the functioning of other brain
systems.

2. Partial versus complete lesions may differ in more than just degree.

3. Disrupting a brain system has different effects than removing it.

4. Studies of the simplest forms of animal learning may bootstrap us toward
understanding more complex aspects of learning and memory in humans.

5. The best theories and models exemplify three principles: Keep it simple,
keep it useful, and keep it testable.

These five themes represent the core message of this book. In the ten chapters that follow, we will elaborate on these themes as they are exemplified in a variety of specific research programs. Through this story we hope to communicate to the broader scientific community how and why computational models are advancing our understanding of the neural bases of learning and memory.

Many questions about hippocampal function in learning still remain unanswered. Some of these open questions are empirical, and we will suggest, at several places throughout the book, what we think are some of the more pressing empirical issues that need to be resolved by further experimentation. Other open questions are of a more theoretical nature, and we will suggest several new modeling directions for future efforts. Although we have aimed this book primarily at non-modelers, we hope that we may excite a few of our readers to go on to become modelers themselves, or to incorporate computational modeling into their own research programs through collaboration with modelers.

2 The Hippocampus in Learning and Memory

2.1 INTRODUCTION

The human hippocampus is a small structure, about the size and shape of a crooked pinkie finger and lying under the cerebral cortex (figure 2.1). There is one hippocampus on each side of the brain, and the two hippocampi come near to joining at the back. The word *hippocampus* is Latin for "seahorse," and

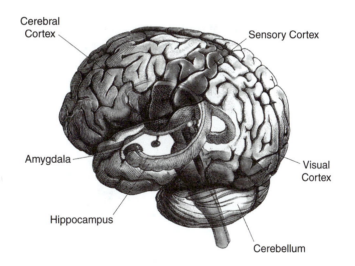

Figure 2.1   The human brain. The cerebral cortex is the wrinkled gray sheet (actually a thin layer of neurons) that covers most of the brain's surface; different areas within the cortex process and store different kinds of information. For example, sensory cortex is specialized to process tactile information, while visual cortex is a primary area for processing visual information. Near the base of the brain is the cerebellum, which is involved in coordination and fine control of movement. Buried under the temporal (or side) lobe of the cortex are the hippocampus and the amygdala, two structures that are involved in the acquisition of new memories. Whereas the amygdala seems critical for the emotional content of memories, the hippocampus may function as a memory gateway, determining which particular episodes and facts enter into long-term storage in cortex. (Adapted from Bloom, Lazerson, & Hofstadter, 1985, Figure 7.5, p. 185.)

the earliest known written description of the structure notes the similarity in appearance: "In its length [the structure] extends toward the anterior parts and the front of the brain and is provided with a flexuous figure of varying thickness. This recalls the image of a Hippocampus, that is, of a little sea-horse."[1] Indeed, the human hippocampus does look like a seahorse, as shown in figure 2.2.

The hippocampi lie on the inner side of the temporal lobes—just below the temples along the sides of the head—in an area called the **medial temporal lobes** (figure 2.3A,B). In cross-section (figure 2.3C), the hippocampus appears as a pair of interlocking C-shaped structures (figure 2.3D). Some early neuroanatomists noted that this shape bore a resemblance to the horns of a ram. In fact, another name for the hippocampus is *cornu ammonis*, or "Ammon's horn," after the Egyptian god Amon, who was often represented with a ram's head. This nomenclature survives in the current names for the subfields of the hippocampus, which are known as fields CA (*cornu ammonis*) 1 through 4. The close-up in figure 2.3D also illustrates important nearby structures, including the **dentate gyrus, subiculum, entorhinal cortex, perirhinal cortex, parahippocampal cortex,** and **amygdala.**

Primates have medial temporal lobes roughly similar to humans', while other mammalian species have analogous structures that are laid out somewhat differently. For example, rats and rabbits, whose cerebral cortex is proportionally much smaller than humans', have a hippocampus that begins near the top of the brain and curves around toward the base (almost like a large-scale version of the ram's horn analogy). Thus, the medial temporal

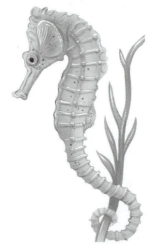

Figure 2.2   A seahorse.

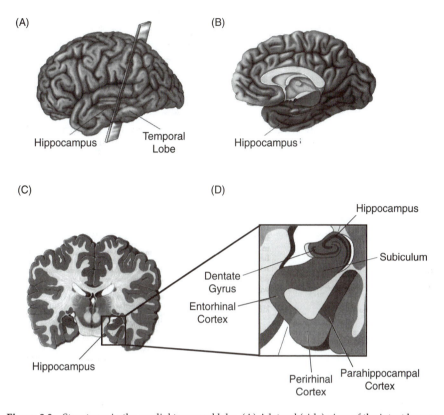

Figure 2.3 Structures in the medial temporal lobe. (A) A lateral (side) view of the intact human brain, showing one temporal lobe. The hippocampus is located on the inner (or medial) side of the temporal lobe. (B) A medial view, showing what the brain would look like if it were sliced down the middle and split into two halves. (C) If the brain were sliced as shown by the plane in (A), the hippocampus would be cross-sectioned, revealing (D) a series of interlocking C-shaped structures. The outer "C" is the hippocampus; the inner "C" is the dentate gyrus. Beyond the hippocampus lie the subiculum, entorhinal cortex, and other associated cortical areas. (Adapted from Bear, Connors, & Paradiso, 1996, Figure 19.7, p. 531.)

concept doesn't apply so well to these animals. In this book, *we use the term **hippocampal region** to refer to a subset of medial temporal structures: hippocampus, dentate gyrus, subiculum, and entorhinal cortex.* The **fimbria/fornix,** a fiber pathway connecting the hippocampus to subcortical structures, is often included as part of the hippocampal region as well. This definition of the hippocampal region applies equally well to any mammal, regardless of the specific anatomical layout of the individual structures. However, the exact functions of the hippocampal region remain a subject of contentious debate. Most neuroscientists now agree that the hippocampus has something to do with learning and memory, but there is little consensus about what exactly the hippocampus is doing when we learn and store new memories.

In this chapter, we review current knowledge about hippocampal-region function. We start with a brief description of the memory impairments in humans with damage to the hippocampal region and then describe some classic behavioral impairments in animals with analogous brain damage. Some commonalities emerge to unify human and animal studies, but there are as many open questions as apparent answers.

It is important to note at this point that what follows is *not* a comprehensive review of the empirical literature on the hippocampal region. Rather, it is a selective review of those aspects of this literature that are most relevant to the subsequent discussion of computational models of the hippocampus and learning.

2.2   HUMAN MEMORY AND THE MEDIAL TEMPORAL LOBES

Much of our understanding of the hippocampal region's role in learning and memory comes from individuals who have suffered damage to the medial temporal lobes. In some rare cases, this damage is so circumscribed that it is almost possible to consider these individuals as having localized damage to the hippocampal region. More often, the damage is diffuse and involves other nearby structures, clouding the picture. By looking at a variety of individuals with a variety of patterns of damage, scientists are trying to build up a picture of what specific impairments follow hippocampal-region damage.

Medial Temporal Lobe Damage and Memory Loss

One of the most famous individuals with hippocampal-region damage was a young man who, to protect his privacy, is publicly known only by his initials, HM.[2] HM suffered from severe epilepsy, which was not ameliorated by drugs. The seizures were so frequent as to be incapacitating and life-threatening. In 1953, when HM was 27 years old, his doctors decided to try an experimental procedure: Since HM's seizures originated in his hippocampi, there was a possibility that surgical removal of the hippocampi would stop seizures from occurring. Doctors removed an 8-centimeter segment from each of HM's temporal lobes, including two-thirds of each hippocampus, as shown in figure 2.4. HM's seizures were indeed alleviated by the surgery, but it soon became apparent that there was a terrible cost: HM's ability to acquire new information had been devastated.

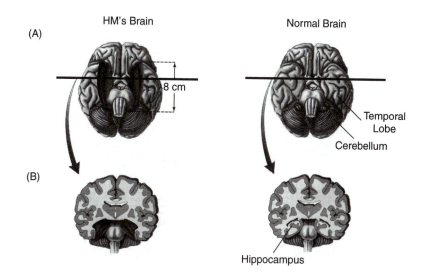

Figure 2.4 (A) A view of the brain from below, showing HM's lesion (left) and a normal brain (right). HM's lesion, involved removal of the medial temporal lobe from both sides of the brain. (B) A cross-section through the brain, with the cut at the position indicated in (A), shows HM's lesion (left) and a normal brain (right). (Adapted from Bear, Connors, & Paradiso, 1996, Figure 19.6, p. 529.)

Although HM's intelligence, language skills, and personality are largely as they were before the surgery, he has essentially no memories for any events from the last five decades. HM does have a reasonably normal memory for events that occurred at least two years before his surgery, but he does not remember subsequent events, such as the Vietnam War or the death of his father in 1967. Although he can participate in a conversation, a few minutes later he will have lost all memory of it. He cannot learn the names or faces of people who visit him regularly. Even the doctors and psychologists who have worked with him for over 45 years must reintroduce themselves to HM each time they meet. Since HM himself has aged since his surgery, he does not even recognize his own face when he is shown a current picture of himself. HM is painfully aware of his own problems and has described his life as constantly waking from a dream he can't remember: "Every day is alone in itself, whatever joy I've had and whatever sorrow I've had."[3]

HM's condition is known as **anterograde amnesia,** the inability to form new memories. In the years since HM was first tested, it has also become clear that some kinds of learning have survived, particularly his ability to learn new skills. We now know that although HM's damage included much of the temporal lobes, it is the damage to his hippocampus and the surrounding brain regions that is responsible for his anterograde amnesia.

The effects of HM's surgery were so debilitating that bilateral temporal lobe removal is now no longer used as a treatment for epilepsy. Unilateral removal, which removes the hippocampus and other parts of the medial temporal lobe from only *one* side of the brain, may still be done in cases of severe epilepsy; this usually results in a much milder memory impairment than seen in HM.

There are, however, other syndromes (also called **etiologies**) that can cause bilateral damage to the hippocampal region. For example, another famous patient, known by his initials RB, became amnesic following a loss of oxygen to his brain during heart bypass surgery. He showed the same general pattern of memory impairments as HM, although RB's amnesia was much less severe.[4] RB died a few years later, and he donated his brain to research so that scientists could better understand the cause of his amnesia. RB's hippocampus did indeed show extensive cell death, but this was limited to the CA1 subregion of the hippocampus (figure 2.5). The case of RB suggested that damage limited to the hippocampus was sufficient to disrupt

(A) Cross-section through a
"normal" brain

(B) "Normal" hippocampus

(C) RB's hippocampus

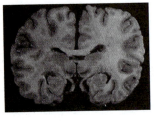

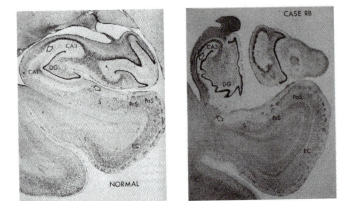

Figure 2.5 RB's lesion was limited to subfield CA1 of hippocampus. (A) A cross-section through the normal brain. (B) A close-up of a cross-section of the hippocampus in a normal brain. Information-processing cells, called neurons, are visible as dark areas. Cells in the dentate gyrus (DG) form one interlocking "C"; the hippocampus (including CA1 and CA3) forms another. CA1 neurons are in the area between the two arrowheads. (C) In RB's hippocampus, CA1 neurons have degenerated, visible as a lack of dark areas between the two arrowheads. The dentate gyrus, hippocampal field CA3, and the nearby subiculum (S) are largely intact, though warped slightly out of position. (Reprinted from Gazzaniga, Ivry, & Mangun, 1998, Figure 7.15.)

memory. Larger lesions do generally cause larger disruptions, accounting for the relatively worse amnesia in HM, who had a much larger lesion than did RB.

Transient loss or reduction of oxygen (called **anoxia** or **hypoxia**) is a frequent cause of amnesia, because hippocampal cells seem particularly sensitive to oxygen deprivation. This can occur during stroke and cardiac arrest, as well as near-drowning, near-strangulation, and carbon monoxide poisoning. Another etiology that can result in amnesia is **herpes encephalitis,** which occurs when the common herpes virus enters the brain and attacks nerve cells there; again, the hippocampal region appears especially vulnerable. A small degree of hippocampal damage occurs in the course of normal aging, and this damage is accelerated and magnified in the early stages of Alzheimer's disease, leading to memory failures. Damage to other parts of the brain can also sometimes cause anterograde amnesia,[5] possibly because damage to these structures interferes with the normal working of the hippocampus; we will return to this issue in later chapters.

In all these cases, *damage to or disruption of the hippocampal region may cause anterograde amnesia: a devastating loss of new memory formation, with relative sparing of intelligence, personality, skill learning, and old memories.* This is why we and others have characterized the hippocampal region as functioning much like a gateway to memory.

Anterograde Versus Retrograde Amnesia

Even a person with normal memory does not remember everything that has ever happened to her. She may have excellent memory for everything that happened to her today and relatively complete memory for everything that happened this week. But ask her what she had for lunch last Thursday or where she was on the morning of May 29, 1986, and unless those events were somehow significant, chances are she will have forgotten. Figure 2.6A schematizes this pattern of normal memory and forgetting: near complete memory for recent events and a gradual decrease in memory of progressively older events. Most people have only a few memories from as far back as infancy.

Using this schematic, figure 2.6B shows one way to schematize pure anterograde amnesia: The individual has normal memory for events from birth through childhood up to the time of the trauma; no memories are formed after the time of the trauma. Note that this does not imply that a person with anterograde amnesia remembers 100% of his childhood—just that he remembers it fully as well as a person with no memory problems.

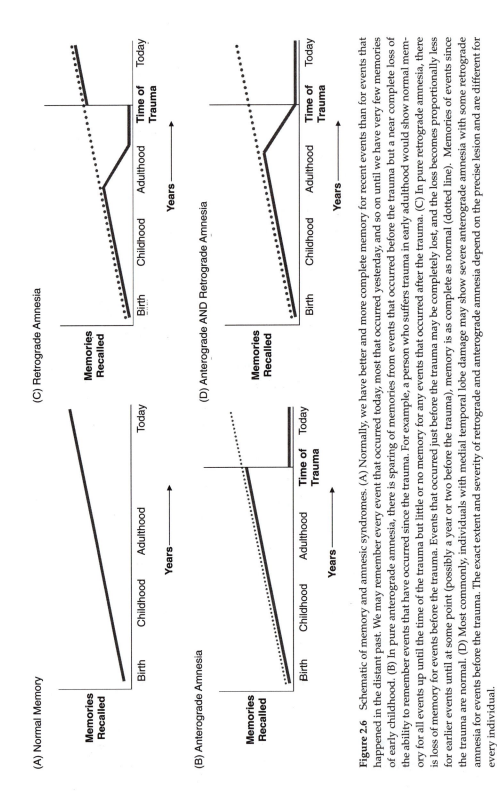

Figure 2.6 Schematic of memory and amnesic syndromes. (A) Normally, we have better and more complete memory for recent events than for events that happened in the distant past. We may remember every event that occurred today, most that occurred yesterday, and so on until we have very few memories of early childhood. (B) In pure anterograde amnesia, there is sparing of memories from events that occurred before the trauma but a near complete loss of the ability to remember events that have occurred since the trauma. For example, a person who suffers trauma in early adulthood would show normal memory for all events up until the time of the trauma but little or no memory for any events that occurred after the trauma. (C) In pure retrograde amnesia, there is loss of memory for events before the trauma. Events that occurred just before the trauma may be completely lost, and the loss becomes proportionally less for earlier events until at some point (possibly a year or two before the trauma), memory is as complete as normal (dotted line). Memories of events since the trauma are normal. (D) Most commonly, individuals with medial temporal lobe damage may show severe anterograde amnesia with some retrograde amnesia for events before the trauma. The exact extent and severity of retrograde and anterograde amnesia depend on the precise lesion and are different for every individual.

An alternative kind of memory impairment is **retrograde amnesia,** a loss of memory from before the trauma, with relative sparing of new memory formation. The slope in figure 2.6C illustrates the specific kind of forgetting in retrograde amnesia: There is little or no memory for events that happened immediately before the trauma, relative sparing of events from the distant past, and a smooth gradient in between.

It is important to note that retrograde amnesia is not the kind of memory loss that is often dramatized in movies, such as Alfred Hitchcock's *Marnie,* in which someone forgets not just events but her very identity. This kind of forgetting (sometimes called **fugue**) is extremely rare in real life. More commonly, memory loss may be restricted to a particular period of time, such as the duration of a violent crime; this is called event-specific amnesia. Both fugue and event-specific amnesia are examples of **psychogenic amnesia:** memory loss due to psychological, not physical, trauma, which often resolves in time, particularly with the help of therapy.[6] Some cases of pure retrograde amnesia resulting from physical brain injury have been reported,[7] but more often, some degree of retrograde amnesia co-occurs with anterograde amnesia, as schematized in figure 2.6D.

HM, for example, shows poor memory for events during the few years prior to his surgery as well as for all events afterward. Figure 2.7A shows the results of a study testing remote memory in several individuals who became amnesic following anoxia or a similar event between 1976 and 1986.[8] The study took place in 1986 and 1987, when the amnesic individuals were all about 50 years old. When the amnesic subjects were asked to recall details of news events that had occurred during the 1950s, the amnesics showed good recall of old information, remembering about as much information as same-age subjects with normal memory. Asked about the 1960s and 1970s, the amnesic subjects recalled progressively less information. Finally, asked about events from the 1980s, the amnesic subjects showed very poor memory; and, of course, they would remember little or nothing about more recent events that had occurred since the onset of amnesia. By contrast, the normal subjects tended to recall about 50% of the news events tested, and this performance was about the same for every decade. Figure 2.7B shows the same pattern of performance in normal and amnesic subjects who were asked to recognize faces of people who had become famous between 1940 and 1985.

The severe anterograde amnesia that follows hippocampal-region damage led to the hypothesis that the hippocampus was needed for the formation of new memories but not for the maintenance of older memories. The presence of retrograde amnesia in patients such as HM challenged this hypothesis;

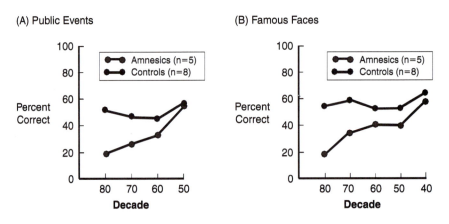

Figure 2.7 Individuals with anterograde amnesia also often show some degree of retrograde amnesia. (A) Five individuals with severe anterograde amnesia and eight control subjects with normal memory were tested for recall of public events during the years 1940–1985. All subjects were about 50 years old. Control subjects showed about 50% recall of the events from each decade. Amnesic subjects showed good recall for the earliest events (1950s) and progressively worse recall for later events. Events that occurred after the onset of amnesia (which varied between the years 1976 and 1986 for these five people) would show effectively no recall. (B) The same pattern of results is shown by these control and amnesic subjects when they were tested for recognition of faces of people who became famous during the various decades. (Adapted from Squire & Zola-Morgan, 1988, Figure 1.)

apparently, some older memories are indeed disrupted after hippocampal-region damage. However, this retrograde amnesia follows a reliable pattern: Memories formed just before the trauma are most likely to be disrupted; older memories are increasingly likely to survive. This suggests that while memories eventually become independent of the hippocampus, there is some **consolidation period** during which newly formed memories still depend on the hippocampus. Hippocampal-region damage during this time may devastate these newly acquired memories.

This idea of the consolidation period does not contradict the idea of the hippocampus as a gateway; it simply means that memories do not pass through the gateway instantaneously. There is some period of time during which recent memories still depend on the hippocampus; thus, destruction of the gate may impair recently acquired memories as well as preventing new learning. This pattern is common enough that, from now on, we will use the general terms **amnesia** and **amnesic** to refer to a syndrome involving severe anterograde amnesia with varying degrees of retrograde amnesia, usually produced by damage to the medial temporal lobes in humans, and corresponding to the effects of hippocampal region damage in animals.

Preserved Learning in Amnesia

There is yet another complication in the hypothesis that hippocampal-region damage disrupts new learning: Some kinds of memory can indeed survive hippocampal-region damage. For example, **short-term memory** is the kind of memory that lets us remember a seven-digit telephone number by constant rehearsal, although any interruption may result in loss of information from short-term memory. Short-term memory tends to be intact in HM and others with anterograde amnesia. This may be enough to allow HM to carry on an intelligent conversation with someone; but if the other person leaves the room and returns five minutes later, HM is likely to have no memory of the conversation.

Even within the domain of **long-term memory,** the kind of memory that lets us remember information over a period of weeks or years, individuals with anterograde amnesia do show some learning. For example, HM was trained on a new motor task, mirror drawing, in which he was asked to trace a figure like that shown in figure 2.8A while viewing the figure and his hand only through a mirror (figure 2.8B). This means that every time his hand moved left or right, it appeared in the mirror to go the opposite way.

Mirror drawing is quite difficult at first, although most people get progressively better with practice. HM became proficient at mirror drawing, and

(A)   (B)

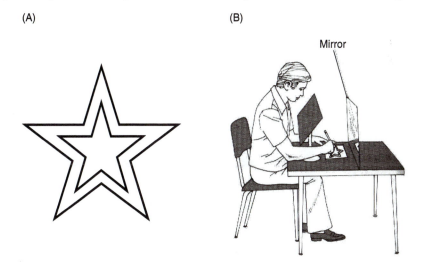

Figure 2.8   The mirror-drawing task. (A) Subjects are given this pattern and asked to trace it, keeping within the borders. (B) A screen is placed above the hand so that the subject can view progress only by watching a mirror, which reverses the apparent motion of the hand. (B is reprinted from Carlson, 1997, Figure 15.5, p. 457.)

his improvement was maintained over many days.[9] Despite this evidence of learning, HM had to have the task explained to him each time he started, because he would claim that he had never done such a thing before. While he remained unaware of his learning and of his past experiences with the task, HM's speed and accuracy in mirror drawing improved with each practice trial, much like those of a person with normal memory. Other individuals with anterograde amnesia show the same kind of improvement with practice,[10] suggesting that motor skill learning is generally spared after hippocampal-region damage.

Other kinds of skills can also be learned by individuals with amnesia. One example is the **figure completion task.** Subjects are shown a fragmented version of a line drawing and asked to name the object; if they fail, they are shown successively more complete versions of the figure until they can name it (figure 2.9). If subjects are retested an hour later, normal subjects will recognize the figure earlier—based on a more incomplete drawing—than they did previously. This effect holds even if there is an interval of many months between test sessions.

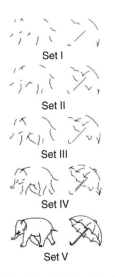

Set I

Set II

Set III

Set IV

Set V

Figure 2.9 One test of perceptual learning (priming) involves picture fragments. Subjects are shown fragmented pictures (top) and asked to name the figure. If the subject cannot, progressively more complete versions are shown until the subject's guess is correct or the complete picture is shown (bottom). Later, the procedure is repeated; subjects tend to recognize the figure earlier (on the basis of a more fragmented picture) even if several months have passed since the original testing session. This implies some memory of the original figure, and this kind of learning is often preserved in amnesic subjects. (Reprinted from Gollin, 1960, Figure 1, p. 290.)

When HM was given this test and was then retested an hour later, he also showed considerable improvement from his first testing session, despite having no explicit recollection of having seen the figure before. Four months later, he still showed improvement over his initial performance. Although HM's testing performance at both intervals was worse than normal performance, it is clear that even in the absence of explicit recall of the experimental task HM showed unmistakable evidence of learning.

The figure completion task is a form of learning known as **priming,** which occurs when people find it easier to process a particular stimulus that they have seen before. Many different forms of priming have been shown to be intact in amnesic individuals, including priming for novel geometric patterns, faces, and the melodies and words of songs—all without a conscious memory of ever having seen or heard the stimuli before.[11]

All these kinds of learning that are spared in amnesia seem to have two features in common: First, they are incrementally acquired with practice. Second, they can be viewed as skills or habits that involve executing a procedure. This general class of learning is often called **procedural memory.** It includes everyday skills such as tying a shoelace that are well-learned and easy to perform but quite hard to describe verbally. Procedural memory is largely spared in anterograde amnesia.

By contrast, the kind of memory that is lost in HM and other amnesic individuals is called **declarative memory** because it is easily accessed by verbal recall. Declarative memory is often further subdivided into **episodic memory,** which is memory for specific (often autobiographical) events, and **semantic memory,** which is memory for facts such as vocabulary items or general knowledge about the world.

A simple heuristic is to define declarative memories as *knowing that* something happened, while procedural memories involve *knowing how* something is done. The cases of HM and others like him suggest that declarative memory depends critically on medial temporal lobe structures (such as the hippocampal region), while procedural memory may depend more on other brain structures. This distinction can be schematized as in figure 2.10, and it has been suggested that each kind of memory may depend primarily on a particular brain structure (or set of structures).*

*Recent studies have suggested that while episodic memory may depend primarily on the hippocampus, semantic memory may depend more on other, nearby structures such as the parahippocampal cortices (Funnel, 1995; Gaffan, 1997; Vargha-Khadem et al., 1997; Mishkin, Vargha-Khadem, & Gadian, 1998, cf. Squire & Zola, 1998).

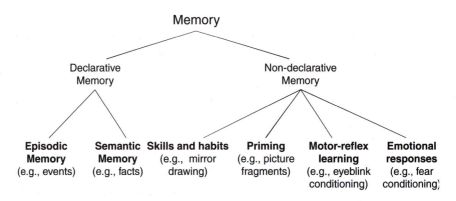

Figure 2.10 Taxonomy of memory proposed by Larry Squire and colleagues (after Squire & Zola-Morgan, 1988; Squire & Knowlton, 1995). Declarative memory consists of items that are easy to verbalize and generally accessible to conscious recall; this includes episodic memory of autobiographical events and semantic memory including vocabulary and general knowledge of the world. Nondeclarative memory is everything else, including skill and habit learning, priming, and conditioning—learning of reflexive or emotional responses to stimuli that habitually predict reward or punishment. Medial temporal lobe damage may devastate the acquisition of new declarative memory, while nondeclarative memory may be largely spared. This leads to the proposal that the medial temporal lobes are critical for forming new declarative memories, while nondeclarative memories may depend on other brain structures.

However, yet again, the picture is not quite as simple as it sounds. Increasingly, studies suggest that some kinds of procedural learning are indeed disrupted after hippocampal-region damage.

2.3   ANIMAL LEARNING STUDIES OF HIPPOCAMPAL FUNCTION

Neuropsychological studies of human memory impairments are based primarily on examinations of those rare individuals who have sustained brain damage to the medial temporal lobes. However, damage in these cases is seldom limited to just a single region of the brain. Although the hippocampal region is especially vulnerable to injury through stroke, anoxia, and encephalitis, these etiologies can cause diffuse damage. Thus, an individual may have memory impairments that reflect damage to regions beyond the medial temporal lobe. Further, even within the medial temporal lobe, damage is rarely complete. Some amnesic individuals have partial sparing of behaviors that do depend on the medial temporal lobes. Thus, no two amnesic individuals are exactly alike, either in their memory disorders or in the exact extent of their brain damage.

However, by also doing research on animals, scientists are able to create precise lesions and be certain to remove certain brain regions completely while causing little or no damage to other brain regions. Thus, animal models of amnesia can avoid some of the problems inherent in human research.

It is important to note that most careful studies compare lesioned animals against specific **control** animals, not against normal animals. A control animal is one that has undergone the same surgical procedure as the lesioned animal—but without the actual lesion; the result is sometimes called a "sham lesion," and the animal is referred to as a **sham control**. For example, a brain lesion may be created by anesthetizing an animal, opening the skull, and removing small pieces of the brain by **ablation** (cutting out brain tissue) or **aspiration** (sucking out brain tissue). Since the hippocampus is buried under the cortex, this kind of procedure usually entails damage to some of the cortex that lies between the skull and the hippocampus. Thus, a control procedure for a hippocampal lesion might be to operate on a second animal in the same way but stop just short of damaging the hippocampus. Thus, any abnormal behavior in the lesioned animal would reflect hippocampal damage, not merely damage to overlying brain tissue, or else the control animals would show the same effect. A more modern lesion technique involves lowering a syringe into a precise brain location and injecting a **neurotoxin** that destroys neurons (brain cells) near the injection site. A sham control for this lesion would involve anesthetizing the animal, lowering a syringe, and injecting a comparable amount of harmless saline. Thus, the lesioned and sham control animal should be identical in every way except for the loss of neurons in the lesioned animal. In this case, any abnormal behavior in the lesioned animal can be safely attributed to the loss of neurons rather than to the general effects of anesthesia and surgery.

The use of proper controls is another advantage of animal research over human research. Humans generally experience hippocampal-region damage as a result of stroke, disease, anoxia, or other brain trauma. It is difficult to envision a proper control for such a subject, so researchers often make do by comparing amnesic subjects against individuals of the same sex and age who have never had any brain injury. But this leaves open the possibility that memory impairments in the amnesic subjects might be the result of damage outside the hippocampal region.

However, animal research presents its own problems. The most obvious deficit in human amnesia is a failure of declarative memory that is usually evaluated by asking subjects to recall or recognize information they have seen previously. It is not so easy to assess declarative memory in animals; obviously, a researcher cannot ask a rat whether it remembers what it did a few hours ago.

One approach to evaluating animal memory has been to test whether animals have something like an episodic memory for specific events. This has been a major focus of study in nonhuman primates and, more recently, in rats. Another approach has been to observe animals with hippocampal damage and assess what behaviors are most devastated; researchers then try to understand what these behaviors have in common with the amnesic syndrome in humans. A third approach is to consider simple learning behaviors that are common to humans and other mammals and attempt to understand the pattern of impairment after hippocampal-region damage across species. We give some examples of each kind of approach below.

Episodic Memory in Animals

Many studies of learning have been conducted using monkeys because they are more similar to humans than any other animal, in terms of both cognitive abilities and brain anatomy. Therefore, if any animal can be argued to have episodic or declarative memory, it should be monkeys.

One of the most commonly used tests of memory in the monkey is called **delayed nonmatch to sample (DNMS),** and it is illustrated in figure 2.11.[12] The monkey faces a table that has three small wells. First, the monkey sees a sample object, such as a red ball, covering the center well. Then a screen covers the wells for a short delay. When the screen is removed, there are two

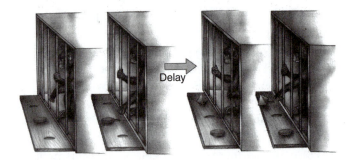

Figure 2.11   The delayed nonmatch to sample (DNMS) task. The monkey sees three wells; the center is covered with a small object (far left); the monkey displaces this object to get a food reward (center left). Next, there is a short delay, usually 5 to 60 seconds, during which the wells are hidden by a screen. When the screen is removed, the two outer wells are covered (center right). One well is covered with the previously seen (sample) object; the other is covered with a new object. The monkey is allowed to displace one object. If it displaces the new object, it obtains a small food reward. The nonmatch to sample task is performed well by monkeys with hippocampal-region lesions if the delay is short. With increasing delays, lesioned monkeys show impairments. (Reprinted from Bear, Connors, & Paradiso, 1996, Figure 19.9, p. 532.)

objects on the table, covering the left and right wells. One of the objects is the sample object that was previously seen, and one is new. There is a food reward under the new object. The monkey must learn to choose the new object to get this reward. In other words, the monkey learns to choose the object that does not match the sample object (hence the task's name).

With extensive training, normal monkeys can learn this task quite well, even when the task involves delays of up to ten minutes. Because the monkey's choice depends on a single event from several minutes before, this task appears to require episodic memory of the sample presentation. Thus, it seems to be a good example of the kind of task that might be disrupted by hippocampal-region damage, based on related deficits in amnesic humans with similar brain damage.

Indeed, DNMS is severely impaired in monkeys with lesions of the hippocampal region, including hippocampus, dentate gyrus, subiculum, and the adjacent entorhinal and parahippocampal cortices.[13] Interestingly, lesioned monkeys are impaired at the task only if there are delays longer than a few seconds. If there is no delay between sample and choice, the lesioned monkeys are practically normal. Thus, the lesioned monkeys, like human amnesics, appear to have intact short-term memories but an impaired ability to form new longer-term memories that span delays of many minutes. In fact, when the same DNMS task was applied to human amnesics, the same pattern of results appeared: The amnesic subjects performed as well as normal subjects when there was little or no delay, but performance grew much poorer at longer delays.[14]

Later, a variety of different monkey studies showed that the exact lesion extent was critical; in fact, lesion limited to the hippocampus alone produced little or no impairment on DNMS, except at the longest delays.[15] These findings highlighted the importance of knowing which structures were damaged and suggested that different structures within the hippocampal region might be performing subtly different functions. We will return to this topic in chapter 9.

Recently, several studies have attempted to demonstrate episodic learning in other species, including rats.[16] In a rodent version of DNMS, a rat is given sample exposure to an odor and later presented with a choice between the same odor and a novel odor; response to the novel odor is rewarded. Again, lesion of the hippocampus does not impair this task, although lesions of the surrounding cortices do lead to an impairment if there is a long delay between sample and choice.[17]

Together, these studies suggest that, in animals and humans, the hippocampus itself may not be strictly necessary for recognition, at least with short delays. It is possible, however, that other more complex forms of recognition memory do require the hippocampus.

Spatial Navigation and the Hippocampus

Given the difficulties in developing direct analogs of episodic memory tests for animals, an alternative approach is to determine which kinds of learning are most severely disrupted by hippocampal-region lesion in animals and then attempt to relate that back to human amnesia.

In rats, one of the most striking features of the hippocampus is the existence of **place cells,** neurons that exhibit electrical activity when the animal is in a particular region of space.[18] For example, suppose a rat is allowed to wander a small, square chamber while an experimenter records the activity of place cells in hippocampal subfield CA1. One cell may become strongly active when the rat is along one edge of the chamber (figure 2.12A), while another nearby cell might become strongly active when the rat is on the opposite side of the chamber (figure 2.12B). With enough place cells, the entire

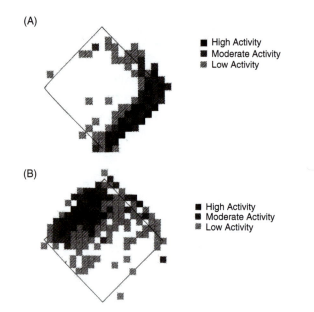

Figure 2.12   Place cell recordings: traces of activity of individual neurons in hippocampal subfield CA1. (A) A rat was allowed to wander freely through a square chamber, and at each point, the degree of activity was recorded from a single CA1 neuron. Dark spots show locations where the neuron was very active; white areas are locations where the neuron was essentially inactive. The neuron was most active when the rat was in a particular area (near the southeast wall) and nearly inactive when the rat was on the far side of the chamber from the preferred location. (B) Another nearby neuron responded most strongly when the rat was near the northwest wall. Given recordings from enough CA1 neurons, it would be possible to deduce the rat's position just on the basis of the pattern of activity. (Adapted from O'Keefe, 1983, Figures 2 and 3.)

chamber is covered, and it is possible to deduce where the animal is simply by monitoring the pattern of cell activity.[19] These and similar findings lead to the hypothesis that the hippocampus is involved in building a spatial map of the environment, which an animal can use to navigate through its surroundings.[20]

If this is so, then spatial learning should be severely disrupted by hippocampal-region damage. In fact, rat data show just this. One technique for studying spatial learning in rats, developed by Richard Morris, involves a **water maze**[21] in which a rat is placed in a circular pool filled with opaque liquid (often water with a little powdered milk). Hidden somewhere in the pool is a small platform, just under the surface of the water. As the rat swims, it will eventually stumble across the platform and escape from the water. On each trial, the experimenter puts the rat into the pool at a new starting position and records how long it takes the rat to locate the escape platform. Normal rats will quickly learn to take short, relatively direct paths to the hidden platform (figure 2.13A). Further studies showed that the normal rats were navigating on the basis of visual cues around the room; if the cues were removed or moved, the rats would not be able to locate the platform.

By contrast, rats with hippocampal lesions never seem to learn the location of the platform.[22] Instead, on every trial, they swim around randomly until they happen upon the platform (figure 2.13B). The lesioned rats can learn that there is an escape platform; if the platform is raised slightly so as to be visible above the water, the lesioned rats swim to it quickly.[23] What the

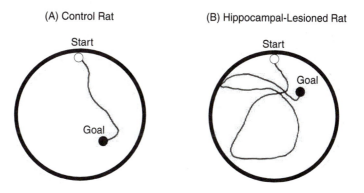

Figure 2.13 The water maze: Rats are placed in a pool at a start location (light circle) and swim to a hidden escape platform (dark circle). (A) After 28 trials, a normal rat swims to the hidden platform by a nearly direct route. (B) After 28 trials, the hippocampal-lesioned rat still swims randomly around the pool until it happens to find the platform. Apparently, the lesioned rat is unable to use visual cues around the room to navigate to the location of the hidden platform. (Adapted from Morris, 1983, Figure 4.)

lesioned rats seem unable to do is to integrate visual information to figure out where they are relative to the hidden platform and how to navigate from one point to the other.

These results and results from other spatial tasks, such as maze learning, show that spatial learning is devastated in rats with hippocampal-region damage. How does one reconcile this result with human data? What do spatial learning in rats and declarative memory in humans have to do with each other? One answer is that each is a task of paramount importance to the species. Rats are, by nature, foraging animals. The ability to navigate to a food source and return home afterward is critical to the rat's survival. By contrast, the ability to form declarative memories of autobiographical events seems to be at the very core of human existence, which focuses on our experiences and the ability to communicate these experiences to others.

But there is another way of looking at things, and that is to question the very nature of spatial learning. What is a place? One definition is that a place is a collection (or configuration) of views. When we stand in one spot and look north and stand in the same spot and look south, those two views should be integrated into a unified percept of the current location so that the next time we approach that spot (from any angle), we recognize where we are. In addition to visual cues, there may be auditory, olfactory and tactile cues, as well as memory of the route by which we reached the spot and what happened when we got there. All this information should be combined into the memory of a "place." Thus, spatial learning may be a special case of configural learning: the ability to bind elements together into a single complex memory.

Viewed in this way, there is a certain parallel with declarative memory. A declarative memory also consists of many separate components that are unified into a single complex memory. For example, the memory of a party might include representations of the locale, the food served, the attendees, some interesting conversations, and so on. These components are collected (configured) into the declarative memory of the event. Thus, declarative memory and spatial memory may share some important features, such as the need to configure information into complex memories and to retrieve them later on the basis of just a subset of the original information (such as a fragment of an autobiographical memory or a view from only one starting point in the pool). Several prominent theories of hippocampal-region function have focused on this idea, and we will review some of these in the context of hippocampal models in chapter 6.

For now, it is important to note that the same neurons that show spatial responses during a spatial task (e.g., figure 2.12) will also respond during a nonspatial task, such as learning to respond to one odor but not another.[24] Thus, it seems that hippocampal neurons encode whatever information is important to the current task, be it spatial or otherwise. Some kinds of task, such as spatial learning and declarative learning, depend critically on this information encoded in the hippocampus; thus, they appear to show the largest deficit following hippocampal lesion. Therefore, even if the hippocampus is not a spatial processor *per se*, spatial learning remains an important domain for studying dysfunction after hippocampal-region damage.

Importance of Well-Characterized Learning Behaviors

Studies of delayed nonmatch to sample in primates and spatial navigation in rodents have yielded a tremendous data bank of information on the role of the hippocampus in memory. But to fully understand the role of the hippocampus in a specific memory task, we need to begin with a clear understanding of how an animal solves the task normally; only then can we characterize and measure what has changed once the hippocampus is damaged.

Unfortunately, in such complex tasks as episodic memory, DNMS, and spatial navigation, neither the behavioral nor the neurobiological mechanism is well understood. While these types of memories are among the most clearly devastated following hippocampal-region damage, the problem for modeling is that psychological studies of these behaviors have not yet led to detailed mechanistic theories or models. That is, psychologists don't really understand how declarative or spatial memories are stored and recalled. Without a good theory of these behaviors to begin with, it is difficult to imagine how they could be mapped onto brain circuits. For this reason, many researchers have argued that it is advantageous to study the hippocampus through simpler forms of learning in which we *do* have a clearer and deeper understanding of both the behavioral strategies used by animals and the essential brain structures involved. The next section discusses one example: classical conditioning.

2.4 CLASSICAL CONDITIONING AND THE HIPPOCAMPUS

One of the most basic forms of memory is **associative learning:** learning relationships between stimuli such as which stimulus predicts another or which pairs of stimuli tend to co-occur. One kind of associative learning is **classical conditioning,** often called **Pavlovian conditioning** after Ivan

Pavlov, the Russian scientist who first described it. Pavlov was a physician who was using dogs to study digestion. Each day, before feeding the dogs, Pavlov rang a bell. Soon, Pavlov noticed that the dogs would begin to salivate as soon as they heard the bell, even if no meat was given. Pavlov reasoned that the bell was a stimulus sufficient to produce salivation in anticipation of feeding—simply because the dogs had learned to associate the bell with the expectation of food. Since Pavlov's time, classical conditioning has received extensive study in normal animals and humans, as well as in animals and humans with various kinds of brain damage. The neural mechanisms for this kind of learning are relatively well understood, which means that it is possible to build precise theories of how memories are created and stored.

Classical conditioning can be obtained with a wide range of stimuli. All that is required is that there is a biologically significant stimulus, such as food or an electric shock (called the **unconditioned stimulus,** or **US**), that elicits an automatic, reflexive response (called the **unconditioned response,** or **UR**). A previously neutral stimulus, such as a tone or a light (called the **conditioned stimulus,** or **CS**), is repeatedly presented just before the US, until the CS alone can elicit a preparatory response (called the **conditioned response,** or **CR**). Figure 2.14 shows this concept schematically.

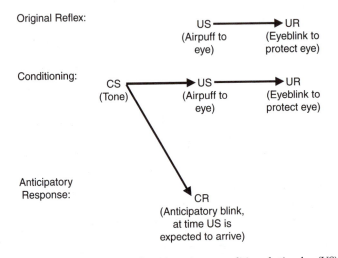

Figure 2.14 Schematic of classical conditioning. An unconditioned stimulus (US), such as an airpuff to the eye, elicits a reflexive, protective response, such as eyelid closure. This is the unconditioned response (UR). If the US is repeatedly preceded by a neutral stimulus, such as a tone or light (the conditioned stimulus, or CS), an association forms in which the CS predicts the US, and there is a conditioned response (CR) to the CS, such as an anticipatory eyeblink, timed so that the eye is fully closed at the expected time of US arrival.

All animals, including humans, exhibit classical conditioning, and the properties of this behavior are similar across all species. One popular form of classical conditioning is the rabbit eyeblink preparation.[25] The experimental apparatus is shown in figure 2.15A. The rabbit is given a mild airpuff or shock to the eye (the US), which elicits a reflexive, protective eyeblink (the UR). This US is repeatedly preceded by a neutral stimulus, such as a tone or a light (the CS). With enough CS-US pairings, the CS itself comes to elicit an anticipatory protective blink (the CR). Over time, the eyeblink CR will be timed so that the eyelid is maximally closed at the exact time of anticipated US arrival, as seen in figure 2.15B.

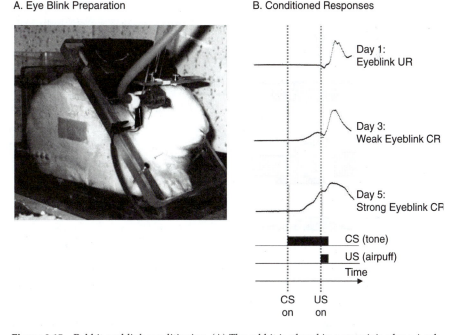

A. Eye Blink Preparation

B. Conditioned Responses

Day 1:
Eyeblink UR

Day 3:
Weak Eyeblink CR

Day 5:
Strong Eyeblink CR

CS (tone)

US (airpuff)

Time

CS   US
on   on

Figure 2.15   Rabbit eyeblink conditioning. (A) The rabbit is placed in a restraining box. A rubber hose delivers precisely timed puffs of oxygen to the right eye (US); these elicit protective eyeblinks (UR). If a previously neutral tone or light CS reliably precedes the US by a few hundred milliseconds, the rabbit develops an anticipatory eyeblink CR to the CS, so that the eye is closed at the time of expected US arrival. An infrared device measures reflectance off the eye, giving an index of eye closure. (B) On the first day of CS-US training, presentation of the CS evokes no eyeblink, but there is a strong blink UR in response to the airpuff US. By the third day of training, there is a small eyeblink CR in response to the tone, which partially closes the eye just before expected US arrival. By the fifth day of training, there is a strong CR, protecting the eye at the time of US arrival. (B is adapted from CR traces shown in Zigmond et al., 1999, Figure 55.13, p. 1430.)

Rabbits are often used for eyeblink conditioning experiments because they are content to sit quietly in a small restraining chamber for long periods of time during the procedure. In contrast, rats are more active animals and do not take well to such restraint. Lately, new procedures have been developed for rats in which the animal is allowed to move freely around a cage during conditioning.[26] Humans are also good subjects for eyeblink conditioning, since a human can be asked to sit still and is often given a movie to watch as entertainment during the experiment.[27] The procedure has even been adapted for monkeys.[28] In all cases, conditioning appears very similar across species, and so results found in one species can reasonably be expected to apply to others.

An obvious next question is whether conditioning survives hippocampal-region damage in animals and humans. On the surface, classical conditioning seems to be nondeclarative: It can be acquired over many iterative trials without any conscious memorization of the rules. In fact, all species tested so far, including invertebrates such as the octopus and the sea snail that do not even have a hippocampus, can display classical conditioning.[29] Therefore, it seems reasonable to expect that hippocampal-region damage should not eliminate classical conditioning. To a first approximation, this is indeed the case; however, it appears that the hippocampus, when present, does play an important but subtle role.

Hippocampal Lesions and Simple Conditioning

Early studies of the hippocampus and conditioning yielded puzzling, seemingly contradictory results. In rabbits, bilateral hippocampal lesions did not retard the rate at which the animal learns to give an eyeblink response to a single CS (figure 2.16).[30] In fact, in one study, the lesioned rabbits actually learned faster than normal rabbits![31] Nor did hippocampal lesions slow acquisition of an eyeblink CR in humans with hippocampal-region damage.[32] These results argued that the hippocampus is not necessary for eyeblink conditioning.

While behavioral studies were suggesting that the hippocampus did not mediate eyeblink conditioning, neurophysiological recordings were suggesting just the opposite. When the activity of single neurons in the hippocampus was recorded during conditioning, the neurons' activity became stronger as the CR was being learned (figure 2.17).[33] Not only did this hippocampal activity mimic the CR, but it also preceded the CR by about 40 milliseconds, suggesting that the hippocampus might be responsible for generating the signal that caused the eyelid to close in anticipation of the airpuff

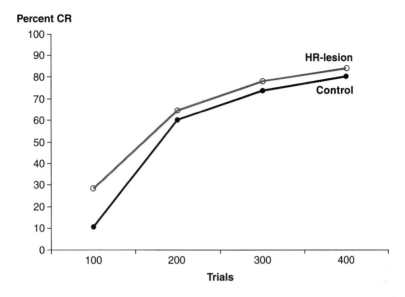

Figure 2.16   Eyeblink conditioning in rabbits is not slowed by hippocampal-region (HR) lesion. (Drawn from data presented in Allen, Chelius, & Gluck, 1998.)

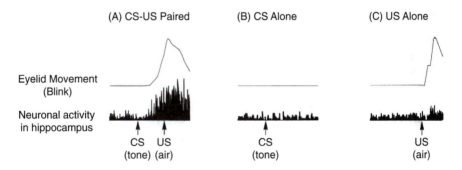

Figure 2.17   Pattern of activity of single neurons in the rabbit hippocampus during eyeblink conditioning. (A) After repeated pairing of a CS and US, the rabbit gives a blink (CR) to the CS, which precedes onset of the US and continues into the US period. Hippocampal neurons show increased activity during this CR and sustain that activity during the blink response. (B) By contrast, in an untrained rabbit, the CS evokes no blink response and no hippocampal activity. (C) If the US is presented alone, there is a reflexive eyeblink (UR) but no change in hippocampal activity. Thus, the hippocampal neuronal activity seems specifically to code for a CR: reflecting the CS prediction of US arrival. (Adapted from Berger, T. W., Rinaldi, P. C., Weisz, D. J., and Thompson, R. F. *Journal of Neurophysiology*, 1983, *50*, 1197–1219, as reprinted in Carlson, 1986, Figure 14.39, p. 586.)

US. Yet the hippocampus could be completely removed without impairing conditioning, as the behavioral studies had shown. So what was the purpose of this hippocampal activity?

One interpretation is that there is a subtle difference between whether a brain structure normally contributes to a particular behavior and whether it is actually necessary for that behavior. On the one hand, the ability of hippocampal-lesioned animals to acquire a CR indicates that the hippocampus is not *necessary* for eyeblink conditioning. On the other hand, the neurophysiological data show that, in the normal brain, the hippocampus is indeed *involved* in eyeblink conditioning.

This difference—between whether the hippocampus is actively involved and whether it is strictly necessary—turns out to be critical in understanding a great deal of data. It also emphasizes one of the dangers of basing too much theory on lesion data: Just because a behavior (such as eyeblink conditioning) *survives* lesion of a brain structure does not mean that that brain structure ordinarily plays no role. As a simple example, when walking, we normally integrate both visual cues and vestibular cues (our sense of balance) to keep upright. When we shut our eyes, we can still stand upright. Vision is not *necessary* for this behavior, but it normally contributes. The same seems to be true of the hippocampus: *The hippocampus may normally contribute to all learning, even those kinds of learning (such as simple classical conditioning) for which its help is not strictly needed.*

The Hippocampus and Complex Conditioning

What is the hippocampus doing during classical conditioning if its contributions appear to be irrelevant to learning a simple tone-airpuff relationship? Later studies showed that although the hippocampus was not needed for simple conditioning—learning that one CS predicted one US—it was indeed needed if the experimental procedure grew a little more complex. In the sections to follow, we describe two variations on the basic CS-US learning described above: trace and long-delay conditioning and sensory preconditioning. In each case, there is evidence that the hippocampal region plays an important role during Pavlovian conditioning.

Trace and Long-Delay Conditioning.   One example of hippocampal-dependent conditioning is the trace conditioning procedure. In ordinary conditioning (often called **delay conditioning**), the CS lasts for a short period of time, usually about 300 milliseconds. At the end of that period, the US occurs, and the CS and US coterminate (figure 2.18A). In **trace conditioning,**

the CS does not last throughout the whole period until US arrival (figure 2.18B). Instead, there is a short interval between CS offset and US onset. To time the CR to coincide with US arrival, the subject must maintain a memory, or *trace*, of the CS during this interval. Trace conditioning generally takes an animal longer to learn than delay conditioning, but normal animals eventually master it.[34]

However, hippocampal lesion greatly impairs the ability to learn trace conditioning. If the trace interval is short (e.g., 300 milliseconds), lesioned animals can learn an eyeblink CR at the same speed as normal animals.[35] However, if the trace interval is increased to 500 milliseconds, the lesioned animals are strongly impaired (figure 2.18C).[36]

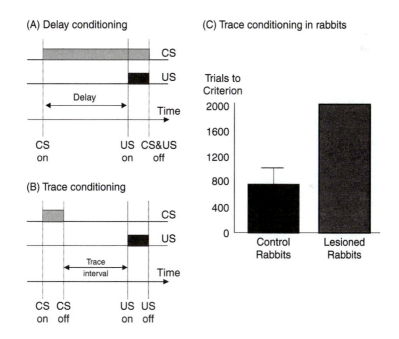

Figure 2.18   (A) In delay conditioning, the CS comes on some time before the US (e.g., 300 milliseconds) and remains on during the delay until US arrival. The CS and US coterminate. (B) In trace conditioning, CS offset occurs some time before US arrival. Some memory, or trace, of the CS must be maintained during the interval to allow generation of the CR at the time of expected US arrival. (C) With a long trace interval (500 milliseconds), control rabbits can reach criterion performance, responding to the CS on over 80% of trials, after about 800 CS-US training trials. By contrast, hippocampal-lesioned rabbits never reach this performance criterion, responding on only about 22% of trials, even after some 2000 training trials. (C is adapted from Figure 5 of Moyer, Deyo, & Disterhoft, 1990.)

Thus, the hippocampus appears to be involved in learning temporal relationships between CS and US, and this may be especially critical in trace conditioning, in which there is a gap between CS and US. This bears a resemblance to the finding in monkey DNMS studies that hippocampal lesions lead to impairments with long delays but not with short ones. Although DNMS and eyeblink conditioning seem superficially very different, the pattern of hippocampal-lesion impairments in each may reflect similar underlying mechanisms and a reliance on hippocampal-mediated temporal processing.

Sensory Preconditioning.   **Sensory preconditioning** is another conditioning procedure that is disrupted by hippocampal lesion. This procedure involves three phases, as summarized in table 2.1. Animals in the Compound Exposure group are first given exposure to a compound of two stimuli, such as a tone and a light, presented together. Next, the animals are trained that one of the stimuli (say, the light) predicts a US (such as a blink-evoking airpuff); eventually, the animals give a blink CR to the light CS. Finally, in phase 3, the animals are tested with the tone. Normal animals will give a modest but detectable response to the tone in phase 3 (figure 2.19). This transfer depends critically on the exposure to the tone and light compound in phase 1; animals that are given separate (unpaired) exposure to the tone and light in phase 1 show little or no transfer and virtually no responding in phase 3.[37] Apparently, the compound exposure in phase 1 allows the animals to make a link between tone and light, so that the learning about the light transfers to the tone in phase 2.

The story is different for animals with hippocampal damage. Rabbits with hippocampal disruption (specifically, lesion of the fimbria/fornix) show no sensory preconditioning (figure 2.19).[38] Animals that are exposed to the compound show no more transfer in phase 3 than animals that are given exposure to the tone and light separately. It seems that the hippocampus is needed for learning the association between tone and light in phase 1.

Table 2.1   Sensory Preconditioning

Group	Phase 1	Phase 2	Phase 3: Test
Compound Exposure	Tone and light (together)	Light → airpuff ⇒ blink!	Tone ⇒ blink!
Separate Exposure (control group)	Tone, light (separately)	Light → airpuff ⇒ blink!	Tone ⇒ no blink

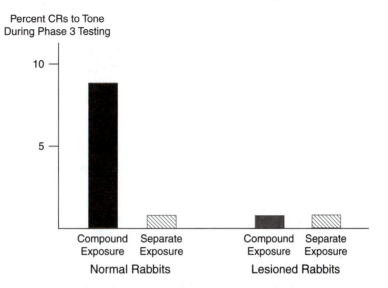

Sensory Preconditioning

Percent CRs to Tone
During Phase 3 Testing

Compound Separate   Compound Separate
Exposure Exposure   Exposure Exposure
Normal Rabbits   Lesioned Rabbits

Figure 2.19 In sensory preconditioning, animals are given phase 1 exposure to a compound stimulus consisting of tone and light, presented together. In phase 2, animals are trained to respond to the light. In phase 3, animals are tested for their response to the untrained tone stimulus. Normal rabbits that are given compound exposure in phase 1 show some responding to the tone in phase 3. By contrast, normal rabbits that are given separate exposure to tone and light in phase 1 show little or no responding to the tone in phase 3. Rabbits with hippocampal-region damage (specifically, lesion of the fimbria/fornix) do not show sensory preconditioning; rabbits there are given compound exposure to tone and light in phase 1 show no more transfer than rabbits given separate exposure. (Drawn from data presented in Port & Patterson, 1984.)

Studies of sensory preconditioning and related phenomena suggest that the hippocampus is especially critical for learning that takes place in the absence of reinforcement (e.g., a US), even within a domain such as classical conditioning. Other conditioning studies have suggested that the hippocampus is critical for learning about *context* and about *configurations of stimuli. What all these tasks have in common is the need to represent relationships between stimuli that are independent of the associations between stimuli and reinforcement.* This idea has formed the basis for many influential theories of hippocampal-region function.[39] We will discuss these theories more fully in chapter 6.

2.5   IS A UNIFIED THEORY OF HIPPOCAMPAL FUNCTION IN LEARNING POSSIBLE?

The wide range of impairments following hippocampal-region damage—declarative memory in humans, spatial learning in rats, stimulus-stimulus learning in classical conditioning—has created a major puzzle for neuroscientists who are interested in specifying a precise function for the hippocampal region. This confusing state of affairs has led to many different theories or descriptions of hippocampal function. Unfortunately, many of these "theories" amount to little more than a description of some or all of the behaviors that are impaired by hippocampal-region damage. They tend to focus on one kind of behavior at the expense of explaining others. Claiming that the hippocampal region is involved in only declarative memory doesn't account for hippocampal-lesion impairments in sensory preconditioning, a behavior that clearly falls within the definition of nondeclarative motor learning. Claiming that the hippocampal region is a spatial processor doesn't account for the monkey data showing impairments in DNMS at long intervals—a task with no particular spatial component.

Attempts to relate lesion studies to particular behavioral functions have, in the past, been fraught with frustration. One prominent memory researcher, Richard Thompson, voiced this frustration when he and his colleagues wrote:

In our view, this question [What is the function of the hippocampus?], as it is phrased, is not likely to be meaningful. Brain structures do not exist in isolation. . . . If the brain as a whole has any one function, it is information processing. . . . Whether or not any given brain "structure" like the hippocampus plays any particular or specialized role . . . it seems very unlikely that a single phrase from the English language, such as "behavioral inhibition" or "spatial map," can serve adequately to characterize its functions.[40]

This suggests that a profitable approach to brain modeling would be to study how the hippocampus interacts with other brain structure to produce behaviors. Such models focus on how information is processed in each region of the brain before being stored or passed on to the next region. This kind of information-processing theory should provide a blueprint for creating a computer program or model to simulate the brain, and this should include recognizable components that perform the functions of the hippocampus and other brain structures. The entire system should show behavior comparable to that of normal animals and humans. When the computer model's "hippocampal region" is damaged, the model should show the same pattern of deficits—and of spared learning—as animals and humans with hippocampal-region damage.

To understand the methods of information-processing theories of brain function in general, and of the hippocampal-region in particular, the next three chapters provide an introduction to the fundamentals of neural network modeling. Chapter 3 serves as an initial introduction to simple neural network models, focusing on the learning rules used for the formation of associations and the application of these rules to understanding the cerebellum. For continuity with the rest of the book, these networks will be illustrated through their application to classical conditioning. Chapter 4 introduces the key issues of stimulus representation—the problem of how to capture within a formal model the events of interest in the natural learning situation, such as the tones, lights, and airpuffs described above. Chapter 5 considers how animals and people learn from mere exposure to stimuli—as in the first phase of the sensory preconditioning task described above—and what kinds of neural networks can capture this type of learning.

Chapter 5 is the last of the tutorial chapters making up part I of this book. Beginning in chapter 6, part II introduces several neural network models of the interactions between the hippocampus and other brain regions during learning.

SUMMARY

• The hippocampal region includes the hippocampus (subfields CA1-CA4), the dentate gyrus, the subiculum, and the entorhinal cortex. The hippocampal region is sometimes defined as including the fimbria/fornix, a fiber pathway that connects the hippocampus to subcortical structures. In humans, the structures of the hippocampal region are located in the medial temporal lobes.

• Most neuroscientists now agree that the hippocampus plays an important role in learning and memory, but there is little consensus as to what that role is.

• Patients such as HM and RB with damage to the medial temporal lobe (hippocampal region) show anterograde amnesia, which is characterized by inability to form new declarative memories—memories such as autobiographical episodes and facts that are easily verbalized. There may be relative sparing of older memories, intelligence, attention, and personality. Anterograde amnesia is often accompanied by some degree of retrograde amnesia, loss of memories formed just before the trauma. Etiologies that can result in anterograde amnesia include stroke, anoxia or hypoxia, herpes encephalitis, normal aging, and Alzheimer's disease, all of which can damage the hippocampus and nearby structures.

• Nondeclarative or procedural learning, such as perceptual learning and motor skill learning, may be spared in amnesia.

• Animal studies have concentrated on developing nonhuman analogs of declarative memory, on identifying tasks such as spatial learning that are especially sensitive to hippocampal damage, and on developing experimental procedures such as classical eyeblink conditioning that are similar across species.

• Eyeblink conditioning is spared after hippocampal lesion, but in the normal brain, the hippocampus does indeed contribute to eyeblink conditioning. Thus, there is a distinction between behaviors for which the hippocampus is needed and those to which it normally contributes.

• The wide range of deficits following hippocampal damage limits the utility of descriptive theories of hippocampal function that focus on a single type of behavior. An alternative approach is to construct information-processing theories of hippocampal function, which attempt to specify how the hippocampus processes information and how the results of this computation are used by other brain regions.

3 Association in Neural Networks

This chapter has two basic purposes. First, it is meant to be a relatively pain-less introduction to neural network models. For this reason, we focus on the simplest possible models and apply them to the most elementary of learning situations: classical Pavlovian conditioning between stimuli (such as tones) and reinforcements (such as airpuffs to the eye). Once such simple models are understood in some detail, it is easier to scale the same principles up to larger models. In fact, many of the more complex models to be discussed in later chapters are simply elaborations of principles that emerge from these smaller systems.

There is a second reason for studying the simplest neural networks: Despite their apparent simplicity, they can provide useful insights into how animals and humans learn, just as the toy airplane models described in chapter 1 can teach us fundamental principles of aerodynamics that apply to full-size planes. Simple network models capture important qualitative ideas about learning and memory expressed within the context of a clearly defined framework for theory development. In chapter 1, we argued that models should be judged not only by how much relevant information they include, but also by how much irrelevant information they leave out. In this chapter, we will introduce one model, the Rescorla-Wagner model, which is in many ways a "model" model. It has stood for nearly thirty years as an example of how it is possible to take a set of complex behaviors, pare away all but the essence, and express the underlying mechanism as an intuitively tractable idea.

Equally important, the Rescorla-Wagner model—for all its apparent simplicity—generates numerous nontrivial predictions that drive empirical studies even to the current day. The Rescorla-Wagner model does not capture all known behaviors, even within its limited domain of classical condition-ing.[1] However, even these limitations of the model have proven useful in understanding which types of learning may depend on different processes and thus possibly arise from different brain regions, as discussed later in this chapter. In these ways, the Rescorla-Wagner model represents a case study for what modeling in the behavioral and neural sciences should aspire to; it is a standard against which the models presented in the rest of this book can be judged.

Section 3.1 reviews the basic properties of nerve cells in the brain and how they communicate with each other. It then introduces the class of models termed **neural networks,** which attempt to capture the essence of this interaction. Section 3.2 discusses how simple (one-unit) models can learn associations between stimuli and reinforcement. Finally, section 3.3 presents the Rescorla-Wagner model of classical conditioning. This model and its variants provide the basis for many of the concepts underlying the more complex models discussed in later chapters.

In this chapter and throughout the book, we present computational principles with a minimum of formalisms; however, some readers may be interested in seeing the formal statements of the models. For these readers, supplemental materials (MathBoxes) are provided with mathematical details and further references. However, the descriptions in the text are sufficient for a reader to understand the material in the rest of the book, without reference to the MathBoxes.

3.1 WHAT IS A NEURAL NETWORK?

Neurons and Information Processing in the Brain

Although the chemical and physical details inside a neuron are exquisitely complex, almost all neurons—in animals and humans—share the same basic architecture and functional principles. Figure 3.1A is a picture of a region of brain tissue with the neurons stained to appear dark. Even within this small region, it is easy to see that neurons vary widely in shape, position, and size. Despite this superficial variation, most neurons have several prototypical features, which are schematized in figure 3.1B. Some of the same basic structure can be seen in the neurons of figure 3.1A.

The prototypical neuron has an **axon,** a primary output pathway by which the neuron sends information to other neurons. The neuron's **dendrites** are treelike branches that collect information sent on by other neurons. In biological jargon, the inputs that arrive at a neuron are called **afferent** inputs (or simply **afferents**).

In most cases, the axon of the afferent neuron comes very close to—but does not touch—the dendrite of the receiving neuron. The gap between neurons is called a **synapse.** Figure 3.2B shows a schematic drawing of a synapse. The afferent neuron releases chemicals, called **neurotransmitters,**

(A)   (B)

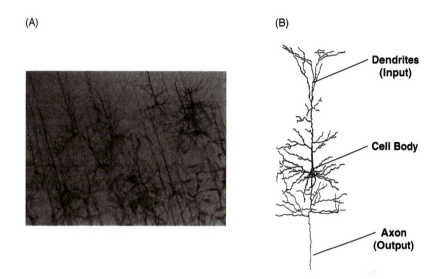

Figure 3.1   (A) Neurons in a small area of brain tissue, revealed through a process known as Golgi staining, in which a random subset of neurons become darkly colored. (Reprinted from Bear, Connors, & Paradiso, 1996, Figure 2.3, p. 25.) (B) A drawing of an individual neuron, in the cortex of a mouse, showing the cell body, dendrites, and axon. The dendrites would be covered with synapses, each a contact from another neuron. The axon is the main output process and may extend some distance before making contact with other neurons. (Adapted from Kuffler, Nicholls, & Martin, 1984.)

into the synapse. The neurotransmitters are picked up by **receptors** in the receiving neuron's dendrites.

The receiving neuron integrates all the information it receives from all its afferents and may produce output in turn, releasing neurotransmitters from its own axon. Some neurotransmitters have an **excitatory** effect on the receiving neuron, meaning that they increase the net activation of the receiving neuron. Other neurotransmitters have an **inhibitory** effect, reducing the net activity of the receiving neuron. Both excitatory and inhibitory inputs can vary in strength, some having a strong effect on the receiving neuron and others having a weaker effect. This depends not only on the particular chemical composition of the neurotransmitters, but also on the strength or efficacy of the synapse itself. Some synapses simply have a greater effect on the overall activity of the receiving cell than others.

Most neuroscientists now believe that a basic mechanism of learning is alteration of synaptic strength. This may occur either by creating new synapses (and deleting defunct ones) or by adjusting the strength of existing synapses.[2]

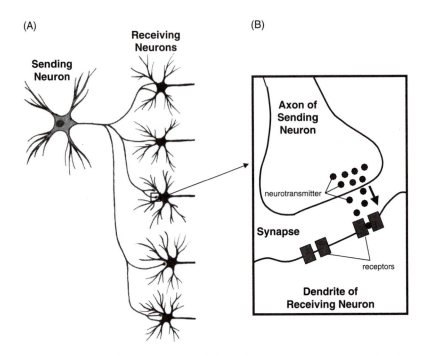

Figure 3.2   (A) An individual neuron sends information via its axon, which may branch to contact many other neurons. The point of contact is called a synapse, a small space between the sending and receiving neuron. (Adapted from Kuffler, Nicholls, & Martin, 1984, Box 1.) (B) Close-up of a synapse. When the sending neuron becomes active, or fires, it releases packets of chemicals, called neurotransmitters, into the synapse. The dendrites of the receiving neuron are covered with receptors, which are specialized to receive different neurotransmitters. The receiving neuron integrates information from all its receptors, and if it receives enough excitatory input, it may become active in turn.

Many subtle details are missing from the preceding description of neuronal processing and communication; some of these will be discussed in later chapters. However, the basic process described above is common to almost all neurons in both animal and human brains. Some of these principles have been known for over a hundred years, and others are still the subject of research. The biggest mystery today is much the same as that pondered by the earliest neuroscientists: How do networks of neurons work together to produce the range of complex behaviors seen in animals and humans?

One approach to understanding how neuronal mechanisms and circuits yield observable behaviors has been to explore simple models of brain circuits. These models allow us to explore the complex behaviors that emerge when neurons are linked together. The study of these model neural networks has gone by many names, including **connectionism** and **parallel distributed**

processing. The study of neural network models has drawn extensively on concepts from neuroscience and psychology, as well as from the tools of mathematics and computer science. Through this interdisciplinary endeavor, modelers have sought an understanding of the general principles by which neuronlike systems can process information and adapt behavior. The next subsection reviews the fundamental principles of modeling neural networks. Later, section 3.2 will discuss the problem of getting networks to learn.

Information Processing in Neural Network Models

Neural network models start with a **node,** a simplified mathematical abstraction of the basic functioning of a neuron. Figure 3.3A shows a network of three nodes, labeled A, B, and C. Each node has inputs (corresponding to a neuron's dendrites) and outputs (corresponding to a neuron's axon). Thus, nodes A and B send output to node C, represented by arrows in the figure.

Nodes A and B do not receive inputs from any other nodes in the figure; they are called **input nodes,** because they are the originators of all input to

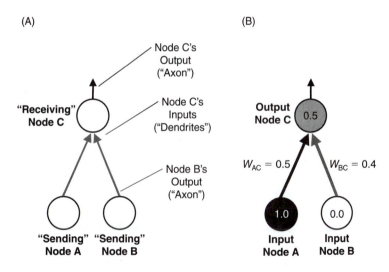

Figure 3.3 (A) Simple model neurons, called nodes. Like neurons, each node has inputs (analogous to a neuron's dendrites) and an output (analogous to a neuron's axon). Here, nodes A and B send output (represented as arrows), which is received and processed by node C. Node C in turn may send output to other nodes (not shown). (B) Each node has an activation level, which determines the probability that the node will fire. These are shown as numbers inside each node. Connections between nodes in a network are often assigned a value, or weight, analogous to the efficacy or strength of a synapse between two neurons. The activation level at node C is determined by the activations of input nodes A and B, multiplied by the connection weights from those nodes. Hence, the activation of node C = $(1.0 \times 0.5) + (0.0 \times 0.4) = 0.5$.

the rest of the network. Node C is called an **output node,** because it does not send output to any other nodes in this network. It may be helpful to think in terms of a rough analogy with the brain: Input nodes might correspond to receptors in the eye or skin that respond to external visual and touch stimuli and send this information on to the rest of the brain. Output nodes might correspond to neurons with axons that leave the brain, such as the nerve cells that guide muscle movement.

Each node in a network has an **activation level,** shown in figure 3.3B as the number inside each node. Activation levels are usually defined to range between 0 and 1. The activation level of a node can be thought of as specifying the probability that the node will generate output of its own. It can also be thought of as approximating the strength of the node's response, on a scale from 0 (not active) to 1 (fully active). In figure 3.3B, we adopt the convention of darkening nodes that are more strongly activated. Thus, input node A is fully active, input node B is not active, and output node C has an intermediate level of activation.

We noted earlier that a combination of excitatory and inhibitory synapses allows one neuron to respond to inputs from a variety of other neurons. Each input can be either excitatory or inhibitory and can be either strong or weak. Within a model neural network, this range of synaptic effects is captured by an **associative weight.** Although most neural network models allow for weights to be both positive (excitatory) and negative (inhibitory), we will begin by confining ourselves to a discussion of positive weights.

Intuitively, associative weights can be thought of as functioning like valves, modulating how much of the activity from one neuron is allowed to flow into the next neuron. If the weights are numbers between 0 and 1, then each weight can be interpreted as a valve that ranges from completely shut (0) to fully open (1), modulating how effective the afferent neuron is in activating the receiving neuron. In figure 3.3B, the weight from node A to C, called W_A, is set to 0.5. This means that 0.5 (50%) of A's activation transfers to C. The weight from node B to C, W_B, is set to 0.4. In the figure, we assume that whatever external stimulus node A responds to is present, so A's activation is 100% or 1.0; B's external stimulus is absent, so B's activation is 0% or 0.0. The activation of C depends on the activation of A and B, modulated by the weights. Since $W_A = 0.5$, half of A's activation gets through; since $W_B = 0.4$, slightly less than half of B's activation gets through. The activation at C is the sum of these amounts:

Activation of C = (Activation of A $\times$ W_A) + (Activation of B $\times$ W_B)
$$= (1.0 \times 0.5) + (0.0 \times 0.4)$$
$$= 0.5$$

In this example, the activation of C is the output or product of the network; more complex scenarios are possible, and we will discuss some in the next chapter. If this network were a model of some behavioral system, then the network output could be interpreted as the strength of a behavioral output in response to a particular set of stimulus inputs: stimulus *A* present, stimulus *B* absent.

The output node C in this network performs an information-processing function roughly comparable to that of a neuron: It collects input from a variety of sources, processes that information (in this case, taking a weighted sum), and then possibly generates a response. This might not seem like a very sophisticated information-processing device, especially when compared to the computational capabilities of personal computers, pocket calculators—or the human brain. However, *the power of nodes in a neural network (and neurons in the brain) comes not so much from their individual power, but from the collective power that emerges when many such devices are interconnected in a network.*

Application of Network Models to Motor-Reflex Conditioning

Chapter 2 introduced the experimental procedure of eyeblink conditioning, and we will continue to use this elementary form of learning as an example. To briefly review: Animals are given mildly aversive airpuffs to the eye (the unconditioned stimulus, or US), which naturally evoke protective eyeblinks. If the US is repeatedly preceded by a stimulus cue such as a tone (the conditioned stimulus, or CS), the animal learns a basic association: that the tone CS predicts the imminent arrival of the airpuff US. Eventually, the animal should come to give an anticipatory blink response to the CS cue alone, timed so that the eye is shut when the airpuff US arrives. Learning is assessed by measuring the strength, reliability, and timing of this conditioned response.

Back in 1943, Warren McCulloch and Walter Pitts demonstrated that such associations could be modeled using a simple neural network much like the one shown in figure 3.4A.[3] A possible CS, such as a tone or light, is assigned to each input node; the activation level of an input node is set to 1.0 when the corresponding cue is present and to 0.0 otherwise. The activation of the output node is interpreted as the strength or probability of a conditioned response, such as an eyeblink. In the example shown in figure 3.4A, the tone is present and the light is absent. Before any training, we assume that all weights between nodes are set to 0.0. Thus, the presentation of the tone does not initially evoke any activation in the output node, and there is no conditioned response.

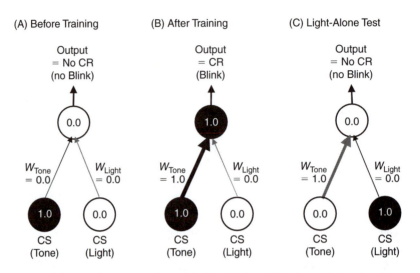

Figure 3.4 (A) A one-layer network model of eyeblink conditioning with input nodes, representing tone and light CSs, and one output node. The activation of the output node is the network's response and corresponds to the strength or probability of a CR (eyeblink). Weights are initially set to 0.0, so activation in either CS node does not produce any activation in the output node nor any CR. (B) The status of the network after being trained that the tone predicts the airpuff. Now the weight from the tone CS has been strengthened to 1.0 (represented by the thicker arrow), and so activation of the tone CS node produces activation in the output node and a blink CR. (C) Since the weight from the light CS has not been changed, activation of the light CS node still does not produce a CR.

Figure 3.4B illustrates what the same network might look like if it had been trained to give a response to the tone CS but not the light CS. In this figure, the weight from the tone node is 1.0 (schematized by a thicker arrow in the figure). Now, whenever that CS is present, the activation of the output node will be $1.0 \times 1.0 = 1.0$; thus, the network generates a strong response to the tone CS. On the other hand, the light CS still has a weight of 0.0; thus, when the light is present (figure 3.4C), the activation of the output node will be $1.0 \times 0.0 = 0.0$, and the network will not respond.

Note that in this very simple model, there are no assumptions about how sensory stimuli such as lights and tones are preprocessed nor how conditioned responses are translated into motor actions. These functions are important, but they take place outside the scope of this model. Like airplane propulsion for the engineer studying aerodynamics in chapter 1, these issues are not directly relevant to the memory processes being studied—and indeed might encumber the model with unnecessary additional complexity, detracting from the model's explanatory power and focus. The model in figure 3.4 is meant to address only one issue: How does one CS come to evoke a response but another does not? The model suggests that this process can be understood by means of associative weights that influence responding.

A reasonable question to ask now is: How does one train the naive network in figure 3.4A so that it becomes the fully trained network of figure 3.4B? The only difference between these two networks is in their weights. *Thus, the key to learning in neural networks is changing the weights between nodes.* As we noted earlier, this is intended to roughly capture what happens during learning in networks of real neurons, in which synaptic strengths are altered, thereby altering the ability of some neurons to cause firing in other neurons.

The earliest approaches to the problem of how to change the weights in a neural network came neither from psychology nor from neuroscience, but rather from engineering. The next section presents an early engineering approach to learning in neural networks.

3.2   NEURAL NETWORK MODELS OF LEARNING

In the late 1950s and early 1960s, Bernard Widrow and Ted Hoff were using neural networks to try to solve some classic problems in engineering and signal processing. These included the automatic transcription of speech, recognizing objects from novel angles, and diagnosing heart defects on the basis of EKG recordings. People can be trained to do all these tasks very well, but it is hard to codify the rules into a traditional computer program. Neural networks offered an alternative approach: Instead of having a programmer tell the computer how to perform a task, the computer could learn for itself.

Widrow and Hoff set up their engineering problems so that each could be represented as a set of input patterns, each of which was associated with a desired output pattern. For example, in speech-to-text transcription, the first step was to preprocess the speech into a set of patterns that could be applied as input to a network. This kind of preprocessing is a complex process and the subject of much research.[4] These input patterns were then paired with output patterns that represented instructions to generate typewritten text. The neural network's job was to take each input pattern and generate the desired output, in this way translating "speech" into "text."

The key problem for Widrow and Hoff was how to teach a network this kind of mapping from input to output. For a simple problem such as eyeblink conditioning, it is often possible to intuit what the fully trained network should look like. For example, in figure 3.4, setting values of 1.0 and 0.0

on the tone weight and the light weight, respectively, made the network respond to the tone but not to the light. In real brains, of course, synaptic strengths are not set "by hand" but learned through repeated exposures to regularities in the environment. Moreover, in very complex problems such as speech transcription, the network might need hundreds or thousands of weights to encode highly complex relationships between the input patterns and the output patterns. In such a case, it is difficult or impossible to choose all the appropriate weights by hand. Thus, Widrow and Hoff needed a **learning rule:** an algorithm that would allow the network to adapt its weights to solve an arbitrary problem.

The Widrow-Hoff Learning Rule

Widrow and Hoff developed a simple but effective learning rule known today as the Widrow-Hoff rule.[5] The rule also goes by several other names, including the LMS (least-mean-squared) or delta rule, for reasons relating to its mathematical underpinnings. These details are presented in MathBox 3.1 for those who wish a deeper understanding of these formal underpinnings; however, they are not essential to understanding the rest of the material in this book. The Widrow-Hoff rule and other related algorithms[6] formed the foundation for tremendous subsequent growth of neural network models in engineering, neuroscience, and psychology.

To train a network to predict or classify inputs correctly, Widrow and Hoff noted that there needs to be an external signal, distinct from the network's actual response, that specifies the desired output. This signal, often called a **teaching input,** is shown in figure 3.5. In the context of eyeblink conditioning, the teaching input specifies whether the airpuff US occurred and thus whether the **desired output** was 1.0 (if the airpuff US was present) or 0.0 (if the airpuff US was absent). Given such a teaching input, the network can compare its own output against the desired output and then adjust the weights so that, in the future, errors are less likely.

Widrow and Hoff proposed that this process should work as follows: First, cues are presented; input nodes corresponding to those cues become fully active (activation level = 1.0). This activation propagates through weighted connections to the output node, producing some level of activation there. This activation becomes the node's output and indicates the strength or probability of a conditioned response.

Next, the teaching signal provides information about desired output. In the case of eyeblink conditioning, this desired output, as shown in figure 3.5, is 1.0 if the airpuff US occurred and 0.0 if the airpuff US did not occur.

MathBox 3.1   The Widrow-Hoff Rule

The Widrow-Hoff rule is an algorithm for training a simple processor to learn arbitrary mappings between input patterns and output patterns.

The basic unit, or *node,* is shown below. Each node j receives a series of inputs i, each of which has a value o_i. In the simplest case, $o_i = 1.0$ if input i is present and 0.0 otherwise, although intermediate values may be assumed. There may be multiple nodes, all operating in parallel and each learning a different relationship from inputs to outputs.

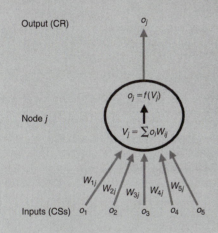

Each node processes its inputs according to an *activation rule.* The total activation V_j of node j is defined as the weighted sum of all inputs i present on the current trial:

$$V_j = \sum_i o_i w_{ij} \tag{3.1}$$

In this rule, w_{ij} is the *weight* or strength of the connection from i to j. If $w_{ij} > 0$, then when input i is present, it increases the total activation of j. If $w_{ij} < 0$, then when input i is present, it inhibits the total activation of j. If $w_{ij} = 0$, then the presence or absence of input i has no effect on j. (Note: In this and other boxes, the terminology has sometimes been changed from the original publication to maintain notational consistency throughout the text.)

Next, an *output rule* is used to convert activation to node output:

$$o_j = f(V_j) \tag{3.2}$$

In the simplest case, the output function f is merely an identity function ($f(x) = x$), so Equations 3.1 and 3.2 combine to yield

$$o_j = \sum_i o_i w_{ij} \tag{3.3}$$

This means that the output of node j is simply the sum of the weighted activations of all inputs i present on the current trial.

Next, the *error* ∂_j for node j is computed as the difference between the node's desired output d_j and its actual output o_j:

$$\partial_j = (d_j - o_j) \tag{3.4}$$

Finally, the weights are changed to reduce this error. For every weight w_{ij} from an input i to node j,

$$\Delta w_{ij} = \beta \delta_j o_i \tag{3.5}$$

Δw_{ij} is the amount by which w_{ij} changes on the current trial. If $\Delta w_{ij} > 0$, then the weight increases; if $\Delta w_{ij} < 0$, then the weight decreases. β is the network's *learning rate.* This is a fixed small number that determines how much a weight may be changed on a single trial. Typically, β might be set to a value between 0.01 and 0.1; in the example in Section 3.2, $\beta = 0.2$ for ease of explanation.

Mathematically, it can be shown that repeated applications of the Widrow-Hoff rule, with a sufficiently small value of β, will improve performance by minimizing the squared difference between actual and desired outputs across all input patterns; for this reason, the Widrow-Hoff rule is also known as the LMS (least-mean-squared) rule. It is also sometimes called the delta rule.

The reader who is interested in further mathematical details may refer to McCulloch & Pitts (1943); Rosenblatt (1958); Widrow & Hoff (1960); Rumelhart, Hinton, & Williams (1986); Gluck & Bower (1988a); Widrow & Winter (1988); Minsky & Papert (1998).

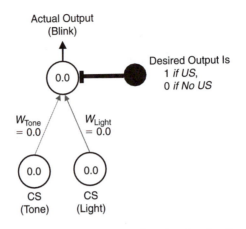

Figure 3.5   A one-layer network for eyeblink conditioning showing the addition of a teaching node indicating the desired output, as suggested by Widrow and Hoff (1960).

Widrow and Hoff defined the network's **error** on a particular trial as the difference between the desired output and the actual output, namely,

OutputError = (DesiredOutput − ActualOutput)

For example, consider the trained network of figure 3.4B. The tone CS is presented, and the output node produces a response (ActualOutput = 1.0). The US will arrive on that trial, so the DesiredOutput = 1.0. Therefore, we can calculate the OutputError as follows:

OutputError = (DesiredOutput − ActualOutput)
             = 1.0 − 1.0
             = 0.0

If the same network is tested on a trial in which the tone CS is absent (e.g., figure 3.4C), the network will not respond (ActualResponse = 0.0), and the US will not occur (DesiredResponse = 0.0). Hence, the Output Error is calculated as

OutputError = (DesiredOutput − ActualOutput)
             = 0.0 − 0.0
             = 0.0

In both these cases, the network's response is perfectly correct, there is no error, and we can conclude that for these trials, the network's weights are as they should be.

However, under other circumstances, there can be an error. For example, consider the untrained network of figure 3.4A: The tone cue is presented, the network does not respond, but the US arrives:

Output Error = (DesiredOutput − ActualOutput)
$$= 1.0 - 0.0$$
$$= 1.0$$

As the network is trained with repeated trials, the error should gradually decrease toward 0.0 (figure 3.4B). Thus, the difference between an untrained network (figure 3.4A) and a trained one (figure 3.4B) is all in the weights, as was noted earlier. Learning is a process of slowly changing the weights to produce appropriate responding—and reduce the error toward 0.0.

In this kind of neural network, the blame for an incorrect response (OutputError > 0) or the credit for a correct response (OutputError = 0) lies in the weights. But there may be many weights in the network, and not all of them may deserve the blame or credit equally. This is a fundamental problem for training neural networks and is often referred to as a credit assignment problem because the issue is how to assign credit (or blame) for a network's output performance to the weights in the network.

Widrow and Hoff's rule provides one solution to the problem of credit assignment. Their approach is called *error-correction learning* because it specifies that each weight should be adjusted according to its particular contribution to the total network error.

The first issue is determining which weights to adjust. Recall that the rule for computing output response is a weighted sum: Each input node contributes to the output node's activation as a function of its own activation multiplied by its weight. If an input node's activation is 0, then it has made no contribution to the output node. Only input nodes with activation > 0 can have any influence.

Thus, if there was some error and the output node's response was wrong, the fault must lie among the weights of those input nodes that were active on the current trial. Under these circumstances, the Widrow-Hoff rule will "punish" or reduce all these weights from the active nodes. This might seem like a rather heavy-handed approach, roughly equivalent to the police arresting all those who were present at the scene of the crime. But each weight is changed by only a very small amount on each trial. A particular weight that is active on one trial when the node's response is wrong will be changed only slightly; but if that same weight is active repeatedly, on many trials when the response is wrong, these changes will accumulate. Over time, the weights that are most to blame for the error will be changed the most; and given enough trials, the network will find an optimal set of weights that minimizes the total error over all types of trials.

To better understand how this learning rule operates, consider the example shown in figure 3.4A, in which the network fails to respond on a trial in which the tone cue is present and the resulting output response is incorrect (Output-Error = 1.0). The fault must lie in the weight from this active tone node but not in the weight from the inactive light node. If there had been other cues present, then the weights from those input nodes would have been changed too.

Now that the blame has been assigned to a subset of the network's weights, the second issue is how much to change each weight. A parameter known as the **learning rate** determines how large the weight changes should be. If there is a large learning rate, then the network as a whole will quickly adapt itself to new contingencies. This can be good or bad; if the learning rate is very high, then random fluctuations in the world (such as noise on the inputs) can lead to large changes in the network, even to the point of disrupting previously stored knowledge. On the other hand, a very low learning rate means that the network will be very stable but will take a long time to adapt to new contingencies. This paradox, called the plasticity-stability trade-off, has been the focus of much study.[7] There is no fixed rule for how to set the learning rate so as to achieve the best balance between stability and plasticity; the optimal learning rate depends on the particular problem being learned. We will return to the topic of learning rates in chapter 10 when we discuss possible neurobiological mechanisms for adjusting learning rates in the brain.

One way to improve a network's performance (that is, to minimize the likelihood of errors) is to make the weight changes depend not only on a fixed learning rate, but also on the current error. If the error is high, then there is good cause to make large changes in the network—even if some prior learning is disrupted as a result. On the other hand, if the error is small, then the network is performing relatively well, and changes should be smaller to preserve the prior learning.

Widrow and Hoff argued that weight changes should depend on both a fixed learning rate and the current error. Thus, for all nodes active on a given trial, weights are corrected for the next trial according to the following:

NewWeight = OldWeight + (LearningRate × Error)

An example may help to clarify how this works. Figure 3.6A is a copy of the untrained network of figure 3.4A. Weights from both input nodes are initially set to 0.0. On the first trial, the tone is presented. The output node's activation is the sum of the weighted activation of each input: 1.0 × 0.0 from the tone and 0.0×0.0 from the light. The activation is therefore 0.0, and the output is also 0.0. Since the airpuff US was present on this trial,

$$\text{OutputError} = (\text{DesiredOutput} - \text{ActualOutput})$$
$$= 1.0 - 0.0$$
$$= 1.0$$

Now, according to the Widrow-Hoff rule, this error should be distributed among active input nodes—only the tone in this case—as follows:

$$W_{\text{Tone}} = 0 + (\text{LearningRate} \times 1.0)$$

Suppose the learning rate is defined as 0.2; then the result of the first tone-airpuff pairing should be

$$W_{\text{Tone}} = 0 + (0.2 \times 1) = 0.2$$

Figure 3.6B shows the updated weight. The network has just taken its first step toward learning the correct response.

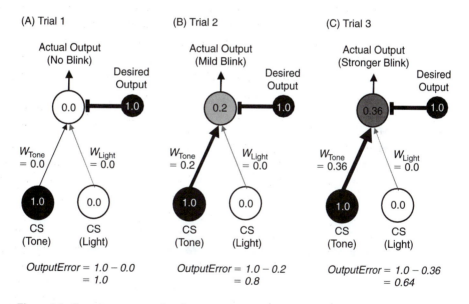

Figure 3.6 Learning to respond to the tone CS. (A) The untrained network before any training. The tone CS is presented, but since its weight is 0.0, there is no activation of the output node, and there is no response. Since the airpuff US always follows the tone CS, the desired output was 1.0, so the output error is 1.0. (B) Assuming a learning rate of 0.2, the weight from the tone CS is adapted to 0.2. On trial 2, the tone CS is presented again. This time, the actual output is 0.2, so the output error is reduced to 0.8. (C) Again, the weight is updated, and on trial 3, the actual output is 0.36, and the output error is only 0.64.

On the second trial (figure 3.6B), the tone occurs again. But this time, weight from the tone is 0.2, so the output node's activation is $1.0 \times 0.2 = 0.2$. This means that the output node is giving a weak response, at 20% of maximum strength (or, alternatively, has a 20% probability of firing). This is clearly better performance than on the last trial, although there is still room for improvement. On the next trial the error is calculated as

$$\begin{aligned} \text{OutputError} &= (\text{DesiredOutput} - \text{ActualOutput}) \\ &= 1.0 - 0.2 \\ &= 0.8 \end{aligned}$$

Once again, the Widrow-Hoff rule specifies that the weight from the active input node should be adjusted as

$$W_{\text{Tone}} = 0.2 + (0.2 \times 0.8) = 0.36$$

On the third trial (figure 3.6C), the output is $1.0 \times 0.36 = 0.36$. Again, the response is better than before; the network is improving, slowly, with each trial. If the process is repeated, with more and more pairings of the tone and the airpuff US, the output response will gradually increase toward 1.0 while the output error will gradually decrease toward 0.0. The error is also decreasing $(1.0 - 0.36 = 0.64)$. Figure 3.7A shows how the output response increases across 15 repeated trials, and figure 3.7B shows how the output error decreases during these same 15 trials.

Figure 3.7A is a **learning curve,** and it is directly comparable to the kind of learning curve generated in an experiment in which animals (or people) are trained to give a conditioned response (e.g., figure 3.7C,D). The most important characteristic is the curve's shape: Early in the acquisition phase, there are large changes in the response between trials, and the network output shows rapid improvement. Later in the acquisition phase, the response levels off near 1.0, and there are only small changes in response from trial to trial. This leveling-off point is called the **asymptote.**

Although all learning curves are roughly the same shape, the labeling and calibration of the axes may be very different. Figure 3.7C shows data from rabbits that are learning conditioned eyeblink responses. On average, the rabbits take some 300 trials to acquire the response. By contrast, figure 3.7D shows data from dogs that are learning that a light predicts arrival of a food US when the conditioned response measured is the degree of anticipatory salivation. Dogs learn the response in about twelve trials. These two kinds of learning occur at different speeds, but the overall shape of the acquisition curves are remarkably similar. Similarly, in the model data (figure 3.7A), the speed of learning can be adjusted upward or downward to change the speed

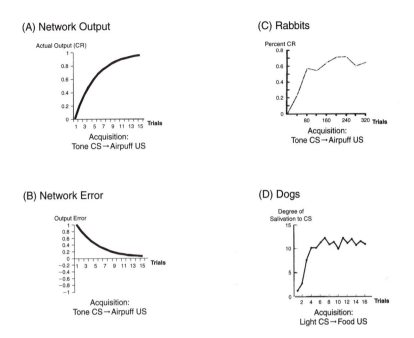

Figure 3.7 (A) Learning curve for the network shown in figure 3.6, given 15 acquisition trials pairing CS and US. Initially (trial 0), the network does not respond to the CS at all, but response increases with repeated pairings; the strength of the response (CR) climbs quickly over the first few trials and then levels off near 1.0. This leveling-off point is the asymptote. (B) The output error corresponding to the learning shown in A. Early in acquisition training, when the actual response is low, the error is high; as the actual response grows, error drops off to zero. (C–D) The learning curves for CS-US acquisition training in rabbits (C) and dogs (D) are similar to the model. (C is adapted from Gormezano, Kehoe, & Marshall, 1983; D is adapted from Hilgard, Atkinson, & Atkinson, 1975, Figure 7.4, p. 197.)

of learning. The actual number of trials required to acquire a response in the model is less important than the fact that the overall shape of the learning curve should be similar to that seen in animal data.

In animals, if the **acquisition** trials (CS-US pairings) are followed by **extinction** trials (CS alone, with no US), the initial learned response will gradually disappear (or *extinguish*). Figure 3.8C,D shows what happens to the learning curves of figure 3.7 when animals are given such additional extinction trials. Similarly, if the network is given CS-US pairings followed by CS-alone extinction trials, it shows similar behavior (figure 3.8A). On the first extinction trial, there is no US, and so the desired output is 0.0. However, because of the previous training trials, the actual output is 0.96 (close to 1.0); the error is computed as follows:

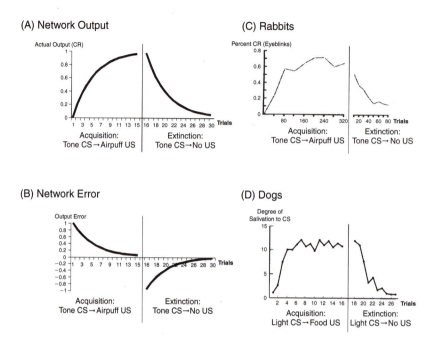

Figure 3.8 (A) After 15 trials of CS-US learning, the network from figure 3.6 is given 15 extinction trials, in which the CS is presented without the US. Again, the response changes quickly over the first few extinction trials, dropping from its previously high levels, then leveling out at a new asymptote near 0.0. (B) The output error is large early in the extinction phase, while the network is still responding to the CS but no US arrives. As the network response in A decreases, the error returns to 0.0. (C–D) Extinction in animals (C = rabbits, D = dogs) shows the same basic form as the model in A. (B is adapted from Gormezano, Kehoe, & Marshall, 1983, Figure 3B; D is adapted from Hilgard, Atkinson, & Atkinson, 1975, Figure 7.4, p. 197.)

$$OutputError = (DesiredOutput - ActualOutput)$$
$$= (0 - 0.96)$$
$$= -0.96$$

Note that now the error is a negative number, indicating that the actual output activation was too high. Intuitively, we might therefore expect that the weight from the active nodes should be reduced, and this is precisely what the Widrow-Hoff rule does:

$$NewW_{Tone} = OldW_{Tone} + (LearningRate \times Error)$$
$$= 0.96 + (0.2 \times -0.96)$$
$$= 0.77$$

The new weight (0.77) is noticeably smaller than the old weight (0.96). Thus, on the second extinction trial, the network's response to the tone CS will be a little weaker. With repeated extinction trials, the response fades away altogether, as is shown in the right half of figure 3.8A. Thus, the Widrow-Hoff error-correcting learning procedure works to adapt the network to the regularities in the environment, even when these regularities are altered. Whereas on trials 1 through 15, the US reliably followed the tone, this has now changed, and the US no longer follows the tone on trials 16 through 30. Tracking these changes in environmental regularities, the network adapts its weights so as to continue to seek an optimal set of weights for correctly predicting the US.

The actual Widrow-Hoff rule was slightly more complex than the foregoing discussion implies. It allowed for the input nodes to be partially active and for a few other complications. Full mathematical details are given in MathBox 3.1.

Widrow and Hoff's work in the late 1950s and early 1960s led to a wide range of computing devices used by engineers for tasks as diverse as weather prediction and the mechanical control of balance.[8] Widrow himself continued to refine the approach and produced networks that could learn difficult problems including recognizing rotated patterns, performing time-series prediction, playing the game of blackjack, and backing a tractor-trailer into a loading dock.[9] Widrow's simple networks also found many practical uses in signal processing applications, including the reduction of noise in computer modems, long-distance telephone lines, and satellite communications.[10] Widrow's collaborator Hoff did not continue to work in this area; he and a handful of fellow Stanford students left academia to start a computer company. They called it Intel. But that's another story.

3.3   RELATIONSHIP TO ANIMAL LEARNING

Widrow and Hoff were engineers, studying machine learning because they wanted to create intelligent computers. They weren't particularly concerned with whether their learning algorithms bore any meaningful resemblance to learning in the brain—any more than an engineer designing airplanes might care whether the designs capture any features of bird flight.

However, a decade after Widrow and Hoff developed their neural network learning rule, psychologists realized that some very fundamental kinds of animal learning could also be described by the same basic error-correcting principle. This insight led to the development of the Rescorla-Wagner model,[11] a simple but elegant description of classical conditioning in animals and humans. As described below, this new model, and the experiments that led to it, challenged some basic axioms of learning that dated back over seventy years.

The Blocking Effect

At the turn of the century, Ivan Pavlov had argued that classical conditioning resulted solely from the pairing of a CS, such as a tone or bell, and a US, such as the presentation of food.[12] That is, as long as the CS and US occurred closely together in time, association would develop between them. By the late 1960s, however, several studies had shown that conditioning wasn't quite so simplistic: It wasn't enough for CS and US to merely co-occur; instead, they had to have some meaningful, predictive relationship.

A classic experiment that demonstrates this principle is the **blocking** paradigm, introduced by Leo Kamin in 1968, which follows the procedure outlined in table 3.1. Kamin originally demonstrated blocking using rats that had been trained to press a lever for food,[13] but the same effect can be obtained in a variety of preparations, including rabbit eyeblink conditioning.[14]

First, the animals are divided into two groups, called the Sit Exposure group and the Pre-Trained group. In phase 1, each animal in the Pre-Trained group is trained that a tone CS predicts an airpuff US. Training continues until the animal learns to give a reliable eyeblink response to the tone. In contrast, the animals in the Sit-Exposure group sit in the experimental chamber for an equivalent amount of time, but they are given no exposure to the tone or the airpuff US. Next, in phase 2, each animal (in both groups) is given presentations of a compound stimulus, consisting of the old tone CS plus a new light CS, presented simultaneously; this compound tone and light stimulus is always followed by the airpuff US. Animals in the Pre-Trained group, having already learned to respond to the tone, continue to respond to the tone and light compound. Meanwhile, animals in the Sit-Exposure group also learn to respond to the tone and light compound. Finally, in phase 3, all animals are tested for responding to the tone alone and to the light alone. Figure 3.9 shows a typical set of results from a blocking experiment in rabbits.[15] Animals in the Sit-Exposure group give reliable responses to either CS.

Table 3.1   The Blocking Experiment

Group	Phase 1	Phase 2	Phase 3: Test
Pre-Trained	Tone CS → airpuff US	Tone CS and light CS → airpuff US	Tone CS → ? Light CS → ?
Sit-Exposure	(*Animal sits in experimental chamber*)	Tone CS and light CS → airpuff US	Tone CS → ? Light CS → ?

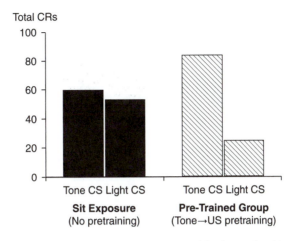

Figure 3.9 Phase 3 responding for a blocking experiment like that outlined in table 3.1. Rabbits in the Sit-Exposure group show strong responding to both the tone CS and the light CS. Rabbits in the Pre-Trained group show strong responding to the tone CS but very little responding to the light CS. Prior training to the tone CS in phase 1 blocks subsequent learning about the light CS in phase 2. (Plotted from data presented in Solomon, 1977.)

By contrast, animals in the Pre-Trained group respond strongly to the tone but give virtually no responses to the light. It appears as if prior learning about the tone blocks subsequent learning about the light.

This blocking effect was problematic for early theories of conditioning, because they expected learning to be determined only by the co-occurrence of the CS and US. If this were true, animals that were given light and US pairings in phase 2 should have learned an association between the light and the US, regardless of prior training. Yet this was not the case: Animals in the Pre-Trained group, which had previously learned to respond to the tone, showed very little responding to the light in phase 3.

Apparently, co-occurrence alone is not sufficient for learning. Instead, blocking suggests that *learning occurs only when the CS is a useful predictor of the US.*[16] In the Pre-Trained group, the tone is a perfectly reliable predictor of the US in phase 1. When phase 2 begins, the tone continues to predict the US; the presence of the light adds no useful additional information. Therefore, there is little learning about the light in phase 2, resulting in weak responding to the light in phase 3.

Blocking also occurs in human learning. For example, in a study by Tom Trabasso and Gordon Bower, college students were trained to categorize objects according to certain predefined rules.[17] The students were presented with geometric figures varying in their color (red versus blue), shape (circle versus triangle), number of lines (one versus two), position of dot (top versus bottom), and position of gap (left versus right). Two example figures are shown in figure 3.10A. Students then had to guess whether each figure belonged to class A or class B; each time, they were told whether they had guessed correctly or not. Given enough trials, subjects deduced the rule determining class membership: for example, all circular shapes belonged in class A, all triangular shapes belonged in class B, and all the other features were irrelevant.

Once this was mastered, the experimenter changed the rules slightly: Now all figures that were circular *and* had the dot on top belonged to class A, while all figures that were triangular *and* had the dot on the bottom belonged to class B. Subjects could continue to perform well by using their old rule of sorting on the basis of shape; the question was whether they would also learn that the dot position predicted class membership.

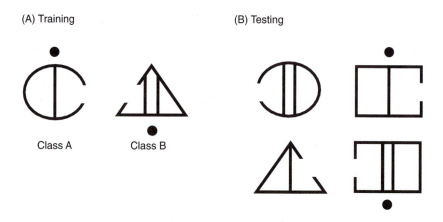

(A) Training

(B) Testing

Class A   Class B

Figure 3.10 Example stimuli used in the human blocking experiment. (A) Subjects were given a set of geometric figures that differed in color (red versus blue in the original experiment), shape (circle versus triangle), number of lines (one versus two), position of dot (top versus bottom), and position of gap (left versus right). In the first phase, all circles belonged in class A and all triangles belonged in class B, regardless of other features. Once subjects acquired this rule, a second feature was made predictive: All figures that were circular *and* had a dot on top belonged in class A, while all figures that were triangular *and* had a dot on the bottom belonged in class B. (Any figures that did not obey this rule were not used.) Since the original rule regarding shape was still predictive, new learning about the dot was blocked. (B) Subjects were given test shapes as shown; given shapes with no dot, subjects were able to accurately sort circles into class A and triangles into class B, demonstrating they had learned the original rule. However, given figures of a new shape (rectangular), subjects were not able to sort on the basis of dot position, demonstrating that learning about the dot had been blocked by prior learning about shape. (Adapted from Trabasso & Bower, 1968, Figure 3.1, p. 74.)

To test this, the experimenter used new figures, shown in figure 3.10B. Given a figure with no dot, all subjects continued to sort the circles into class A and the triangles into class B. However, given a figure with a new shape (rectangular), no subjects were able to correctly sort on the basis of dot position! Thus, prior learning that the shape predicted class membership appeared to have *blocked* subsequent learning that the dot position also predicted class membership. More recent studies have verified that blocking is as pervasive in human learning as it is in animal learning.[18]

The Rescorla-Wagner Model of Conditioning

The blocking effect posed a challenge for simple theories of classical conditioning. It suggested that cues do not merely acquire strength on the basis of their individual relationships with the US; rather, *cues appear to compete with one another for associative strength.* Thus, in the blocking experiment of table 3.1, the light competes with the tone during phase 2; in the case of the Pre-Trained group, the light loses this competition: Since the tone already accurately predicts the US, the light provides no additional predictive information.

This study and others like it led to a growing view among psychologists that to produce effective conditioning, a stimulus cue (CS) must impart reliable information about the expected occurrence of the outcome (US). Moreover, even if a given cue is predictive of a US, it might not become conditioned if its usefulness has been preempted by another co-occurring cue that is a better predictor of the US or that has a longer history of successfully predicting the US. The result of all these findings was to show that "simple" Pavlovian conditioning was not nearly as simple as had once been thought! Instead, animals appear to be very sophisticated statisticians, calculating measures of reliability, usefulness, and predictive value among the stimuli they encounter. In other words, they are acutely sensitive to the **informational value** of stimuli.

It turns out that there is an elegantly simple way to formalize this process developed by Robert Rescorla and Allan Wagner in the early 1970s.[19] The key idea behind the Rescorla-Wagner model is that changes in CS-US associations on a trial are driven by the discrepancy (or error) between the animal's expectation of the US and whether or not the US actually occurred. Sound familiar? Rescorla and Wagner's model of classical conditioning incorporated the same error-correcting principle developed ten years earlier by the engineers Widrow and Hoff. Ironically, it took a decade before two other researchers, trained in both engineering and psychology, realized that the

MathBox 3.2   The Rescorla-Wagner Model

The Rescorla-Wagner model assumes that the change in association between a CS and the US depends on the associative strength of all cues present on that trial. Formally,

$$\Delta w_{ij} = \alpha_i \beta (\lambda_j - V_j) \tag{3.6}$$

where i is a CS and j is a US, w_{ij} is the strength of the existing association between i and j, and Δw_{ij} is the increment to w_{ij} on the current trial. The size of this increment is proportional to three factors: the salience (e.g., amplitude) of CS i (α_i), the learning rate (β), and the difference between the asymptote of conditioning to that US (λ_j) and the total associative strength of all cues present (V_j).

On each trial, the total associative strength is computed as

$$V_j = \sum_i w_{ij} \tag{3.7}$$

for all CS i present on the current trial.

In most cases, the conditioned response CR is simply defined as

$$CR = V_j \tag{3.8}$$

According to the learning rule in Equation 3.6, the changes in associative strength w_{ij} are thus proportional to the difference between the CR and the asymptote λ_j. The asymptote λ_j is generally taken to be 1.0 on those trials in which a particular US j is present and 0.0 on those trials in which no US is present.* Therefore, the learning rule in Equation (3.6) can be restated as

$$\Delta w_{ij} = \alpha_i \beta (US - CR) \tag{3.9}$$

In their original formulation, Rescorla and Wagner noted that the learning rate (β) might differ for different USs; for example, learning might be greater on trials in which the US is present than when it is absent. Additionally, Rescorla and

*In principle, it would theoretically be possible for different USs j to be relatively weaker or stronger, and hence be assigned different values of λ_j.

Wagner assumed that CS salience (α_i) might differ for different stimuli. Many later researchers simplified the model by assuming that all CSs in an experiment have equal salience ($\alpha_i = 1.0$), thus,

$$\Delta w_{ij} = \beta (US - CR) \tag{3.10}$$

This is the version of the learning rule that is presented in the text.

Learning in the Rescorla-Wagner model is formally equivalent to the Widrow-Hoff (1960) rule, presented in MathBox 3.1. First, the computation of associative strength (Equation 3.7) can be restated as

$$V_j = \sum_i o_i w_{ij} \tag{3.11}$$

assuming that $o_i = 1.0$ when input i is present and $o_i = 0.0$ otherwise. Thus, this is the same as the activation level computed in the Widrow-Hoff rule (Equation 3.1 in Math Box 3.1).

Second, learning in the Rescorla-Wagner model is mathematically equivalent to the Widrow-Hoff (1960) rule. MathBox 3.1 stated that weight change in the Widrow-Hoff rule was calculated by

$$\begin{aligned}\Delta w_{ij} &= \beta \delta_j o_j \\ &= \beta (d_j - o_j) o_i \end{aligned} \tag{3.12}$$

Again assuming that $o_i = 1.0$ when input i is present and $o_i = 0.0$ otherwise, the rule reduces to

$$\Delta w_{ij} = \beta (d_j - o_j) \tag{3.13}$$

Note that node output o_j is the CR, while the desired output $d_j = \lambda_j = US$. Thus, the Widrow-Hoff rule can be rewritten as

$$\Delta w_{ij} = \beta (US - CR) \tag{3.14}$$

This is the same as Equation 3.10.

The reader who is interested in further mathematical details, as well as description of the successes and failures of the Rescorla-Wagner model, may refer to Rescorla & Wagner (1972); Wagner & Rescorla (1972); Walkenback & Haddad (1980); Sutton & Barto (1981); Gluck & Bower (1988a); Siegel & Allan (1996).

Widrow-Hoff rule and the Rescorla-Wagner model embodied the same error-correcting principle.[20] MathBox 3.2 provides a formal statement of the Rescorla-Wagner model for the mathematically inclined.

A critical property of the Rescorla-Wagner model of conditioning (and of the Widrow-Hoff training rule for neural networks) is that the weights associated with one cue can indirectly influence the weights accruing to other co-occurring cues. That is, if a tone and light are both present on a trial, they will compete for associative weight. This competitive property of the Rescorla-Wagner model allows it to account for many important conditioning phenomena, especially those with complex stimuli involving the presentation of multiple stimulus elements (such as tones and lights paired together).

For example, the Rescorla-Wagner model (and the Widrow-Hoff rule) can account for the blocking effect. Consider the network in figure 3.11A; this represents the state of affairs after phase 1 training in which a tone predicts an airpuff US. Now, at the start of phase 2, the light and tone are presented

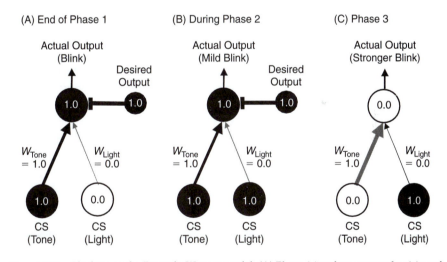

Figure 3.11 Blocking in the Rescorla-Wagner model. (A) Phase 1 involves repeated pairing of the tone CS with an airpuff US. At the end of this phase, there is a strong weight from the tone input node, which in turn can activate the output node. (B) Phase 2 involves presentation of both tone and light CSs, paired with the US. Since the tone already perfectly predicts the US and the output node is fully activated, there is no output error, and no learning occurs. Hence, the weight from the light input node remains at 0.0. (C) Finally, in phase 3, the network is tested with presentations of light alone. Since the weight was never changed from 0.0, there is no activation of the output node, and no behavioral response occurs. Hence, the Rescorla-Wagner model correctly shows blocking.

together (figure 3.11B). The output node receives activation from both input nodes, multiplied by their weights: $1.0 \times 1.0 = 1.0$ from the tone and 1.0×0.0 from the light for a total of 1.0. This is the output node's activation. Since the airpuff US is present on this trial, the response is correct—and the error is 0.0. Since weight change is determined by the error and the error is 0.0, there is no learning on this trial—or, indeed, on any other phase 2 trial. By the end of phase 2, the network weights will still be the same as they were at the beginning of phase 2: The tone is strongly weighted, and the light is not. A subsequent test presentation of the light in phase 3 is shown in figure 3.11C: There is no weight from the light input node, so there is no activation of the output node—so there is no response to the light alone. Thus, the network will show blocking—just like the Pre-Trained animals in figure 3.9.

The blocking effect is only one of numerous subtle conditioning phenomena that are addressed by the Rescorla-Wagner model. Later in this chapter, we will return to the blocking effect and the way in which it has helped to elucidate the neural mechanisms of conditioning.

Broad Implications of the Rescorla-Wagner Model

One of the most important lessons to be learned from the Rescorla-Wagner model is that it is possible to understand a large body of data via a relatively simple mathematical rule. An equally important implication is that learning in many different experimental procedures and many different species— including humans—shares some fundamental characteristics.

A quarter century after its publication, the Rescorla-Wagner model is generally acknowledged as the single most powerful and influential formal model of learning ever produced by psychology.[21] The model gained such wide acceptance because it was simple, it was elegant, and could explain a wide range of previously puzzling empirical results. This is one hallmark of a successful model: *The model should show underlying order among a series of results initially seem unrelated or even contradictory.*

The Rescorla-Wagner model also made novel and surprising predictions about how animals ought to behave in new experimental procedures, and experimenters rushed to test these predictions. This is another feature of a successful model: *It should generate subtle predictions that were not intuitively obvious before.* Ideally, modeling and empirical work should cycle; the model should make predictions that, when tested, provide new data. If the data match the predictions, the model is supported. If not, then the model must be revised. This revised model then generates new behavioral predictions, and the cycle begins again.

By virtue of its simplicity, the Rescorla-Wagner model does not account for all kinds of learning. Many researchers devoted themselves to showing how one or another addition to the model allows it to account for a wider range of phenomena[22]—but with too many additions, the model loses some of its simplicity and appeal. In the next chapter, we will focus on some important limitations of the model and mechanisms that have been proposed to circumvent these limitations. However, these limitations need not be considered shortcomings of the Rescorla-Wagner model *per se*. Rather, these limitations are more appropriately understood as lying outside the model's stated domain.

Within its domain, the Rescorla-Wagner model combines explanatory power with mathematical simplicity. It takes an intuitively tractable idea—namely, that learning is driven by error—pares away all but the most essential details, and explores implications of this idea that were not obvious before. The Rescorla-Wagner model is also a starting point from which many subsequent models were built; some of these newer models will be described in the chapters to come.

Error-Correction Learning and the Brain

Currently, most neuroscientists believe that an important mechanism of biological learning is the alteration of synaptic strength. There is an obvious parallel between this idea and the idea of weight adjustment in the Rescorla-Wagner model. So it is tempting to jump to the conclusion that the Rescorla-Wagner model describes a rule for synaptic changes between individual neurons.

However, there is good evidence that this is *not* the case. The Rescorla-Wagner model requires a teaching signal, to provide information about the desired output. If there were more than one output node, as could happen in a more complicated network, there would need to be a different teaching signal for each output node. The brain, with its immense number of neurons, would require an equally staggering number of teaching signals if it were to implement the Rescorla-Wagner model of learning at each synapse.

Our current understanding of the way in which neurons form and alter connections is incomplete. An extensively studied candidate mechanism is **long-term potentiation (LTP)**.[23] In one form of LTP (called **associative LTP**), simultaneous activity in two neurons leads to a strengthening of the synapse that connects them to each other. This learning process was anticipated by Donald Hebb in the 1940s, long before the technology existed to observe activity in individual neurons,[24] and the basic idea harks as far back as the psychologist William James in the nineteenth century.[25] LTP is a mechanism for synaptic change that depends on neuronal correlation but does not require a teaching input. Thus, this form of synaptic learning (also known as *synaptic plasticity*) does not implement error-correction as embodied in the Rescorla-Wagner model.

Nevertheless, while the Rescorla-Wagner model of learning probably does not take place at the cellular level, error-correction mechanisms do appear to emerge from brain circuits. Certain brain regions have very strong inputs that do appear to act as teachers, specifying desired outputs for the entire region, if not for individual cells. One example is the cerebellum, an essential brain region for the storage and expression of learned motor reflexes, such as classical eyeblink conditioning.[26]

Figure 3.12 shows a very simplified schematic of the cerebellar pathways for eyeblink conditioning, based on the work of Richard Thompson and colleagues. Information about a CS, such as a tone or light, enters through primary sensory processing areas in the brain and eventually reaches the cerebellum. Information about a US, such as a corneal airpuff, travels through a way station known as the **inferior olive.**

Climbing fibers carry this information from inferior olive to cerebellum, where they make very powerful synapses onto cerebellar neurons. The output from the cerebellum is a signal that is related to the strength of the conditioned eyeblink response; this information travels to brain structures that are responsible for executing the motor commands to close the eyelid.* Conditioned response information also travels along a feedback pathway to inhibit the inferior olive.

The feedback pathway from cerebellum to inferior olive is inhibitory, which means that when a conditioned eyeblink response is generated, inferior olive activity is depressed. The other input to the inferior olive, carrying US information, is excitatory. Various neurophysiological studies have suggested that the inferior olive activity reflects the difference between US and the conditioned response, which can be formalized as

InferiorOliveActivity = US − CR

Note that the US here is equivalent to information about the desired output. When the US is present, the animal should have blinked. When the US is not present, the animal should not have blinked. Thus, this subtraction of US and

---

*In fact, the relationship between cerebellar output and CR generation is complicated, since the output of cerebellar Purkinje neurons is inhibitory; CRs are generated when Purkinje cells decrease their activity.

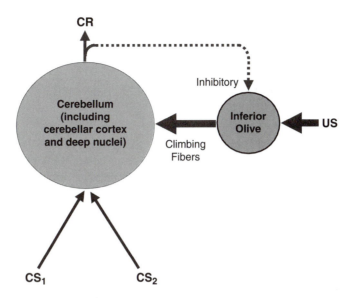

Figure 3.12   The cerebellum (including cerebellar cortex and deep cerebellar nuclei) receives information about auditory CSs via a connection from early sensory processing centers in the brain. It also receives information about airpuff USs via a pathway that passes through the inferior olive. The inferior olive also receives an inhibitory feedback connection from the cerebellum. As the CR develops, inhibition increases in the inferior olive, reducing the amount of US information that reaches cerebellum. In effect, the output of the inferior olive is proportional to (US – CR). This is analogous to the error term in the Rescorla-Wagner model. Thus, the inferior olive could provide the error signal to drive cerebellar learning in motor-reflex conditioning. The cerebellar-inferior olive system may implement error correction learning in this circuit.

conditioned response information is essentially the same as the error computation in the Rescorla-Wagner model, namely,

$$OutputError = DesiredOutput - ActualOutput$$
$$= US - CR$$

In fact, inferior olive activity during acquisition starts off high, before the conditioned response is reliably generated, and gradually drops back to baseline as the conditioned response is acquired (figure 3.13A,B).[27] This activity pattern is basically the same as the pattern of output error generated by the Rescorla-Wagner model during learning (figure 3.13C,D). This suggests that the inferior olive could be computing output error, providing the information necessary to implement error-correction in the cerebellum.

Once the error is computed, the next step in the Rescorla-Wagner model is to update weights accordingly, to reduce the error on subsequent trials. To do this, the error signal must be transmitted to the connections between input

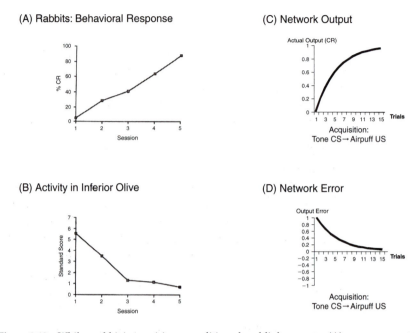

Figure 3.13 While a rabbit is acquiring a conditioned eyeblink response (A), measurements are taken from the inferior olive (B). Activity in the inferior olive is high early in training, when the CR is low, and decreases as the CR develops. Activity in the inferior olive is given as standard scores, representing the activation during the presentation of the CS relative to baseline activity. The decrease in inferior olive activity as a function of training is similar to the decrease in network error in the Rescorla-Wagner model (D) as a function of learning (C). This has led to the suggestion that the inferior olive might be calculating response error. (A and B are adapted from Sears & Steinmetz, 1991, Figure 3.)

and output nodes. In the cerebellum, the same neurons that receive sensory information are also contacted by climbing fibers, carrying information from the inferior olive (figure 3.12). Synapses carrying sensory information to the cerebellar neurons are known to be modified depending on the presence or absence of climbing fiber activity.[28]

On the basis of these data, we have proposed a model of the cerebellum as a circuit for implementing the Rescorla-Wagner model of learning.[29] The basic idea is as follows: When a tone CS is presented, sensory information reaches the cerebellum, but no conditioned response is elicited. If the US appears, this information travels to the inferior olive, which computes the error as $US - CR = 1.0 - 0.0 = 1.0$. This error information is carried via climbing fibers to the cerebellar neurons, and initiates synaptic change. Over many

CS-US pairings, the net effect is to make the cerebellum more likely to generate a response when the CS appears.[30] As the conditioned response begins to emerge, the feedback pathway from cerebellum to inferior olive becomes active. This inhibits activity in the inferior olive. Eventually, when the response is completely learned, there is no activity in the inferior olive (since US − CR = 1.0 − 1.0 = 0.0). At this point, the climbing fibers are silenced, and learning stops. Thus, error-correction might be implemented at the level of the cerebellar-inferior olive circuit.

The power of the simple cerebellar model shown in figure 3.12 can be illustrated by its application to behaviors such as blocking.[31] As was described earlier, a blocking procedure involves several phases. In phase 1, a cue such as a tone predicts an airpuff US (see table 3.1). This is followed by phase 2, in which a tone-light compound is paired with the US. In phase 3, there should be little or no response to a test of the light. This, according to the Rescorla-Wagner model, is because prior learning to the tone blocked learning about the second stimulus. The cerebellar model of figure 3.10 expects that, during phase 1, the tone will eventually come to elicit a conditioned response, at which point the output error is 0, and inferior olive activity will be fully inhibited. When tone-light conditioning begins, there is still no error—since the tone elicits a strong conditioned response—and so there is no learning about the light.

This interpretation assumes that blocking depends on low output error, and hence low inferior olive activity, during phase 2. Thus, blocking should be disrupted if inferior olive activity is inflated during phase 2. A recent study by Thompson and colleagues confirmed this prediction.[32] In their study, rabbits were first trained to give reliable eyeblink responses to a tone CS. Next, the rabbits were given injections of a drug (picrotoxin) that temporarily disabled the feedback pathway from cerebellum to inferior olive (figure 3.14). With this pathway disabled, the inferior olive's activity should reflect the US, without any information about the conditioned response:

InferiorOliveActivity = US − 0

The rabbits were then given phase 2 training of blocking, in which the compound of tone CS and light CS was paired with the US. In these rabbits, inferior olive activity was high whenever the US was presented, whether or not a conditioned response was generated. Thus, learning continued; in phase 3, the rabbits gave a strong response to the light CS: Blocking had been prevented.

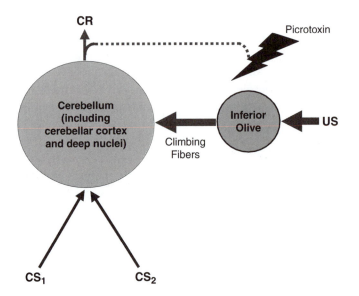

Figure 3.14 The cerebellar circuit model of figure 3.12 predicts that error-correction learning depends on the inferior olive computing the difference between US and CR. If the CR feedback pathway is interrupted, then the inferior olive output should always mirror the US, regardless of the CR. Blocking and other behaviors that depend on an error signal should also be disrupted. In fact, when the CR feedback pathway is disrupted by injection of the drug picrotoxin to the inferior olive, blocking is indeed disrupted in rabbit eyeblink conditioning.

These and related results provide strong support for the interpretation of the cerebellar-inferior olive circuit as implementing error correction.[33] The cerebellum is not the only place in the brain where such error-correction learning may take place; just as the strong climbing fibers may serve as teaching inputs to cerebellum, there may be analogous systems in the hippocampus and elsewhere. For example, similar error-correcting circuits may exist in the brain structures that are responsible for learning fear responses to threatening stimuli.[34] Brain chemicals, such as dopamine, may also play a role in broadcasting error signals throughout the brain.[35]

Still, error correction, as assumed in the Rescorla-Wagner model, may be the exception rather than the rule in brain systems. Teaching inputs may have evolved to serve very specialized functions in a few critical brain regions. It is important to note that error correction is only one behavioral principle of learning; other brain mechanisms may be devoted to implementing other principles, and some of these will be introduced in later chapters. The next, and final, section of this chapter, reviews some of the limitations of error-correction learning.

3.4   LIMITATIONS OF ERROR-CORRECTION LEARNING

In the Rescorla-Wagner model, all weight changes depend on the prediction error at the output node. This means that learning in the network is governed by the degree to which network output (conditioned response, or CR) deviates from desired output (US). No other learning occurs. Thus, if the network is simply exposed to a stimulus, without any US, then US = CR = 0, output error is zero, and there is no learning. However, several studies with animals and humans suggest that individuals can learn about stimuli just from exposure to those stimuli, without any explicit reinforcement (US) or response (CR). This general class of phenomena—often called perceptual learning, or learning through mere exposure—can be accommodated in neural networks only by making additional assumptions about the network architecture or the learning algorithm. In chapters 5 and 6, we will review some of these possible solutions and argue that they are relevant to understanding different kinds of learning in the brain. For now, we will discuss two simple conditioning procedures that involve learning without explicit reinforcement.

Sensory Preconditioning

Back in chapter 2, we introduced a behavioral phenomenon called **sensory preconditioning.** Table 3.2 reviews the experimental procedure, using the example of eyeblink conditioning. In sensory preconditioning, rabbits are assigned to one of two groups. In the Compound Exposure group, rabbits first receive unreinforced exposure (that is, no US) to tone and light stimuli, presented together in a compound. In the Separate Exposure group, rabbits receive equivalent unreinforced exposure to the tone and light, presented separately. In phase 2, all rabbits are then trained that the light predicts a blink-evoking airpuff US. Once a conditioned response is learned to the light, all rabbits are then tested for their response to the other, tone stimulus. Rabbits in the Separate Exposure group give little or no response to the tone. By contrast, rabbits in the Compound Exposure group give a significant response to

Table 3.2   Sensory Preconditioning

Group	Phase 1	Phase 2	Test
Compound Exposure	Tone and light (together); no airpuff	Light → airpuff ⇒ **blink!**	Tone ⇒ **blink!**
Separate Exposure	Tone, light (separately); no airpuff	Light → airpuff ⇒ **blink!**	Tone ⇒ no blink

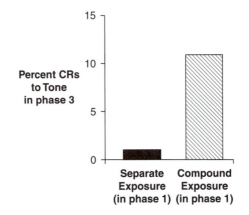

Figure 3.15 Sensory preconditioning in rabbit eyeblink conditioning. One group of rabbits is given exposure to the tone and light, separately, in phase 1. These rabbits are then trained to respond to the light in phase 2. In phase 3, the rabbits are presented with the tone and show very little transfer of learned responding. A second group of rabbits is given phase 1 exposure to the tone and light, presented together as a compound stimulus. These rabbits are then trained to respond to the light; when tested with the tone in phase 3, they give a strong response. (Plotted from data presented in Port & Patterson, 1984.)

the tone (figure 3.15). In effect, prior exposure to the tone-light compound causes these two stimuli to be "chunked" or compressed; later learning to one stimulus then tends to generalize strongly to the other stimulus.

Now consider what happens with a network, such as the one in figure 3.6, given the same training. Initially, all network weights are set to 0.0. This means that the network will not respond to any stimulus or combination of stimuli. During phase 1 (the exposure phase), if the network is given exposure to the tone-light compound, it will not generate a response. Since there is no US during phase 1, this nonresponse is correct: There is no output error, and so there is no learning. The weights do not change during this phase. Thus, pre-exposure in the absence of reinforcement has no effect on the network. The weights at the beginning of phase 2 are the same for a network given compound exposure as for one given separate exposure—or no exposure at all. In all three cases, phase 2 learning about the light transfers minimally to the tone. Thus, the Rescorla-Wagner model does not account for sensory preconditioning.

Latent Inhibition

Another example of learning through mere exposure is **latent inhibition,** which has been developed and extensively studied by Robert Lubow.[36] Table 3.3 schematizes a latent inhibition procedure, again using a rabbit

Table 3.3   Latent Inhibition

Group	Phase 1	Phase 2
CS-Exposure	Tone CS	Tone CS → airpuff US **...Slow learning**
Sit-Exposure	*(Sit in experimental chamber)*	Tone CS → airpuff US **...Normal learning**

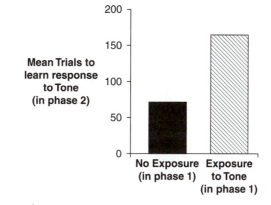

Figure 3.16   Latent inhibition in rabbit eyeblink conditioning. One group of rabbits is given exposure to the tone, while a second group is given an equivalent amount of time in the experimental chamber, but not exposed to the tone. Next, both groups of rabbits are trained to respond to the tone. The nonexposed rabbits learn the association quickly; the exposed rabbits are significantly slower to learn. (Plotted from data reported in Solomon & Moore, 1975.)

eyeblink conditioning example. Rabbits in the CS-Exposure group are given phase 1 presentations of a CS (e.g., a tone) without any reinforcement. For comparison, rabbits in a Sit-Exposure group are allowed to sit in the conditioning chamber for an equivalent amount of time with no exposure to any CS. In phase 2, both groups receive training in which the tone is paired with the US until the rabbit gives a reliable conditioned response. Rabbits in the Sit-Exposure group learn this response at normal speed; rabbits in the CS-Exposure group, previously exposed to the tone, show much slower learning, as is seen in figure 3.16.

Latent inhibition is a complex and intriguing phenomenon that may reflect the contribution of many different processes in the normal brain. We will discuss some of these in chapters 7 and 9. For now, we just note that the Rescorla-Wagner model learns only when there is output error, that is, when the CR does not equal the US. In phase 1 of latent inhibition, the CR is initially 0—and there is never any US, so the output error is always 0. Thus, both the CS-Exposed and Sit-Exposed conditions undergo no learning in phase 1 and hence are expected by the Rescorla-Wagner model to perform identically in phase 2. Thus, the Rescorla-Wagner model fails to capture the robust and widely demonstrated behavior of latent inhibition.

Implications of the Limitations of Error-Correction Learning

Section 3.3 argued that the error-correction principle of the Rescorla-Wagner model is a powerful model that can account for a wide range of conditioning behaviors in a relatively simple and elegant way. Further, it appears to have some biological relevance: Cerebellar circuitry is sufficient to implement the kind of error computations required by the model and to use error signals to drive learning. Thus, the Rescorla-Wagner model may be more than a psychological description of learning; it may be a model of how the cerebellum implements conditioned learning.

However, the Rescorla-Wagner model has several limitations, most notably its failure to account for mere exposure effects such as latent inhibition and sensory preconditioning. It is interesting to note that sensory preconditioning and latent inhibition are among the behavioral paradigms that are disrupted by damage to the hippocampal-region.[37] This suggests that something about mere exposure effects might be especially sensitive to hippocampal-region mediation, while other effects—such as those captured by the error-correcting principle of the Rescorla-Wagner model—might not depend on hippocampal-region mediation but, rather, depend on the cerebellum and other extrahippocampal structures.

Thus, it might be possible to model a full range of conditioned behaviors by considering a system that has a "cerebellar" module, which implements simple error-correction learning, and a "hippocampal" module, which includes other capabilities such as mere exposure learning and representational compression.

This leads to the question of what kind of a model the hippocampal module might be. Clearly, it must have additional capabilities beyond error correction. Perhaps the chief requirement is the ability to form new stimulus representations: ways of representing stimulus information independent of their association with the US. The next chapter, chapter 4, explores how these representational issues can be addressed through network models that are elaborations of the error-correction networks presented in this chapter.

SUMMARY

• Most neuroscientists now believe that the basic mechanism of learning is alteration of synaptic strength.

• The power of nodes in a neural network (and neurons in the brain) comes not just from their individual power, but from their collective power, which emerges only when many such devices are interconnected in a network.

• The key to learning in neural networks is changing the weights.

• Researchers in both psychology (Rescorla and Wagner) and engineering (Widrow and Hoff) argued that weights should be changed proportionally to output error, the difference between actual and desired responses. A teaching signal provides information about the desired response. This kind of learning is called error-correction learning, because over many trials, it tends to minimize the output error.

• The Rescorla-Wagner model (and the Widrow-Hoff rule) can account for some simple forms of learning, including acquisition of a conditioned eyeblink response, and more complex training procedures, such as blocking. It does not account for results such as latent inhibition and sensory preconditioning, which involve learning after mere exposure to stimuli in the absence of reinforcement (such as a US).

• There is evidence that error correction takes place in some places in the brain. For example, during eyeblink conditioning, the inferior olive may provide a teaching signal to allow cerebellar neurons to reduce the difference (error) between their output (the CR) and the desired response (a prediction of the US). This is a circuit-level instantiation of the Rescorla-Wagner model. Error-correction circuits may also underlie some fear learning. However, error correction may be the exception rather than the rule in brain systems.

4 Representation and Generalization in Neural Networks

When we look out at the world, reflected light enters each eye, falls on the retina, and activates some of the neurons there. If we were to record the complete pattern of activated and inactivated retinal neurons, the resulting pattern would be a recoding, or **representation,** of the visual scene. The activated retinal neurons send output that leaves the eye and eventually reaches the visual cortical areas, at the rear of the brain. Again, a pattern is created there, consisting of activated and inactive neurons. The visual scene has been rerepresented. In fact, the visual scene (or any sensory stimulation) goes through an arbitrary number of rerepresentations as it is processed by the brain.

Representations are not unique to the brain. We use representations throughout our daily life. The letters in written words are representations of sounds, and the words themselves represent ideas and concepts. The federal government may represent a person by her nine-digit Social Security number; her friends may represent her in conversation by a name; and the Department of Motor Vehicles may represent her by a sequence of letters and numbers on her driver's license. Each of these representations was chosen to suit a particular need. When we refer to our friends, for example, it is easier to use a short name than to memorize an arbitrary numerical code. However, the government, which must organize records on millions of people, needs a unique way to represent each one—hence, the Social Security number.

The neural network models that we presented in the preceding chapter all assumed a simple representational scheme for relating events in the world to components of the model. The scheme was as follows: Each distinct stimulus event, such as a tone, a light, or an airpuff, was represented by a single input node in the network; the occurrence of that stimulus event was modeled by activating the corresponding node. This activation propagated through the network, and the output node's activity represented the probability (or strength) of a response.

*A representation that relates one stimulus (or stimulus feature) to one node (or component) of the model is referred to as a **component representation** (or a **local*** *representation*). Although simple in conception, component representation has been sufficient for a broad range of applications in psychology, neuroscience, and engineering. However, this component representation has serious limitations, and neural network modelers—as well as animal learning theorists—have been grappling with these limitations for years. In this chapter, we review the key limitations of component representation in learning theories and discuss how psychologists and neural network modelers have addressed these limitations.

Section 4.1 introduces the general concepts of representation and generalization. A fundamental challenge for learning is as follows: On the one hand, people and animals often infer that similar stimuli should be associated with similar outcomes; on the other hand, when necessary, people and animals can learn that similar stimuli should be associated with different outcomes. There is always a trade-off between the former process (generalization) and the latter process (specificity) in learning. Section 4.2 discusses some modeling approaches to implementing generalization, and section 4.3 discusses ways to preserve specificity. One way to balance the generalization-specificity trade-off is to use multilayer networks, which incorporate one or more layers of nodes between the input and output nodes. These multilayer networks can develop new stimulus representations during learning. In later chapters, we will argue that this kind of adaptive representation is a primary function of the hippocampal region.

4.1   REPRESENTATION AND GENERALIZATION

Psychologists have long understood that *a fundamental property of animal and human learning is* **generalization,** *the degree to which learning about one stimulus transfers to other stimuli.* One classic generalization study involved training pigeons to peck at a key when a yellow light was present.[1] In this study, yellow light was the stimulus cue, and responding was measured in terms of how many times the pigeons pecked at the key while the light was on. Because the perceived color of light depends on its wavelength, usually given in nanometers (nm), or billionths of a meter, the "yellowness" of the light can be quantified by noting that the wavelength was 580 nm. After training, the pigeons were tested to see how they would respond to other wavelengths (colors) of light, including 560 nm (yellow-green), 520 nm (green), 600 nm (yellow-orange), and so on.

Not surprisingly, the pigeons responded most strongly to the yellow light on which they were trained, as shown in figure 4.1. However, the pigeons also responded to other colors of light, and the strength of their response

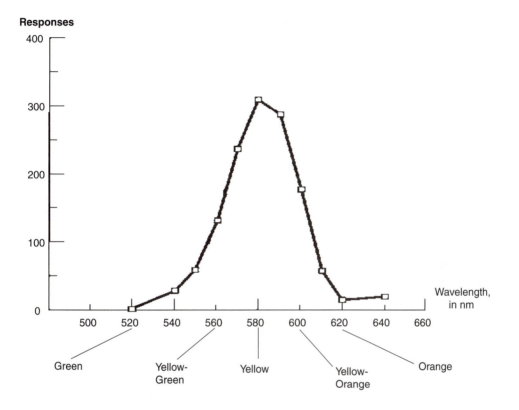

Figure 4.1 Stimulus generalization gradients in pigeons that were trained to peck at a key when illuminated with yellow light but not when dark. Yellow light has a wavelength of about 580 nanometers (nm). When the pigeons were tested with other colors of light, their response rates decreased as the test light colors got farther away from the trained color. Thus, a 560-nm light (yellow-green) still produced a strong response, but a 520-nm light (green) produced little or no responding. Similarly, 600-nm light (yellow-orange) produced more responding than 620-nm light (orange). This general shape, in which response falls off with increasing distance from the trained stimulus, is characteristic of generalization in a wide range of tasks and species. (Adapted from Guttman & Kalish, 1956, pp. 79–88.)

depended on how close (in terms of wavelength) the new color was to the trained yellow light. The less similar a test color was to the trained color, the less the pigeons pecked. The bell-shaped curve in figure 4.1 is known as a **generalization gradient,** and it is a common feature of generalization studies in a variety of modalities (e.g., using tones, shapes, brightnesses, or textures) in species ranging from honeybee to octopus to rabbit to human.[2]

Generalization based on physical similarity is fundamental to learning and allows us to apply prior learning to new instances. For example, an animal that eats a mushroom and becomes sick may generalize from this experience and avoid other mushrooms in the future. Similarly, a person who has learned to drive a Chevrolet is likely to be able to generalize all or most of this skill to driving a Toyota, even though the two cars have slightly different layouts for their steering wheels and gearshifts. *Generalization is thus critical for applying prior experience to new situations, without requiring fresh learning about every new instance.*

Generalization in One-Layer Networks

The one-layer networks that were introduced in chapter 3, with their component representation of features in the world, have serious limitations for capturing the natural patterns of animal and human generalization. Figure 4.2 shows a network with input nodes representing different colored lights. Like the pigeons in the experiment described above, this network can be trained to respond when the yellow light is present (the middle of the five input nodes). This training results in strengthening the weight from the yellow

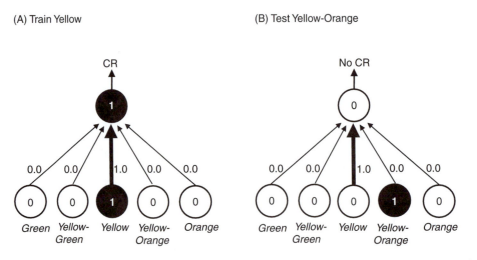

Figure 4.2 A network to implement the stimulus generalization experiment schematized in figure 4.1 could have one input node for each possible color of light. In effect, each color of light represents a different conditioned stimulus (CS). (A) The network is trained to respond to a yellow light. At the end of training, the weight from the "yellow" input node to the output node is strong. (B) When a yellow-orange light is presented to the network, it activates a different input node. This input node has never had its weight strengthened, so it does not activate the output node. The network gives no response to the yellow-orange light, despite the similarity in color to the previously trained yellow light.

input node to the output node, so that a response is generated in response to the yellow light, as shown in figure 4.2A.

Now consider what happens when, for the first time, the network is presented with a slightly different stimulus: a yellow-orange light (figure 4.2B). Although the yellow-orange input node is just to the right of the yellow input node, its weight has never been strengthened. Accordingly, the network does not respond at all to the yellow-orange light—or to any other novel color. Thus, a generalization gradient for this network, as shown in figure 4.3, would reflect strong responding to the trained stimulus but no responding to any other stimulus. This is in striking contrast to the gently sloping generalization gradient shown by animals and humans illustrated in figure 4.1.

The problem with the network in figure 4.2 is that it treats two physically similar stimuli—such as yellow and yellow-orange lights—exactly the same as it treats two dissimilar stimuli, such as the tone and light described in chapter 3. Clearly, however, animals and people do not treat the tone/light distinction equivalently to the yellow/yellow-orange distinction; we are far more likely to generalize what we know about a yellow light to a very similar yellow-orange light and far less likely to generalize what we know about a tone cue to a light cue. *A major challenge for learning theorists has been to understand how differences in stimulus similarity affect learning and generalization behaviors.*

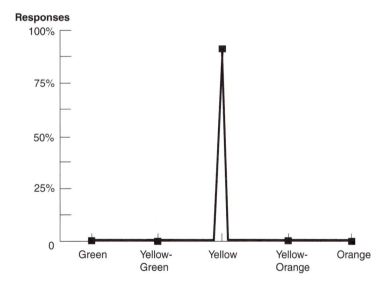

Figure 4.3 The stimulus generalization gradient for the network shown in figure 4.2A,B. The network responds strongly to the yellow input but does not respond to any other input. By contrast, animals and humans typically have smooth generalization gradients in which responses decrease as a function of increasing distance from the trained stimulus (refer to figure 4.1).

Two Challenges for Generalization in Networks

The problem with the simple network models from chapter 3, illustrated in figure 4.2, is that they miss an essential feature of how animals and people respond to stimuli that are similar to those they have experienced before. *In general, animals and people tend to assume that two stimuli that are physically similar will have similar consequences and generalize accordingly.*[3]

Of course, generalization does have its costs. Consider again the animal mentioned earlier that has encountered one mildly poisonous mushroom. If this animal generalizes from this one bad experience with a particular mushroom to every other similarly colored food, it will deprive itself of many perfectly satisfactory food sources. Likewise, a child who has one frightening experience with an aggressive dog may overgeneralize and develop a fear of all dogs. Thus, *there is also a need for specificity in learning, to allow superficially similar stimuli to be associated with different responses.*

How much generalization is appropriate depends on the particular situation, and it may be difficult to determine this in advance. In general, *there is always a trade-off between generalization and specificity in learning.* Understanding how people and animals balance these two competing forces has been a major concern of psychological learning theorists for many years. The sections to follow discuss some of the main psychological issues concerning generalization and similarity and review how these have informed or anticipated subsequent theories of brain function.

4.2   WHEN SIMILAR STIMULI MAP TO SIMILAR OUTCOMES

Given the importance of stimulus generalization in learning and the poor generalization shown by simple network models such as the one in figure 4.2, many researchers have sought methods to incorporate appropriate stimulus generalization. Central to this work was the realization that the component representation shown in figure 4.2 might be a convenience but probably bears little relation to how stimuli are encoded in the brain.

In addition to its problems with inappropriate generalization, a component representation also has serious limitations for representing larger-scale problems: It requires that one node be dedicated to each possible stimulus. Given the vast number of unique stimuli in the universe and the relatively low number any one individual could experience in a single lifetime, component representation is wasteful, if not impossible.

We now know that the brain generally represents information using **distributed representations,** in which each stimulus is encoded by many different neurons and each neuron may respond to conjunctions of features that may be present in many different stimuli.[4] This does not mean that neurons are not specific: An individual neuron in visual cortex may respond maximally to the sight of a particular bar rotated to a particular angle moving at a particular speed in a particular direction, while another neuron in sensory cortex might respond to a touch stimulus on a particular part of the body surface. But each of these neurons will be activated by any stimulus that shares the relevant features. Distributed representation (also called **coarse coding**) is efficient because a large number of stimuli can be processed by a smaller number of neurons, each of which encodes some features of the stimuli. Distributed representations also have the advantage that if some of the units are lost or degraded, the remaining units may be able to provide enough information to represent the stimuli adequately. The cost of a distributed representation is that recognizing a particular stimulus may require integrating information from the many different neurons that encode the stimulus features.

In the late 1950s W. K. Estes, a mathematical psychologist, showed that just this sort of encoding scheme could account for a wide range of stimulus generalization behaviors in animals and humans.[5] At around the same time, neuroscientists such as Karl Lashley and Donald Hebb were coming to similar conclusions, based on experimental and theoretical analyses of the brain.[6] Like Estes, they concluded that the brain most likely uses distributed representations to encode information. But they had only indirect evidence for this assumption. More recently, however, neuroscientists have found explicit empirical evidence for distributed representations in the visual system, sensory and motor cortex, and other brain regions.[7] As with the learning theories of chapter 3, behavior-driven and physiology-driven research converged on similar principles.

Application of Distributed Representations to Learning

To illustrate how a distributed representation uses a set of overlapping elements to encode input stimuli, turn back to the problem of training pigeons to peck at differently colored lights. Figure 4.4A shows a distributed representation for encoding the discrimination among colored lights.

Each color activates a subset of the nodes: Yellow activates the three centermost nodes, orange activates the three rightmost nodes, and so on. *The pattern of activated and nonactivated nodes is the representation of each color input.*

In figure 4.4A, the nodes are laid out **topographically,** meaning that nodes responding to physically similar stimuli—such as yellow and yellow-orange lights—are physically next to each other in the network. Actually, the physical layout itself is not really what is important. Rather, what is important is that *the degree of overlap between the representations of two stimuli reflects their*

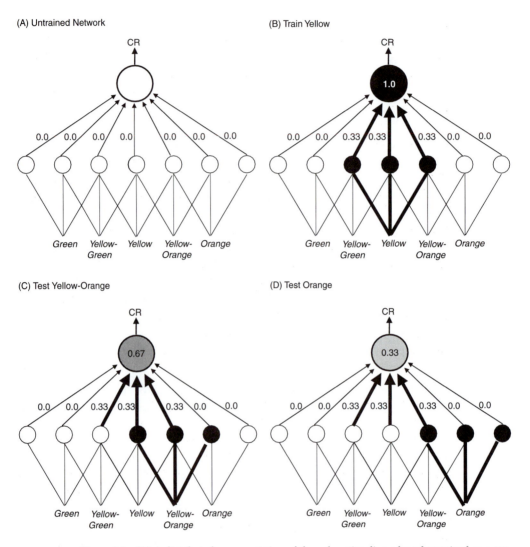

Figure 4.4   (A) A distributed representation of the color stimuli can be schematized as a network with a large number of input nodes connected to a single output node. One stimulus, such as yellow light, will activate a subset of these inputs nodes. A similar stimulus, such as yellow-orange light, will activate a subset of nodes that overlaps highly with the nodes activated by yellow. Orange light will activate a subset of nodes that overlaps minimally with the nodes activated by yellow. (B) When the network is trained to respond to yellow light, this corresponds to increasing the weights to the output node from all the input nodes that were activated by yellow light. (C) If this network is then tested with a new stimulus, such as yellow-orange light, the response will generalize depending on the overlap between the input nodes activated by yellow and by yellow-orange. (D) Increasingly different colors, such as orange, overlap still less with the representation of yellow and evoke correspondingly less response.

physical similarity. Thus, in figure 4.4A, there is more overlap between the representations for yellow and yellow-orange than between those for yellow and orange. There is no overlap between the representations of very different colors, such as green and orange.

Now suppose that this network is trained on the problem of responding to a yellow light. This is done within this distributed network by increasing the weights from the nodes that are active in response to yellow light (figure 4.4B). One way to do this would be with the Rescorla-Wagner learning rule from chapter 3, whereby each of the weights from the three active nodes would eventually equal one-third (approximately 0.33, as indicated in the figure). The weights from the two inactive nodes would remain at 0.

It is instructive to compare the distributed network in figure 4.4B, which was trained to respond to a yellow light, with the local-representation network from figure 4.2A, which was trained in the same way. The distributed network in figure 4.4B has the learning distributed across three weights of 0.33 each; in contrast, the component network in figure 4.2A has this same yellow→response rule localized as one single weight of 1.0. When tested on the original yellow light, these two networks yield identical behaviors: Both give a maximal response when this yellow light is presented.

However, the difference between the distributed and local versions of this associative rule becomes apparent when the networks are presented with other, similar stimuli. The distributed network's generalization behavior can be tested by presenting it with a yellow-orange light, as illustrated by figure 4.4C, where yellow-orange activates a representation that has considerable overlap with the trained yellow light. As a result, there is a reasonably strong response of 0.67, proportional to the two-thirds degree of overlap between the representations for yellow and yellow-orange lights. If the same network were tested with orange light, there would be less overlap and a weaker response of 0.33, as shown in figure 4.4D.

Figure 4.5 shows that the pattern of responding to a whole series of novel lights produces a stimulus generalization gradient that decreases with distance to the trained stimulus—just like the gradient seen in studies of stimulus generalization by animals and humans (figure 4.1). This is in marked contrast to the generalization gradient in figure 4.3, which was produced by the network with only a local component representation.

It is worth noting that the gradients in figure 4.1 and 4.5 are not identical—the network responds more strongly to orange light than the pigeons do—but this is less important. The exact width and shape of the generalization gradient can be manipulated by varying the number and overlap of nodes in the network. What is important is the overall shape: A network that uses

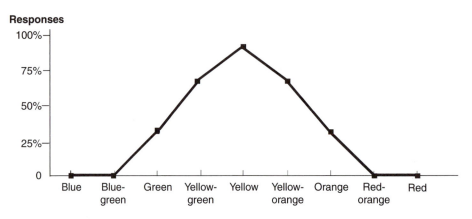

Figure 4.5   The trained network in figure 4.4 generates this stimulus generalization gradient, which shows decreasing responses as a function of distance from the trained stimulus. Responding is highest for the trained stimulus (yellow), decreases for slightly different colors (yellow-orange and yellow-green), and is still less for more distant colors (green and orange). Colors that do not overlap at all with the representation of yellow (e.g., blue, red) would evoke no response at all. This generalization curve is similar in shape to that seen in animals and humans (e.g., figure 4.1). The exact width and shape of the generalization gradient depend on how input nodes are allocated between and among different input patterns.

distributed representation tends to generalize much more realistically than one that uses a local representation.

Stimulus Generalization and Distributed Representations in Multilayer Networks

The distributed representation of the network in figure 4.4 can be viewed as an intermediate layer of nodes, which lie in between the original inputs (yellow, yellow-orange, and orange light) and the output. In effect, the original inputs have simply been left out of the drawing. Figure 4.6 shows what the network would look like if these original inputs are included; the distributed representation now falls in an **internal layer** of nodes (sometimes called a **hidden layer** in neural network jargon).

As before, there is an upper layer of associative weights connecting these nodes to the output, and changing these weights alters the network's output response. But now there is also a lower layer of representational weights that determines what representation is evoked by the inputs. In figure 4.6, yellow inputs again activate the leftmost internal-layer nodes, orange inputs again activate the rightmost internal-layer nodes, and yellow-orange inputs activate the center nodes. Again, there is more overlap between similar stimuli—such as yellow and yellow-orange—than between less similar stimuli, such

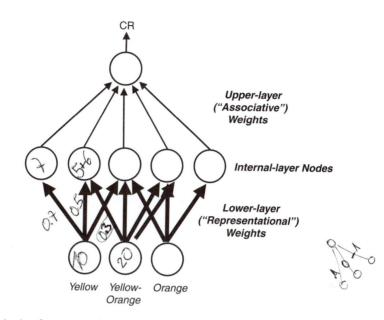

Figure 4.6   Another way to schematize the distributed representation is to consider a multilayered network. For simplicity, only the input nodes corresponding to yellow, yellow-orange, and orange are shown. Between the input nodes, which become active in response to particular stimulus inputs, and the output node is a third internal layer of nodes. Weighted connections from input nodes to internal-layer nodes activate a distributed representation across the internal-layer nodes. Weighted connections from internal-layer nodes to the output node determine the network's response to a given input. The lower layer of weights are *representational*, since stimulus representations in the internal layer depend on how those weights are set. The upper layer of weights are *associational*, since stimuli are associated with responses on the basis of how the internal-layer representations activate the output node.

as yellow and orange. For now, we assume that the weighted connections between input units and internal units are fixed, so that the representation of a particular stimulus is "hard-wired" and unalterable. Later, in section 4.3, we will discuss how these weighted connections might be modified to change representations.

Integrating Distributed Representations with Error-Correction Learning

A multilayered network that incorporates distributed representations (figure 4.6) can be used to illustrate and explain several very counterintuitive empirical results regarding generalization. For example, it might seem logical to expect that the optimal way to train an animal (or a network) to respond to a yellow light would be simply to present the yellow light over many training trials and provide reinforcement on each trial. However, Rescorla noted that the Rescorla-Wagner model, when applied to a network with distributed representations, leads to a different prediction.[8]

Rescorla's analysis of his model as applied to this kind of training paradigm can be understood as follows: First, the network is trained to respond to yellow light (figure 4.7A). As usual, this means that those internal-layer units that are activated by the yellow input have their connections to the output node strengthened. Using the Rescorla-Wagner learning rule, each of the connections from the leftmost internal nodes will have a weight of 0.33 at the end of training. When yellow light is presented, the response will be the sum of the activated internal nodes times their weights:

$$\text{Response} = (1.0 \times 0.33) + (1.0 \times 0.33) + (1.0 \times 0.33) + (0.0 \times 0.0) + (0.0 \times 0.0)$$
$$= 1.0$$

This is the maximal response; further training with the yellow light will not result in any further weight changes because there is no more error to correct, and therefore the Widrow-Hoff (Rescorla-Wagner) rule indicates no further weight changes.

Suppose that the network is next trained to respond to an orange light. On the first trial (figure 4.7B), the network will give a small response to orange, proportional to the small overlap between the trained yellow and novel orange inputs. The Rescorla-Wagner rule states that the connections from each active weight should then be increased so as to reduce the error in response to the orange stimulus. After several training trials, the weights will be adjusted so that the network gives a strong response to orange (figure 4.7C):

$$\text{Response} = (0.0 \times 0.33) + (0.0 \times 0.33) + (1.0 \times 0.56) + (1.0 \times 0.22) + (1.0 \times 0.22)$$
$$= 1.0$$

Notice that the weights from the two rightmost nodes have increased from zero—and the weight from the central node has increased too. Now, if the yellow light is presented again (figure 4.7D), the response is the sum of the weighted connections from all active internal units:

$$\text{Response} = (1.0 \times 0.33) + (1.0 \times 0.33) + (1.0 \times 0.56) + (0.0 \times 0.22) + (0.0 \times 0.22)$$
$$= 1.22$$

Note that this is stronger than the originally trained response to a yellow light! This seems paradoxical. However, when Rescorla conducted a similar experiment with rats, this is exactly what he found,[9] just as the Rescorla-Wagner model predicted.

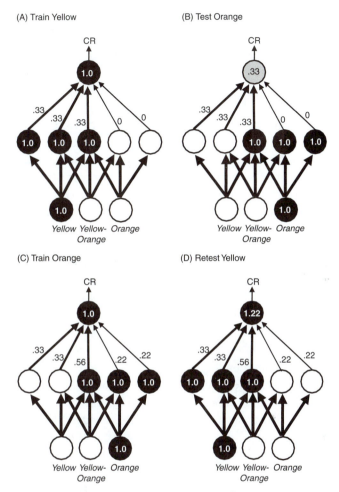

Figure 4.7 The use of a distributed representation can explain some counterintuitive generalization results, including one predicted by Rescorla (1976) and later confirmed in animals. (A) The network is trained to respond to yellow light. This is done by applying the Widrow-Hoff learning rule to the upper layer of weights. The internal nodes that are activated by yellow have their connections to the output strengthened. With sufficient training, the network gives a strong response (1.0) to yellow. Further training with yellow light will not result in any further increases in connection weights or response strength. (B) If an orange stimulus is presented, the network gives a weak response, proportional to the relatively low overlap between the representation of orange and that of yellow. (C) The network is now trained on orange. The weights from internal nodes that are activated by orange are strengthened. Note that the weight from the center internal node, activated by both yellow and orange, increases beyond its original level. (D) When yellow is presented once again, the increase in the center internal node weight causes a stronger response (1.22) than was originally trained. Thus, additional generalization training on a similar (orange) light increased the response to yellow light beyond what could have been achieved by training to the yellow light alone.

These and other findings demonstrated that distributed representations provide a framework for capturing empirical data on stimulus similarity and generalization, especially when combined with the error-correcting learning procedure from the Rescorla-Wagner model (also known as the Widrow-Hoff rule).

The Limits of Similarity-Based Generalization

So far, this chapter has focused on how generalization to novel stimuli is affected by the manner in which a network (or brain) represents information. Generalization allows efficiency in learning: It is not necessary to explicitly learn a response to each different stimulus if learning about one stimulus can generalize to other, similar stimuli. However, generalization can have its costs: It hinders the ability to make fine discriminations among similar stimuli that are to be mapped to different responses.

For example, a child learning to read must discriminate between the letters "G" and "C," which have very different meanings, even though their appearance may differ by only a single serif. Conversely, "G" and "g" may look dissimilar, yet they encode the same letter and, in many situations, should be treated the same way. Ideally, the letter stimuli should be represented somewhere in the brain so that there is considerable overlap between the representations for the letters "G" and "g," which have the same meaning, but little representational overlap between "G" and "C," despite their superficial physical similarity. Thus, *the optimal degree of generalization depends not only on the physical similarity between stimuli but also on the similarity (or difference) between their meanings, or consequences.*

4.3   WHEN SIMILAR STIMULI MAP TO DIFFERENT OUTCOMES

Suppose that an animal is trained that either a tone or a light predicts an unconditioned stimulus (US) (such as a shock or airpuff to the eye) but that there will be *no* US when the tone and light appear together. Thus, the animal must learn to respond to the individual tone or light cues but to withhold responding to the tone and light compound. Naturally, there should also be no response when no stimulus is present, that is, when neither the tone nor the light is present. This task is known by two different names: Psychologists call it **negative patterning,** while mathematicians and neural network researchers call it the **exclusive-OR** (or XOR) task. By either name, it is an extremely difficult task.

Because both the tone and the light cues are part of the tone-and-light compound, there is a natural tendency to generalize from the component cues to the compound and vice versa. However, such generalization will interfere with learning because the components and the compound are associated with very different outcomes. Thus, negative patterning is difficult because it requires suppressing the natural tendency to generalize among similar stimuli.

With extensive training, the negative patterning tasks can be mastered by rats, rabbits, monkeys and humans. Figure 4.8A shows one example of negative patterning in rabbit eyeblink conditioning.[10] After a few days of training, animals learn to give strong responses to either the tone alone (open

(A) Negative Patterning in Rabbits

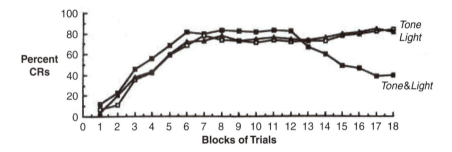

(B) Failed Negative Patterning in One-Layer Network

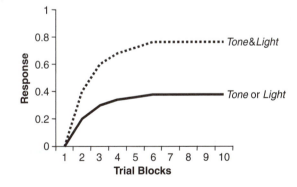

Figure 4.8 Negative patterning involves learning to respond to two CSs (e.g., tone and light) when presented separately but withholding response when the two CSs are presented together. (A) Rabbit eyeblink conditioning data (as reported in Kehoe, 1988): With extensive training, rabbits produce blink CRs to the tone or light separately but not to the compound. (Adapted from Kehoe, 1988, Figure 9.) (B) A simple network, like that shown in figure 4.9A, cannot solve the problem. Trained with the Widrow-Hoff learning rule (and learning rate 0.2), the network comes up with a "compromise" solution: responding partially to the tone or light alone but always responding more to the compound than to the components. Further training will not improve performance.

triangles) or the light alone (open squares). However, the rabbits generalize incorrectly and also give strong responses to the compound tone and light stimulus (solid circles). Only with extensive training do the rabbits begin to suppress responding to the compound while maintaining strong responses to either component alone.

This negative patterning task can be applied to a simple network containing one input node for the tone, one input node for the light, and one output node, as shown in figure 4.9. When this network is trained on the negative patterning task, it can learn to respond appropriately to the individual cues; but it can never learn to do this while also withholding responding to the compound cue, as is illustrated in figure 4.8B.

Figure 4.9 shows the reason for this failure. To produce correct responding to the tone alone, the weight from the input unit encoding tone must be strengthened to 1.0 (figure 4.9A). To produce correct responding to the light alone, the weight from the input unit encoding light must also be strengthened to 1.0 (figure 4.9B). But this means that if the tone and light are presented together, activation will flow through those weighted connections and produce strong responding to the compound—stronger responding, in fact, than to either component alone (figure 4.9C).

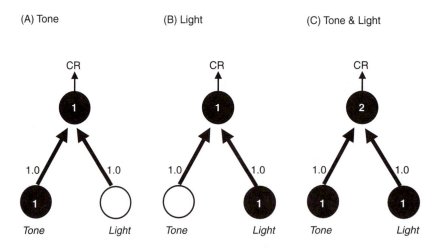

Figure 4.9 A simple, three-node network cannot solve the negative patterning problem. (A) To correctly generate a strong response to the tone CS, there must be a strong weight on the connection from that input to the output. (B) To correctly generate a strong response to the light CS, there must be a strong weight on the connection from that input to the output. (C) But then, when both tone and light CSs are present, the network will incorrectly give a strong response; in fact, the response to the compound (tone and light) will always be stronger than the response to either component cue alone.

All the weights could be decreased, of course, to reduce responding to the compound in figure 4.9C, but this would also incorrectly reduce responding to the components. In fact, there is no way to set connection weights in the network of figure 4.9 so that the network responds correctly to all three different types of training trials.

Multilayered Networks and Configuration

Widrow and Hoff and Rescorla and Wagner were all well aware that their learning procedure could not provide a solution to this type of task. Both sets of researchers were also aware of one possible solution to this limitation: adopting additional nodes to represent cue configurations. This can be done by using internal-layer nodes, as is shown in figure 4.10. One internal-layer node (tone-only) becomes active whenever the tone is present, one (light-only) becomes active whenever the light is present. A third node (tone&light) responds to the configuration, becoming active only when *both* tone and light are present. This is accomplished by specifying that there is a minimum total input (known as a **threshold**) that must be reached before the node can become active.

Figure 4.10A shows that when the tone (alone) is present, the tone-only node becomes active, and this in turn activates the output node. Similarly, in figure 4.10B, the light activates the light-only node, which activates the output node. However, when both tone and light are present (figure 4.10C), all three internal-layer nodes are activated. The tone-only and light-only nodes each send excitatory activation to the output node. However, the configural tone&light node sends an inhibitory signal to the output node, which counteracts the excitatory activation. Activation in the output node is 0, and the network does not respond to the configuration of tone and light. Thus, this multilayer network with configural internal-layer nodes can solve the negative patterning problem.

Negative patterning is just one example of a larger class of problems, involving configurations of stimuli, that single-layer networks cannot solve. *Configural tasks require sensitivity to the configurations (or combinations) of stimulus cues, above and beyond what is known about the individual stimulus components.*

Configural learning also occurs in human learning. It is especially apparent in categorization learning, the process by which humans learn to classify stimuli into categories. In several papers over the late 1980s, one of us (Mark Gluck) and his graduate advisor (Gordon Bower) used simple configural networks to model some aspects of human categorization learning.[11] These

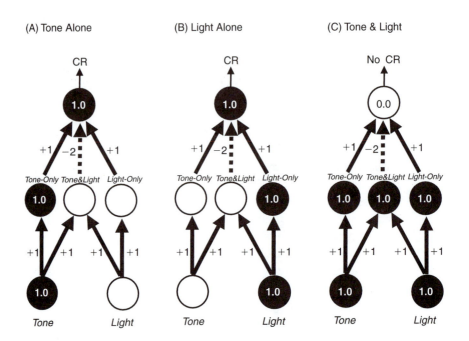

Figure 4.10 A multilayer network with configural internal-layer nodes can solve the negative patterning problem. One internal-layer node (tone-only) becomes active whenever the tone CS is present, one (light-only) becomes active whenever the light CS is present, and one (tone&light) becomes active when both tone and light are present but not when only one is present. (A) When the tone alone is present, the tone-only internal-layer node sends excitatory activation to the output node, and the network generates a response. (B) When the light alone is present, the light-only internal-layer node sends excitatory activation to the output node, and the network generates a response. (C) When both tone and light are present, the tone&light configural node is also activated. This sends strong inhibitory signals to the output node, counteracting the excitatory signals from the tone-only and light-only nodes, so the net output is 0. Thus, the network responds to the components but not to the configuration of tone and light.

models were not meant to capture all of the richness of category learning by people, but they did show that some underlying principles of category learning could be understood as reflecting the same error-correcting principles that are evident in the Rescorla-Wagner model of conditioning.

One of these studies started with an experiment testing human subjects' ability to learn a fictitious medical diagnosis. On each trial, subjects were given the description of a hypothetical patient who had particular symptoms. Subjects were required to determine on the basis of the pattern of symptoms whether each patient had a rare disease. Certain symptom configurations indicated the rare disease; other configurations indicated that the patient did not have the rare disease. The key design principle was that no single symptom was perfectly predictive of the disease or its absence; instead, subjects had to learn about configurations of symptoms. The use of a network with configural nodes can provide a reasonable approximation to human performance in many cases.[12]

For example, figure 4.11A shows a network that can learn to diagnose hypothetical patients on the basis of whether the patients complain of symptoms including fever, ache, and soreness.* By setting appropriate weights from each internal-layer node to the output, the network can learn which symptoms—and which configurations of symptoms—should lead to diagnosis of the rare disease. For example, if a patient reports fever and soreness, this would activate the internal-layer nodes corresponding to these individual symptoms as well as their configuration (figure 4.11B). By setting upper-layer weights appropriately, the network could learn to diagnose this symptom pattern as being indicative of the disease; other symptom configurations could indicate the absence of the disease, much as in the negative patterning problem.

Although this type of simple network model can be applied only to a restricted range of experimental circumstances, it has shown surprising accuracy in predicting human behavior within that range, including data on the relative difficulty of learning various classifications and their responses to generalization tests involving various combinations of cues.[13]

Configuration and Combinatorial Explosion

The previous section argued that networks that incorporate configural nodes can provide additional learning power that enables the solution of the negative patterning problem and other complex tasks. Moreover, this configural-cue representation has been shown to accurately capture some aspects of human categorization and animal learning behaviors.

However, it should be obvious that the approach is inherently limited. The disease-diagnosis network of figure 4.11 has one internal-layer node for each symptom, and one for each possible combination of symptoms. As long as there are only three symptoms, this is acceptable as a psychological model because it requires keeping track of weights on only seven nodes. But suppose the problem required learning about ten symptoms; in this case, more

---

*In their original papers, Gluck and Bower did not draw their networks in the same way as shown in figure 4.11; they showed only the configural (internal-layer) and output nodes. However, the formal properties of the networks were exactly the same as shown in figure 4.11.

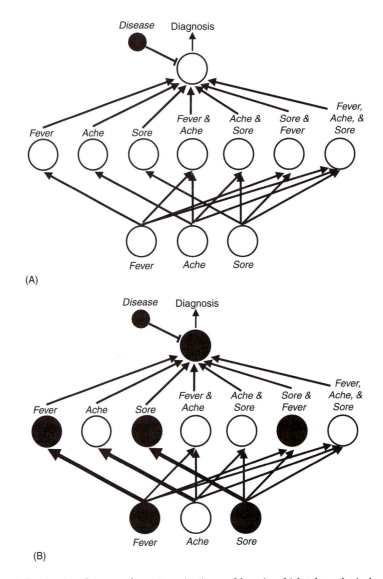

Figure 4.11 A network to encode a categorization problem, in which a hypothetical patient's configuration of symptoms is used to diagnose the presence or absence of a disease. The presence or absence of individual symptoms, as well as combinations of two or more symptoms, may be predictive. For simplicity, the numbers corresponding to weight strengths are not shown in this and subsequent figures; instead, line thickness approximates the strength of connections. (B) For example, the presence of both fever and soreness might predict the presence of the disease, but fever or soreness alone (or in combination with a third symptom, ache) might predict the opposite. This kind of network with configural nodes can mimic many aspects of how humans learn categorization tasks.

than a thousand internal-layer nodes would be required to encode every possible combination of one or more symptoms! And this is only for a "toy" problem; in the real world, there is a potentially unlimited number of stimuli that could occur singly or in combination. If it were necessary to devote one neuron to encode each possible configuration, the requirements would quickly surpass even the vast number of neurons in the brain. This dilemma is called a **combinatorial explosion,** reflecting the rapid expansion of resources required to encode configurations as the number of component features increases.

Even if combinatorial explosion were not a problem, devoting one node to each possible configuration is wasteful. Although there may be a vast number of possible stimulus configurations, any one individual will experience only a small fraction of these configurations in a single lifetime.

At the same time, the power of configural networks argues that this general approach can be very fruitful, both as a computational tool and as a psychological model. What is really needed is a way to harness the computational power of configural nodes without vast numbers of nodes to encode all possible configurations. The simplest way out of this dilemma is to assume that configural nodes are not prewired but, rather, are created as needed. Thus, suppose that the problem is to learn which combinations of ten symptoms predict a rare disease. As was mentioned above, more than a thousand nodes would be required to code every possible configuration of symptoms. If only a few of these thousand symptom configurations actually occur, then only a few configural nodes would be needed—just enough that there is one configural node for each configuration that might appear.

Of course, for most interesting problems, it is impossible to know in advance exactly how many configurations might occur. One possible solution is simply to construct a new internal-layer node each time a new configuration is encountered during learning. Such a network is often called an **exemplar model,** since each internal-layer node responds to one "example" of stimulus configurations that has been experienced so far. Such exemplar models do capture some aspects of human learning.[14] However, an exemplar model will eventually suffer from an accumulation of internal-layer nodes, as more and more examples are experienced. Further, an exemplar model employs a local representation—one internal node for each input pattern— rather than a distributed representation. Section 4.2 described how distributed representations are often better choices when it comes to modeling stimulus generalization, although some exemplar models include strategies to allow generalization.[15]

Fortunately, there is an alternative approach that involves creating configural nodes that are part of a distributed representation. This approach, called the **error backpropagation algorithm,** is one of the most powerful learning algorithms ever developed—and one of the most widely used in neural network applications in psychology and engineering.[16] The next section describes this algorithm.

Learning New Representations in Multilayer Networks

In the previous sections, we discussed how the addition of internal-layer nodes in a network can allow for stimulus generalization and configural learning. In both cases, we assumed that the weights from the input layer to internal layer nodes were preset to allow the internal-layer nodes to respond to useful configurations. This strategy is fine for a very simple problem in which the optimal internal-layer representation is known *a priori*. However, if a problem is even moderately complex, it is rarely obvious how the lower-layer weights should be set.

On the other hand, it turns out to be a very thorny mathematical problem to have the network discover its own lower-layer weights. The Widrow-Hoff rule (embodied in the Rescorla-Wagner model) provides a simple mechanism for changing weights based on the error between actual learned response and the desired output (an accurate prediction of the US). This works fine for the upper layer of weights in a multilayer network because the desired output for these nodes is provided by the presence or absence of the US. However, there is no clear teacher for determining the desired pattern of activations at the internal layer of nodes, and therefore, there is no simple way to train the lower layer of weights using the Widrow-Hoff rule. Thus, *although the Widrow-Hoff rule works very well for networks with only a single layer of weights, it does not apply directly to multilayer networks.*

Widrow and Hoff were well aware of the limitations of their learning rule, but at the time of their original work, no solution was available. In 1969, Marvin Minsky and Seymour Papert published an influential book called *Perceptrons* (an early name for neural networks) arguing that the inability to train multilayer networks was serious enough to make neural networks all but useless as computational tools.[17]

What was missing back then was a way to train multilayer networks. Specifically, how could error correction learning be applied to internal-layer nodes, for which no desired output signal was available? Subsequently, an approach known as the error backpropagation algorithm was developed. It says that the error at a given internal-layer node is a function of the error at all the output layer nodes to which that internal-layer node connects. In effect, the error at the output layer is propagated backward to the internal layer.

The mathematical specification of this algorithm is fairly complex, and an outline of the procedure is given in MathBox 4.1. However, a simple example will suffice to illustrate the general principles. Consider again the negative patterning problem (tone → US, light → US, tone&light → no US), and the network shown in figure 4.12A with four internal-layer nodes labeled A, B, C, and D. The backpropagation algorithm assumes that all weights are initialized to small, random values, represented in the figure by connections of varying thickness. On the first trial, a light is presented (figure 4.12B); it causes some random pattern of activation in the internal-layer nodes, depending on the random weights; in this example, node A is strongly activated, nodes B and D are weakly activated, and node C is only minimally activated. Activation from the internal-layer nodes feeds up to partially activate the output node, producing a response of 0.3.

Now, it is time to train the weights to reduce output error. Since the US was present on this trial, the desired output is 1.0, and—just as in the Widrow-Hoff rule—the error is therefore $1.0 - 0.3 = 0.7$. This error is distributed among the upper-layer weights according to a weight change rule similar to the Widrow-Hoff rule (figure 4.12C): the weight from the most active node A to the output node is strongly increased; the weights from B and D are moderately increased; and the weight from C is increased only a minimal amount.

Now the lower-layer of weights are updated (figure 4.12D). Internal-layer node A was highly active and also has a strong weight to the output node; therefore, it influenced activity in the output node a great deal, so it deserves a large share of the blame for the output node's error. But, A's activation reflects the weights feeding into it, so they should share the blame. As a result, the weights coming into A are changed substantially. In this case, the weight from the active light input node is strengthened. This means that next time the light is presented, node A will be activated more strongly, and it in turn will cause more output activation. This process is repeated for the other internal layer nodes. For example, node C was minimally active and also had a small weight to the output node; therefore, it could not have exerted much influence over the output; the lower-layer weights coming into C are therefore changed only minimally. Once all the lower-layer weights are updated, the trial finishes; a new stimulus is presented, and the cycle begins again.

After a large number of training trials, the network settles into a state in which it gives the correct output to each input stimulus. Figure 4.12E shows one such final state. Presentation of the light alone activates node A strongly, which in turn produces output activation; presentation of the tone alone

MathBox 4.1   Error Backpropagation

The error backpropagation algorithm extends the Widrow-Hoff learning rule to deal with multilayer networks. A canonical version of the backpropagation algorithm was described by Rumelhart, Hinton, and Williams (1986).

Each trial is divided into two phases: a *forward* pass, during which all nodes process inputs and produce outputs, and a *backward* pass, during which nodes compute errors and adapt weights.

In the forward pass, each node computes activation and output, much as in the Widrow-Hoff rule (MathBox 3.1):

$$V_j = \sum_i o_i w_{ij} + \theta_j \tag{4.1}$$

$$o_j = f(V_j) \tag{4.2}$$

Equations 4.1 and 4.2 apply to both internal-layer and output-layer nodes. Equation 4.1 includes a *bias* term θ_j that represents the node's baseline tendency to become active, independent of external inputs. The Widrow-Hoff activation rule (Equation 3.1) is a special case of this rule, in which there is no bias term.

The *output function f* is usually defined as a sigmoid function, for example,

$$f(V_j) = \frac{1}{1 + e^{-V_j}} \tag{4.3}$$

The graphical representation of this sigmoid function is shown below. One implication of a sigmoidal function is that node output is clipped at a maximum 1.0 and minimum 0.0.

Once all nodes have computed their output, the forward phase is completed, and the backward, weight-adapting phase begins.

For output nodes, error ∂_j is defined as

$$\partial_j = (d_j - o_j)f'(V_j) \tag{4.4}$$

Here, d_j is the desired output of node j and o_j is the actual output; f' is the first derivative of the output function f. Using the sigmoidal output function of Equation 4.3, the first derivative is

$$f'(V_j) = V_j(1 - V_j) \tag{4.5}$$

Note that if a different output function is used, that is, $f(x) = x$, then $f'(x) = 1.0$, and Equation 4.4 reduces to the Widrow-Hoff error computation rule (Equation 3.4).

For internal-layer nodes, desired output d_j is not defined. Instead, the error at internal-layer node j is estimated by backpropagating some of the error from output nodes k to which j connects:

$$\partial_j = \left(\sum_k \partial_k w_{jk}\right) f'(V_j) \tag{4.6}$$

Once error is calculated for all nodes, all nodes in both the internal and output layers update weights according to the rule

$$\Delta w_{ij} = \beta \partial_j o_i \tag{4.7}$$

where β is a learning rate (typically between 0.01 and 0.1) and o_i is the output of node i. Again, this is the same as the Widrow-Hoff learning rule (Equation 3.5).

Most implementations of error backpropagation also include a *momentum* term, α. In this case, the weight change on each trial is influenced not only by the current error, but also by previous weight changes:

$$\Delta w_{ij} = \beta \partial_j o_i + \alpha \Delta w_{ij}* \tag{4.8}$$

The momentum α is generally set less than 1.0, and $\Delta w_{ij}*$ is the amount by which the weight was changed on the previous trial. Use of momentum tends to speed overall learning in the network by ensuring that weights change smoothly, in one direction, across trials, rather than zigzagging up and down on alternate trials.

The interested reader should consult the following for a complete derivation of the backpropagation algorithm, its uses and shortcomings: Rumelhart, Hinton, & Williams (1986); Stone (1986); Hinton (1989, 1992); Stork (1989); Minsky & Papert (1998); and Reed & Marks (1999).

activates node D strongly, which in turn produces output activation; presentation of the tone and the light together also activates nodes B and C, which inhibit output activation. Thus, the network correctly responds to the individual cues but not to the compound stimulus, thereby correctly solving the negative patterning task.

There are actually many ways in which the network of figure 4.12 could have solved the negative patterning problem. In the example shown, internal-layer node A was set to respond to the tone and C was set to respond to the light. But the mapping could have just as easily been reversed, and the problem would still have been learned in the same basic way. Very different solutions are possible too. Which particular solution is found depends on the number of internal-layer nodes, the network learning rate, and even the order of stimulus presentation. Even if all these things are held constant, the way in which the random initial weights are set will influence the final outcome. If the network in figure 4.12A is reinitialized with a different set of starting values for the weights and then trained on the negative patterning problem again, it may find a slightly different—but possibly equally valid— solution, such as the one shown in figure 4.12F. As a result, when neural network researchers present a learning curve summarizing the network performance (e.g., figure 4.13), the results are usually an average of the performance of a number of different experiments (called **simulation runs**) with the same network but different initial weights.

Computational Limitations of Backpropagation

The backpropagation algorithm has several shortcomings. First, the algorithm is relatively complex, as a glance at MathBox 4.1 will confirm, and this complexity slows learning. The network of figure 4.12, which includes only two input nodes and three stimulus patterns, may still require about 500 trial blocks, each of which includes one example of each stimulus type, to learn this task.* A network with only two internal-layer nodes can require anywhere from a few hundred to a few thousand training trials to learn the negative patterning problem.[18] Learning can be faster if the mathematical parameters (defined in MathBox 4.1) are set appropriately, but it is sometimes hard to know in advance what is an appropriate setting. By contrast, the configural-cue network in figure 4.10, with its hand-coded lower-layer

---

*The exact learning time for a network that is trained with error backpropagation will vary according to several of the parameters outlined in MathBox 4.1, as well as with the network architecture.

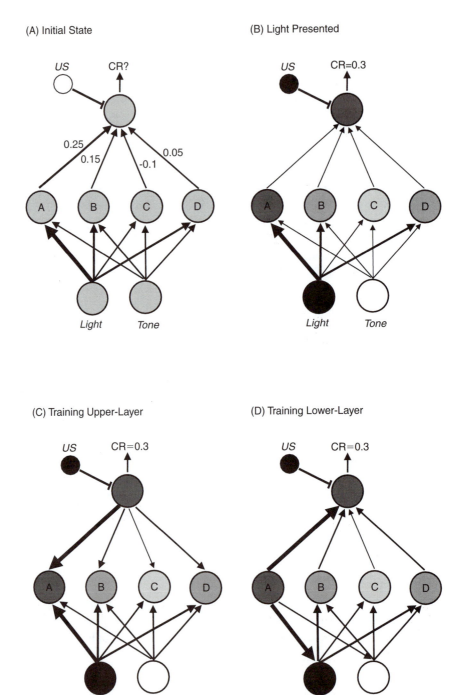

(A) Initial State

(B) Light Presented

(C) Training Upper-Layer

(D) Training Lower-Layer

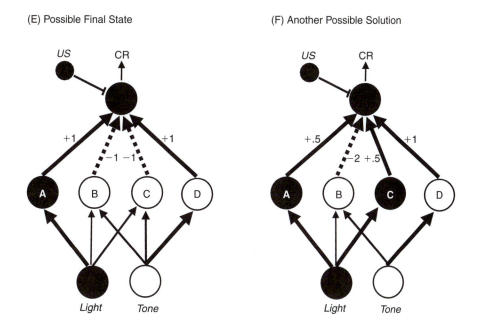

(E) Possible Final State

(F) Another Possible Solution

Figure 4.12   (A) A multilayer network with four internal-layer nodes A, B, C, and D. All weights are initialized to small random values. To avoid clutter, only the weights on the upper layer are shown; small random values are set on all lower-layer weights as well. (B) A light CS is presented. Because of the random weights, this stimulus causes strong activity in internal-layer node A, some activity in B and D, and little activity in C. This pattern of activation feeds into the output node, which produces a response (in this example, the response is 0.3). (C) Training the upper layer weights is similar to the Widrow-Hoff rule. The error is computed as the difference between desired output (US = 1) and actual output (CR = 0.3). A fraction of this error is distributed among all active internal-layer nodes; since A was the most active, it receives most of the weight change. In the future, when node A is again active, it will now produce more activation in the output node. (D) The lower-layer weights are changed by backpropagating error from the upper layer. Node A, which was highly active, receives a large fraction of the error. This is distributed as weight change along the connections feeding into A. In this case, the connection to the active light node is strengthened; the tone node was inactive, so there is no change to this connection. Next time the light stimulus is present, it will cause more activity in A, which will in turn cause a stronger output. A similar process is repeated for each of the remaining internal-layer nodes B, C, and D. (E) After numerous training trials on the negative patterning problem, the network might find a solution as shown: When the tone alone is present, node A is activated and in turn activates the output node. When the light alone is present, node D is activated and in turn activates the output node. When both tone and light are present, configural nodes B and C are also activated, and inhibitory output from these nodes counteracts the excitatory output from A and D; the output node does not become active. This is a similar solution to the one constructed by hand in figure 4.10 except for the presence of two configural nodes (B and C) instead of one. (F) If the same network from figure 4.12A had been initialized with different random weights, it might have developed a different but equally valid solution. For example, the light alone might activate nodes A and C, the tone alone might activate node D, and node B might respond to the configuration. This network might show a learning curve indistinguishable from the one generated by the network in (E).

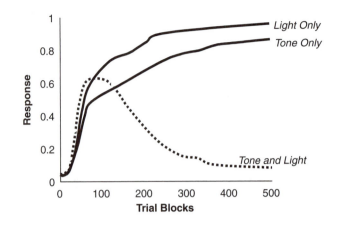

Figure 4.13 Learning curve, averaged over ten simulation runs for a network with the architecture shown in Figure 4.12A, trained on the negative patterning problem (tone → US, light → US, tone & light → no US). Each trial block includes one presentation of each stimulus type. Out of the ten simulation runs, only one failed to learn to respond to light and tone but not the compound; even after 1000 trial blocks, this network was still responding more strongly to the compound than to the components. Compare to the experimental results from rabbits shown in figure 4.8A.

weights, can learn the same problem in a few dozen trials. Thus, there is a cost to flexibility in representations: The more flexible the network, the longer it takes to construct new representations and hence the longer it takes to learn.

A second limitation of the error backpropagation algorithm is that it does not always work. Figure 4.13 shows performance on the negative patterning problem averaged over ten simulation runs. Out of these ten simulation runs, one failed to reach a solution: It persistently responded more to the compound stimulus than to the components, even after 5000 training trials. In such cases, the only solution is to stop the network, wipe its memory by returning all weights to initial random values, and begin training again, hoping for better results. This is not necessarily a fatal problem for the model as a psychological theory of animal and human learning; in most psychology learning experiments, a small number of the subjects (animals or people) often fail to solve complex training tasks. Like the networks, they seem to get stuck and never find a solution.

A further concern about the backpropagation algorithm is that it involves a large number of parameters, including the number of internal-layer nodes, the learning rate, and others (interested readers can refer to MathBox 4.1 for details). Each of these parameters may be adjusted to improve how well the network learns. The optimal values for these parameters are generally different for each task and therefore must often be chosen and fine-tuned by hand. A great deal of research has been devoted to optimizing performance on a particular problem by changing some parameter in the algorithm, but these solutions often apply well to one specific problem (or problem domain) without applying well to other problems (or problem domains).

Despite all these limitations on performance, the backpropagation algorithm has proven extremely useful as an engineering tool. In fact, given enough internal-layer nodes and enough training trials, a network that is trained by backpropagation can, in principle, learn any arbitrary relationship from a set of inputs to a set of outputs.[19]

The backpropagation algorithm has been used to train networks for all kinds of practical applications, including networks that detect forged signatures, pronounce typewritten text, discover faults in mechanical equipment, interpret sonar returns, and diagnose diseases.[20] Backpropagation is probably the single most widely used algorithm for training neural networks in business and engineering applications. Countless algorithmic variations have been developed to address various shortcomings or to speed learning.[21] However, these variations typically increase mathematical complexity while producing only moderate improvements in performance. Therefore, the canonical version of backpropagation described here remains the standard method for training most multilayer networks. In fact, when researchers announce that they are "using a neural network" for a particular application, it is usually a safe bet that they are employing the error backpropagation algorithm.

Psychological and Biological Validity of Backpropagation

Backpropagation's success as an engineering tool does not necessarily imply anything about its validity as a psychological model of learning or as a model of the biological mechanisms underlying that learning. Given that the backpropagation algorithm can produce complex learning behaviors, it is natural to wonder how well this learning procedure succeeds as a psychological or biological model of learning.

On the surface, there is an immediate difficulty with this comparison. The backpropagation algorithm requires that nodes be able to send error information backward to the nodes that originally provided their input (refer to figure 4.12D). This is problematic for models of biological learning: The connections in the brain are so complex and extensive that it seems unlikely that there could be precise reciprocity in neuronal connections; these and other biological features are often conveniently ignored by neural network model-ers.[22] Several authors have suggested ways in which something like back-propagation could be implemented without requiring such precise backward connections.[23] More recent neurophysiological studies have sug-gested that neurons may indeed be able to send information backward to the neurons that activated them.[24] While backpropagation may not be plausible as a literal model of neuronal learning, it may still be useful as a systems-level description of learning in a brain network.

In the next chapter, we will discuss ways in which a slightly different kind of network architecture—the autoassociator and its derivative, the auto-encoder—can capture some aspects of brain anatomy and physiology, partic-ularly in the hippocampus.

SUMMARY

• Generalization refers to the tendency to transfer learning about one stimu-lus to other, superficially similar stimuli. Generalization is critical to apply prior experience in new situations without requiring fresh learning about every new instance. Conversely, specificity allows learning different re-sponses to stimuli that may superficially look very similar. The optimal de-gree of generalization versus specificity therefore depends not only on the superficial similarity of stimuli, but also on their meaning or consequences for a user.

• Component representations relate one stimulus (or feature) to one node in the model. In distributed representations, information about each stimu-lus (or feature) is encoded by many nodes. Distributed representations pro-vide a framework for encoding stimulus similarity and allow stimulus generalization.

• Distributed representations can be implemented by adding an internal layer of nodes to a neural network, between the input and output nodes.

• Although the Widrow-Hoff rule works very well for networks with only a single layer of weights, it does not apply directly to multilayer networks. The error backpropagation algorithm extends the Widrow-Hoff rule to allow changes to the lower layer of weights, thereby changing stimulus represen-tations in the internal layer.

5 Unsupervised Learning: Autoassociative Networks and the Hippocampus

Chapters 3 and 4 described several neural networks that can be trained to associate cues, such as tone and lights, with a reinforcing stimulus, such as the airpuff unconditioned stimulus (US). By definition, a US is something qualitatively different from other cues: Whereas any detectable stimulus can become a conditioned stimulus (CS), USs are prewired to evoke reflexive behavioral responses. Thus, an airpuff US evokes a protective eyeblink, a foot-shock US evokes a reflexive movement of the leg away from the offending site, and a food US evokes feeding behavior in a hungry animal. In human learning, the concept of a US is often broadened to mean any stimulus that is to be predicted. Thus, in the fictitious medical diagnosis task of chapter 4 (figure 4.11), the presence of the rare disease was predicted by subjects on the basis of symptoms, and so the symptoms functioned as CSs that predicted a disease US.

What all these paradigms have in common is that there is a special input, the US, and the job of the animal, human, or computational model is to predict this US on the basis of available cues. The conditioned response is correct insofar as it predicts the US. This principle forms the basis of error-correction rules such as the Widrow-Hoff rule, embedded in the Rescorla-Wagner model. Learning occurs exactly when there is a difference between the prediction of the US (embodied by the conditioned response) and the actual US. In a sense, learning is **supervised** by a system that monitors this prediction error and adjusts associative weights accordingly.

Such error-correction systems have their uses, but—as was described in the previous chapter—they fail on paradigms such as sensory preconditioning and latent inhibition in which learning takes place in the absence of any explicit US and hence in the absence of any prediction error. Such paradigms are sometimes called **mere exposure** paradigms or **latent learning** paradigms. Learning in these paradigms is often called **unsupervised learning,** in contrast to supervised learning that is based on predicting an external reinforcement.

The dichotomy between supervised and unsupervised learning has a long history in psychology. In the first half of the twentieth century, this division defined two different schools of learning research. One school, led by Clark Hull, emphasized the study of supervised learning in which there was an explicit goal, reward, or punishment for an animal or person's behavior.[1] Rescorla and Wagner followed in this tradition in developing their model of classical conditioning.[2]

A second school of researchers, led by Edward Tolman and working at about the same time as Hull, chose to focus on unsupervised forms of learning in which animals were merely exposed to a novel environment but not trained on any particular task.[3] Tolman was especially interested in how animals learned during the exploration of new spatial environments. For example, in one study, rats were placed at the starting point of a maze and rewarded with cheese when they found their way to an endpoint in the maze.[4] The experimenters recorded how often the rats deviated from the most direct path to the goal.

As figure 5.1 shows, rats gradually made fewer and fewer errors in the maze, finding their way to the cheese reward faster and more efficiently. A second group of rats was given the same task but without the cheese. As might be expected, these rats showed no particular tendency to head toward the goal location but instead appeared to wander randomly about the maze. One might assume, therefore, that these unreinforced rats were learning little about the maze. However, after they wandered the maze for ten days, cheese was placed in the goal location starting on the eleventh day. As seen in figure 5.1, these rats made a veritable beeline for the goal: On day 13, they reached the goal faster, on average, than the rats that had been given the food reward all along. Tolman interpreted this result as implying that although the unreinforced rats appeared to be wandering aimlessly through the maze during the first part of the study, they were in fact actually exploring and learning about their environment. Later, when challenged to navigate the maze, the rats used this prior learning to guide their path.

From these and similar experiments, Tolman concluded that animals can and do naturally learn about their environment even when they are not explicitly rewarded for doing so. Tolman argued that the rats in figure 5.1 formed **cognitive maps**—mental models of their environment—during exposure to a maze.

Interestingly, it is exactly this kind of unreinforced learning that seems to be chiefly disrupted by hippocampal-region damage in animals. Recall from chapter 2 that rats with hippocampal-region damage are unable to learn the location of a submerged platform in a milky pool and do not show behaviors

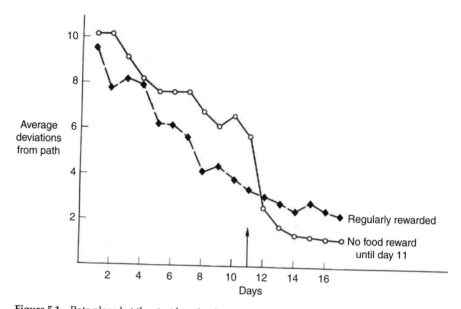

Figure 5.1   Rats placed at the start location in a maze, with a food reward regularly available in a goal location, learn to run directly to the goal, as indicated by fewer deviations from the most direct path. A second group of rats are placed in the maze, allowed to run in the maze without food for ten days, and then placed in the maze with food available from day 11 on; these rats learn very quickly to run directly to the food, quickly outperforming even the rats who received food reward all along. This implies that during the first ten unrewarded days, the rats were exploring and learning about the maze environment; later, when a food reward was available, they were able to use that information to find food efficiently. (Based on Hilgard & Bower, 1975, p. 135, Figure 5.3, adapted from Tolman & Honzik, 1930.)

such as sensory preconditioning and latent learning that depend on learning about cues presented in the absence of a reinforcing US. Thus, to a first approximation, it would seem that unsupervised "Tolmanian" (CS-CS) learning depends on the hippocampal region, while supervised "Hullian" (CS-US) learning does not. To the extent that this mapping holds true, it would suggest that the error-correction networks from chapter 3 may be better descriptions of learning in hippocampal-lesioned animals than in intact animals.

To take this simple mapping a step further, if error-correcting networks can capture supervised (CS-US) learning of the kind seen in hippocampal-lesioned animals, what kind of network architecture is capable of the unsupervised (CS-CS) learning that is seen in animals with an intact hippocampus? There do, in fact, exist network architectures that are capable of the kinds of unsupervised learning that Tolman described. These networks are called **autoassociative networks** and are described below. The autoassociative networks are of particular interest, not only because they capture some features of hippocampal-dependent learning, but also because there is a long tradition in neuroscience of using them as models of how certain circuits within the hippocampus operate.

5.1   AUTOASSOCIATIVE NETWORKS

In an influential 1949 book, Donald Hebb proposed that the brain stores information via a simple rule: *If one cell (or neuron) A connects to a second cell B, and if the two cells are repeatedly active at the same time, then the connection between them is strengthened, so future activity in A is more likely to cause activation in B.*[5] This rule is often called **Hebb's rule,** and the learning it embodies is called **Hebbian learning.**

In contrast to the supervised learning characterized by the Widrow-Hoff learning rule, Hebbian learning is unsupervised, meaning that it does not depend on a special teaching signal, such as a reinforcing US. Weight change is automatic in Hebb's rule and depends only on conjoint activity in pairs of nodes.

Hebb's rule was originally proposed as a theory of how large assemblies of neurons in the brain operate. Later neurophysiological studies verified that Hebbian learning does occur in the brain: Synapses between coactive neurons do grow stronger. This process is called **long-term potentiation (LTP),**[6] because the synaptic change (potentiation) has been observed to last for weeks in the laboratory and may last longer in living animals. This synaptic process (there are several variations) has been observed throughout the brain[7] and is currently believed to underlie many kinds of changes in the brain.[8]

Figure 5.2A shows a simple example of an autoassociative network,[9] trained according to Hebb's rule. Eight nodes are shown, and each has a weak connection to all the others. Each node is *both* an input node and an output node, meaning that it receives input from external sources, while its activation level is part of the final output produced by the network. External inputs arrive and activate some subset of nodes in the network (darkened circles in figure 5.2A); other nodes remain inactive. This pattern of active and inactive nodes represents knowledge to be stored by the network. According to Hebb's rule, connections between coactive nodes are strengthened (figure 5.2B). This is usually done in one massive step, by simply setting all the relevant weights to 1.0. At this point, the pattern is **stored** in the network. A different input pattern, which activates different nodes (figure 5.2C), could be stored in the same way (figure 5.2D).

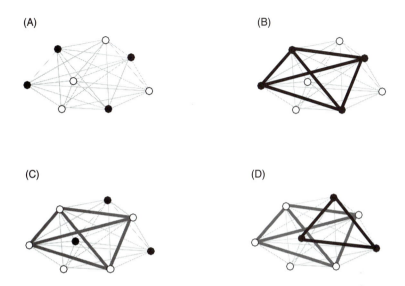

Figure 5.2 Simplified example of an autoassociative network, consisting of a group of nodes (circles). (A) External inputs (not shown) evoke a pattern of activity over the network, resulting in the activation of a subset of nodes (solid circles). (B) Weighted connections develop between coactive nodes; the pattern is said to be stored. (C) Later, a different pattern is presented that activates a different subset of nodes (solid circles). (D) Weights between these coactive nodes are strengthened, and the new pattern is stored.

The ability to remember patterns in this way is one mechanism by which the brain might store memories of past events. Once a pattern has been stored, activation in any one node will produce activation in the other nodes of a pattern. Thus, even after the external input is turned off, the pattern (stored as an assembly of active nodes) remains for some time, until activation gradually dies away. In this way, superficially unrelated but temporally coincident stimuli can be bound together into a unified memory. For example, an episodic memory of meeting a celebrity might include not only the gist of the conversation with that person, but also details of the cocktail party where the meeting occurred, such as the time and place and who else was present. Each of these details could be represented as a node (or a group of nodes) that could then be bound together by synaptic changes between these coactive nodes.

Of course, a stored pattern is no use unless it can be retrieved later. And this leads to the most interesting property of an autoassociative network: *Given a partial or incomplete version of a stored memory, an autoassociative network can retrieve the entire stored pattern.* This is called **pattern completion,** and figure 5.3 shows an example. The network has already stored two patterns, represented

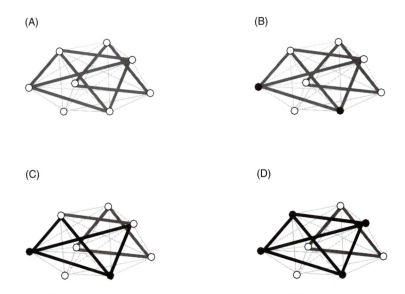

Figure 5.3 Pattern completion in an autoassociative network. (A) The network has stored two patterns by strengthening the weights between nodes that are coactive in each pattern. (B) A partial version of one pattern is presented, which activates a subset of the nodes (solid circles). (C) Activation flows from active nodes along previously strengthened connections (heavy lines), (D) and the entire pattern is retrieved.

by strong connections between the nodes that were coactive (figure 5.3A). Now, a partial version of one stored pattern is presented, which activates only a few of the nodes in the stored pattern (figure 5.3B). Activation then spreads along the previously strengthened connections (figure 5.3C), activating the remaining nodes (figure 5.3D). Finally, the entire pattern is reinstated.

In the previous example of remembering a celebrity, pattern completion means that, given a mention of the individual, spreading activation will activate nodes corresponding to the details of the party where the celebrity was encountered—retrieving the complete memory from a partial cue.

A variant of this process is **pattern recognition,** the ability to take an arbitrary input and retrieve the stored pattern that is most similar to that input. In figure 5.4A, the network has been trained on the same two patterns as in the earlier example. Next, in figure 5.4B, the external inputs present a new pattern that overlaps partially with one of the stored patterns. Activation will spread along weighted connections to activate the other nodes in the stored pattern (figure 5.4C). At the same time, lack of such activity will mean that the extra node that is incorrectly activated will eventually become quiet. In the end, the stored pattern is correctly retrieved (figure 5.4D). The network has "recognized" its input as a distorted version of the stored pattern.

(A)   (B)

(C)   (D)

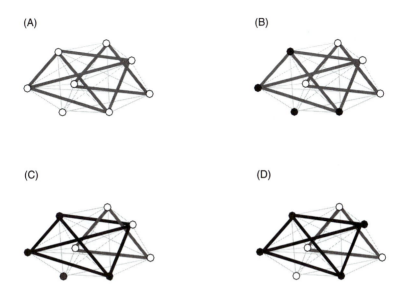

Figure 5.4   Pattern recognition in an autoassociative network. (A) The network has stored two patterns by strengthening the weights between nodes that are coactive in each pattern. (B) External inputs activate nodes (solid circles), some of which are part of a previously stored pattern and some of which are not. (C) Activation spreads along previously strengthened pattern, activating nodes that are part of the stored pattern. Other nodes, which do not receive this input, gradually become inactive until (D) the stored pattern is retrieved. At this point, the network has recognized the input in (B) as a degraded version of the stored pattern retrieved in (D).

In addition to serving as models of memory for events,[10] the twin features of pattern completion and pattern recognition have led to many engineering applications of autoassociative networks. These applications range from interpreting sonar signals to guiding robot navigation to optimizing how tasks are assigned to cooperating units.[11]

5.2   HIPPOCAMPAL ANATOMY AND AUTOASSOCIATION

Traditionally, most theories that have tried to map from hippocampal anatomy to behavioral function have focused on a particular subfield within the hippocampus: field CA3. As shown in figure 5.5, CA3 is roughly the part of the hippocampus enclosed by the dentate gyrus. Hippocampal field CA1 lies next to CA3 and merges into the subiculum and dentate gyrus.

Figure 5.6 shows a schematic of information flow into and out of CA3. One primary input comes from entorhinal cortex, carrying highly processed information about all kinds of sensory input. This pathway is called the **perforant path,** since its fibers physically perforate the dentate gyrus to reach

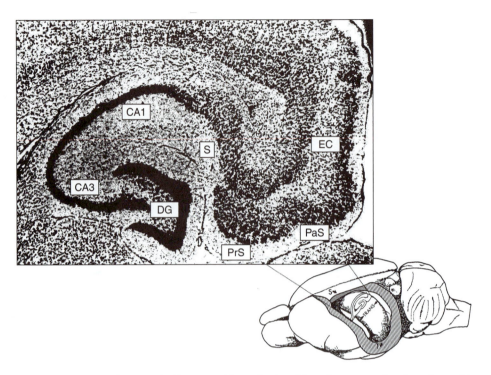

Figure 5.5 Lower right: Drawing of the rat brain, with surface removed to show the position of the hippocampus; the cutaway view shows the internal organization of the hippocampal region. Top left: Photomicrograph of a cutaway section through the rat hippocampus. The hippocampus (including fields CA3 and CA1) is visible as a "C"-shaped line of neurons; the dentate gyrus (DG) is an interlocking "C"-shaped line of cells. Adjacent to hippocampal field CA1 is the subicular complex (including S = subiculum, PrS = presubiculum, PaS = parasubiculum) and entorhinal cortex (EC). (Adapted from Amaral & Witter, 1989, Figures 1 and 2.)

CA3. A secondary path from the entorhinal cortex synapses in dentate gyrus before proceeding on to CA3. The connections from dentate gyrus to CA3 are called **mossy fibers,** and they make sparse, large, and presumably very powerful synapses onto CA3 neurons. CA3 neurons process this information and send their outputs on to hippocampal field CA1 and from there out of the hippocampus.

One of the most striking features of CA3 anatomy is the high degree of **internal recurrency,** meaning that CA3 neurons send axons not only out of CA3, but also back to synapse on other CA3 neurons. Such feedback is a general principle throughout the brain, but it is dramatically heightened in CA3. For example, each CA3 pyramidal neuron in the rat may receive about 4,000 synapses from entorhinal inputs but up to about 12,000 synapses from other CA3 cells.[12] This means that each CA3 pyramidal neuron

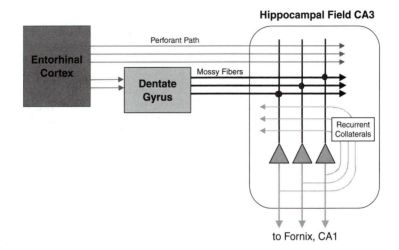

Figure 5.6 Schematic of information pathways into and within hippocampal field CA3. Highly processed, multimodal sensory information from entorhinal cortex travels via the perforant path to contact pyramidal neurons in CA3. There is also an indirect path from entorhinal cortex via the dentate gyrus (the mossy fiber path). CA3 pyramidal neurons have a high degree of internal recurrence, meaning that axons have collaterals that travel back to contact other CA3 neurons, as well as sending information out of CA3 to the fornix, CA1, and elsewhere.

receives inputs from about 4% of all other CA3 pyramidal neurons. This is nowhere near the 100% recurrency that is assumed in the simplified network models of figures 4.2 through 4.4, in which every node is connected to every other node. However, this 4% recurrency is orders of magnitude higher than the degree of internal recurrency that is observed elsewhere in the brain. Furthermore, the connections between CA3 neurons are modifiable by LTP in much the same manner as Hebb proposed. In fact, LTP was originally discovered by researchers studying synapses in the hippocampal region.[13]

Given these anatomical and physiological characteristics, it seems logical to ask whether CA3 could function as an autoassociative network. One of the earliest and most influential models of hippocampus, published by David Marr in 1971, proposed exactly that.[14] In its simplest phrasing, Marr's model assumes that CA3 pyramidal neurons form an autoassociative network in which external inputs (from entorhinal cortex and dentate gyrus) activate a subset of CA3 neurons. Recurrent collaterals between coactive nodes are strengthened, storing the pattern. Since Marr's original publication, a wealth of new empirical data has shown that some additional aspects of his model were incomplete or incorrect.[15] Nonetheless, many of the basic ideas underlying Marr's model have withstood continuing empirical and theoretical analysis and are implicit in most modern models of hippocampus.[16]

Storage Versus Retrieval

One important requirement for an autoassociator, implicit in the above discussion, is that the network be able to operate in two distinct modes: a storage mode and a recall mode. Remember the example of figure 5.2D, in which one pattern has been stored in the network and a second pattern is presented. How does the network "know" whether this second pattern represents new information to be stored (as in the example of figures 5.2C and 5.2D) or a distorted version of an old pattern to be retrieved (as in figures 5.3 and 5.4)?

The simplest assumption is that there is an external input, a "teacher," that guides the network into either a storage state or a recall state. This may not be as unlikely as it sounds; recent evidence has suggested that areas of the brain may be flooded with chemicals (called **neuromodulators**) that encourage the brain either to store new information or to retrieve familiar information. Chapter 10 discusses this idea in more detail, with particular reference to the neuromodulator **acetylcholine.**

However, the anatomy of the hippocampus suggests a second (possibly complementary) way to guide the network into storage or recall mode. Figure 5.6 illustrated the two principal information pathways into hippocampal field CA3: the direct perforant path from entorhinal cortex and the indirect path via dentate gyrus, which terminates in mossy fiber synapses onto CA3 neurons. These mossy fiber synapses are very sparse: In the rat, each CA3 pyramidal neuron receives only about 50 mossy fiber synapses,[17] a mere fraction of the inputs from the perforant path or from recurrent collaterals. However, these mossy fiber synapses are physically much larger and stronger than the other inputs: Whereas input from hundreds or thousands of entorhinal inputs may be required to activate a CA3 pyramidal neuron, coincident activity on a relatively small number of mossy fiber inputs may be sufficient to activate the CA3 neuron.[18]

The implication is that mossy fiber inputs may be strong enough to act as teaching inputs, causing pattern storage. In the absence of mossy fiber activation, the network may perform pattern retrieval and pattern completion, as schematized in figure 5.7. When a new pattern is presented for storage, the strong mossy fiber inputs cause the CA3 neurons that they contact to become strongly active (figure 5.7A). According to Hebb's rule, strong conjoint activity in two neurons causes strengthening of the connections (synapses) between them (figure 5.7B). At this point, the pattern is stored. Later, a partial version of the input is presented along weaker perforant path inputs; this produces partial activation in some of the same CA3 neurons (figure 5.7C).

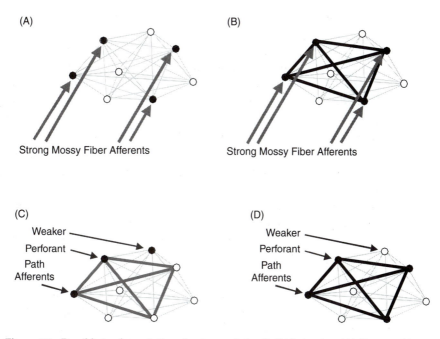

Figure 5.7 Possible implementation of autoassociation in CA3 circuitry. (A) One set of inputs, the strong mossy fibers from dentate gyrus, activate a set of CA3 neurons. (B) In the presence of this strong input, plasticity occurs along connections (synapses) between coactive neurons. (C) Another set of inputs, the perforant path afferents from entorhinal cortex, make relatively weaker synapses onto CA3 neurons, activating a subset of CA3 neurons. (D) This weaker input is enough to spread along previously strengthened connections, retrieving a stored pattern, but not enough to maintain activity in neurons that are not part of the pattern, nor enough to cause new plasticity. Thus, storage occurs when strong mossy fiber inputs are present; pattern retrieval (including pattern completion and pattern recognition) occurs when weaker perforant path inputs are present.

Activation spreads along recurrent connections that were previously strengthened—enough to activate some additional CA3 neurons but not enough to cause additional synaptic plasticity, which requires very strong conjoint activation (figure 5.7D). As a result, the stored pattern is recalled, but no new learning takes place.

This method for implementing an autoassociator in the brain relies on the fact that there exist inputs, specifically mossy fibers, that make unusually strong synapses on target neurons. Such a situation may be the exception rather than the rule, although as we noted in chapter 3, climbing fibers in the cerebellum may share a similar function: forcing cerebellar Purkinje cells to become active and guiding learning.

Capacity, Consolidation, and Catastrophic Interference

One problem with autoassociative networks is that they have very limited capacity; that is, they can store only a small number of unrelated patterns before new information begins to overwrite the old. For example, suppose one memory incorporates nodes A, B, C, and D and creates strong associations between them, such that activation of a subset will spread to retrieve the entire memory (figure 5.8A). Now, suppose a second pattern is presented that incorporates nodes A, B, E, and F and the associations between these nodes are strengthened (figure 5.8B). If the network is presented with a partial memory consisting of E and F (figure 5.8C), activation will spread to A and B (figure 5.8D) and from there to C and D (figure 5.8E), thereby "retrieving" a

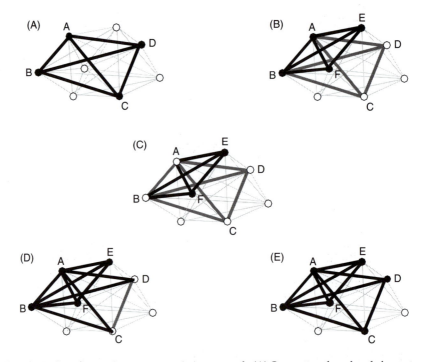

Figure 5.8 Interference in an autoassociative network. (A) One pattern has already been stored in the network by weighting connections between coactive nodes (nodes A, B, C, and D). (B) A new set of inputs is presented to the network, activating a new subset of nodes that partially overlaps with the previous pattern (nodes A, B, E, and F). Connections between coactive nodes are strengthened, and the new pattern is stored. (C) A partial pattern is presented (nodes E and F) that overlaps partially with the second stored pattern. (D) Activity spreads along previously strengthened connections to activate nodes A and B and from there (E) spreads to activate nodes C and D, thus "retrieving" a complex pattern that was never stored.

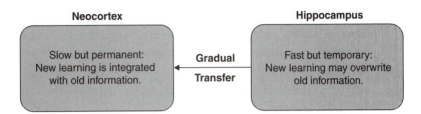

Figure 5.9   General format of many connectionist models of amnesia. The cortex is assumed to be a large-capacity, permanent store for memory associations and to be able to integrate new information with old associations. However, learning is assumed to be slow and possibly to require several iterated presentations. The hippocampus is assumed to be capable of storing memory within as little as a single exposure, but older memories are liable to be overwritten by newer ones. The hippocampus is thus only a temporary store. Over some period of time (known as the consolidation period), memories are integrated into cortex and become independent of the hippocampus.

complex pattern that was never stored! Such **interference** or confusion among stored patterns is a fundamental limitation of autoassociative networks.

Marr noted this potential for interference in autoassociative networks, and he made his second important contribution to hippocampal modeling by suggesting a possible solution.[19] He proposed that memory consisted of two separate but interacting modules (figure 5.9). One, which he located in cortex, was assumed to be a large-capacity, permanent memory store. The second, which he located in hippocampus, was a limited-capacity, limited-duration store. The hippocampal network was conceptualized as an auto-associative network. In brief, the general idea was that a stimulus would enter via the sensory systems and eventually lead to activation of cells in the cortex and hippocampus. The hippocampus would quickly strengthen connections between coactive cells, capturing the memory. Over some period of time, this information would be retrieved and stored in the cortex in such a way as not to interfere with other, earlier information. Eventually, the memory would become independent of the hippocampus, so that when new information overwrote the hippocampal cell assembly, the cortical copy would be safe.

Marr's characterization of the hippocampus as a temporary buffer for memories before they are consolidated into long-term memory provides a compelling account of three key aspects of anterograde amnesia. First, hippocampal damage results in a permanent closing of the gateway for acquiring new memories. Second, hippocampal damage does not disrupt memories that have previously been stored in the cortex. Third, since there is a consolidation period, during which memories are transferred from hippocampal to cortical storage, hippocampal damage may result in time-limited retrograde amnesia for recently stored memories.

Many connectionist models of amnesia have followed Marr in assuming this kind of fast, temporary hippocampal storage and slow, permanent cortical storage.[20] Many nonconnectionist models and theories assume this kind of organization as well.[21]

5.3   AUTOENCODERS: AUTOASSOCIATION WITH REPRESENTATION

Autoassociative models of hippocampus have considerable power for describing the hippocampal region's role in episodic memory formation. However, while autoassociative networks may be a good model of episodic learning and pattern completion—essential components of memory, to be sure—they have little to say about other, equally important kinds of learning. For example, they do not allow error-correction learning, nor do they allow the formation of new representations, such as the multilayer networks of chapter 4.

Fortunately, there is an elaboration on autoassociative networks that combines the latent learning and pattern completion abilities of autoassociators with the error-correction and representational power of multilayered networks. This kind of network is called an **autoencoder.**

A New Interpretation of Autoassociators

So far in this chapter, we have illustrated autoassociative networks as amorphous clusters, with connections drawn between individual nodes. Drawn in this way, they look very different from the associative networks that we presented in earlier chapters.

For example, figure 5.10A shows an autoassociator that interconnects nodes representing light, tone, odor, and texture cues. Each node is connected to each of the other nodes. Each node functions as both an input node and an output node: receiving activation from sources outside the network and producing output that is taken as the network's response. The same network can therefore be redrawn as in figure 5.10B. Here, each cue is represented by an input and an output node. Each input cue activates one input node, which in turn activates a corresponding output node. Input nodes also have modifiable weighted connections to all the other output nodes. The pattern of activation at the output layer is taken as the output of the network.

Here is how the autoassociator works, drawn this way. A pattern is presented for storage and activates several nodes at the input level—for example, light and odor but not tone or texture (figure 5.11A). Each input node causes activity in the corresponding output-level node; that is, the output nodes for light and odor are activated (figure 5.11B). Connections between

(A) Four-Node Autoassociator

(B) Redrawn as Feedforward Network

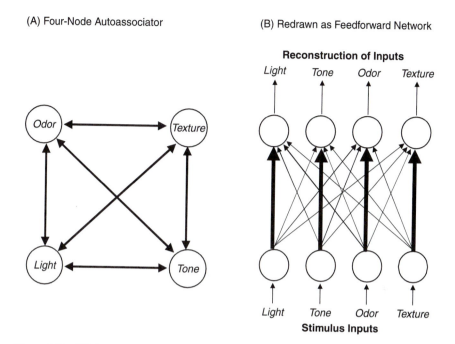

Figure 5.10   (A) An autoassociator, containing nodes representing four cues. Each node is connected to all the other nodes, and each node functions as both an input node and an output node. (B) The same autoassociator can be redrawn with separate input and output nodes for each cue. There is a strong, nonmodifiable weight from each input node to the corresponding output node. Thus, activation of the light input node causes activation of the light output node. There are also modifiable connections from each input node to each output node, so weights between coactive cues can be strengthened.

coactive nodes are strengthened. This means that connection weights between the light input node and the odor output node and those between the odor input node and the light output node are strengthened (figure 5.11C). At this point, the pattern is stored. In effect, the network has learned to associate an input pattern with an output that is the same pattern. Now it may be clear why these networks are called autoassociators: Rather than associating an input pattern with an arbitrary output (such as a reinforcing US), they associate a pattern with itself.

Later, a partial version of the stored pattern may be presented, such as light only (figure 5.11D). The inputs activate their corresponding outputs but also activate those output nodes to which they have previously strengthened connections (figure 5.11F): The output nodes corresponding to light and odor are activated, and the stored pattern is reconstructed at the output level.

This might seem like a more complicated method to picture an auto-associator than the drawings of section 5.2, but it has an important advantage: When it is drawn in this way, there is a clear difference between what portions of the pattern are presented as external input and what portions are reconstructed by the network. In figure 5.11E, the difference between the input activations and the output activations consists of elements of the pattern that the network has reconstructed. The degree of difference between the original input pattern and the output pattern produced by the network is a measure of the error in the reconstruction. If the error is high enough, this implies that the new pattern may be one that has not been seen before. As such, this reconstruction error in an autoassociative network can also be viewed as a measure of the **novelty** of the input pattern: For a familiar (previously stored) pattern, input and output will match perfectly; for a novel (never-stored) pattern, input and output will deviate; for a pattern that contains elements of a previously stored pattern, the input and output may be similar but not identical.

Cast in this way, an autoassociative network can capture some features of latent learning. In the example of figure 5.11, two stimuli (light and odor) were always presented together; strong weights developed between the input and output nodes to reflect this correlation. Later, when the light was presented alone (figure 5.11D), the network output reflected expectation that the odor should also occur (figure 5.11E). Thus, without any explicit reinforcement (i.e., US), the network learned which stimuli reliably co-occur and which (tone and texture) do not.

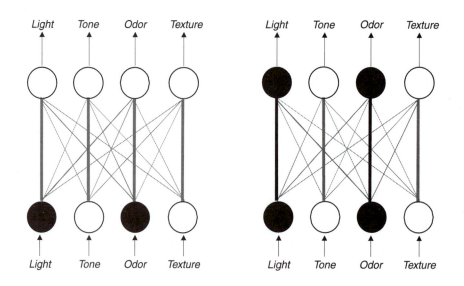

(A) Input Presented

(B) Output Nodes Activated

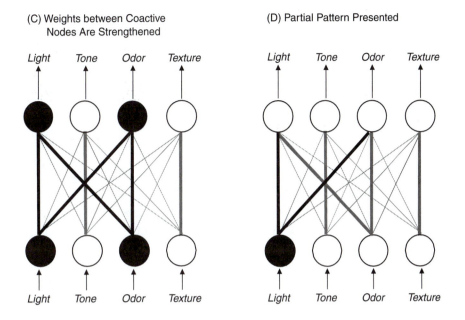

(C) Weights between Coactive Nodes Are Strengthened

(D) Partial Pattern Presented

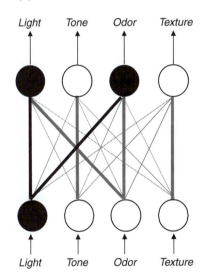

(E) Stored Pattern Is Recalled

Figure 5.11   The two-layer autoassociator in action. (A) Input is presented by activating a subset of the input-layer nodes (e.g., light and odor). (B) This activates the corresponding output nodes (i.e., light and odor). (C) The weights between coactive nodes are strengthened (from light input to odor output and from odor input to light output). (D) Later, a partial version of the stored pattern is presented as input (e.g., light only). (E) Activation spreads along previously strengthened connections to retrieve the stored pattern (i.e., light and odor).

Autoencoders: Multilayer Autoassociators

A second reason for drawing autoassociators with two layers of nodes is that it is fairly easy to see how to extend the network to include an additional, internal node layer between the input and output nodes (figure 5.12). Because the internal-layer representation can be thought of as a recoding of the input pattern, this type of network is sometimes called an **autoencoder.**[22]

Like the autoassociators, the autoencoder in figure 5.12 is trained to reconstruct the input pattern on the output nodes. When the output faithfully matches the input, the autoencoder has stored the pattern. When presented with a partial or distorted version of a stored pattern, the autoencoder will reconstruct the stored pattern on its output nodes. When a novel pattern is presented, the discrepancy between input and output patterns gives a measure of this novelty.

However, just as the Widrow-Hoff rule was insufficient to train a multilayer associative network in chapter 4, Hebbian learning is insufficient to train a multilayer autoencoder—and for exactly the same reason: There is no *a priori* way to determine activations in the internal-node layer so that the

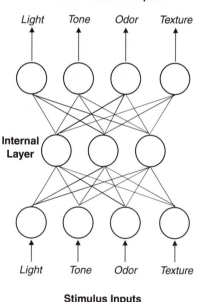

Figure 5.12   An autoencoder is an autoassociative network with an internal node layer.

outputs reconstruct the inputs faithfully. Without knowing these desired activations, there is no way to set the lower layer of weights.

However, once again, error backpropagation provides one way in which this kind of network could be trained. We know the desired responses of the output-layer nodes; they should simply replicate the pattern of activations across the input layer nodes. Knowing this, we can use one application of error-correction learning to train the upper layer of weights. The error at the output layer is backpropagated and distributed among the internal-layer nodes, giving an estimate of the desired activations there. Now, a second application of error-correction learning can be used to train the lower layer of weights. (For details on the error backpropagation algorithm, refer to Math-Box 4.1.) With repeated presentations of an input pattern, the output nodes come to produce the desired responses: an accurate reconstruction of the input pattern.

Usually, autoencoder networks are drawn with the internal layer containing fewer nodes than either the input or output layer, as in figure 5.12. In this case, the autoencoder's task is complicated: In figure 5.12, the network has to accept four stimulus inputs and produce four outputs, but it has only three internal-layer nodes to encode this information. The only way to accomplish this task is if the network can identify regularities and redundancies in the input. For example, in figure 5.11, we discussed an experiment in which light and odor always co-occur. In this case, the autoencoder could make use of these statistical regularities: It would need only one internal-layer node to represent the joint occurrence of light and odor, leaving one node each to represent tone and texture (figure 5.13A). The representations of light and odor have been **compressed,** or made more similar. Later, when the light is presented alone, the network performs pattern completion and activates the output node corresponding to odor as well (figure 5.13B).

The general principle of compression, illustrated in figure 5.13, is analogous to what happens when a computer file is compressed for saving as a smaller file. Information is not lost; rather, it is encoded in a more efficient manner that requires less disk space, analogous to using fewer internal nodes in a network. Similar schemes are also used to compress speech and other sounds for efficient transmission over phone lines.

Predictive Autoencoders

So far, we have shown that autoassociative networks can learn about stimulus relationships through mere exposure to stimuli. The multilayer autoencoders are autoassociative networks that form internal-layer representations that

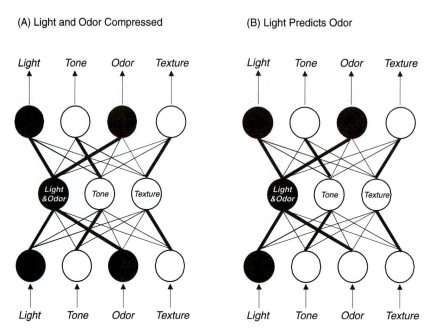

(A) Light and Odor Compressed   **(B) Light Predicts Odor**

Figure 5.13   The autoencoder compresses the representations of redundant (co-occurring) stimuli in its internal layer. (A) For example, if light and odor always co-occur, one internal-layer node may come to encode both. Weights from this node to the outputs ensure that the light and odor output nodes are active whenever the corresponding inputs appear. Other internal-layer nodes encode the presence of tone and texture. The figure shows a local representation; in reality, the representation of a stimulus may be distributed over several nodes. (B) Later, if light is presented alone, the compressed internal-layer representation activates the output nodes corresponding to both light and odor.

compress stimulus redundancies while preserving nonredundant information. There is still one more important feature of learning: learning that combinations of cues predict the US reinforcement and generating an appropriate conditioned response. With one more small variation, this can be achieved.

Figure 5.14 shows a **predictive autoencoder.**[23] This is an autoencoder with one or more additional output nodes trained to predict the reinforcement. Remember that reinforcement is itself just another kind of stimulus. An airpuff US, for example, is felt as a somatosensory (touch) stimulation on the sensitive cornea; a footshock US activates pain receptors in the foot; and so on. Thus, if a tone CS reliably predicts an airpuff US, this really means that the airpuff US is a stimulus that normally occurs in the presence of the tone stimulus. In effect, tone and airpuff are elements of a single pattern that the network should learn to reproduce.

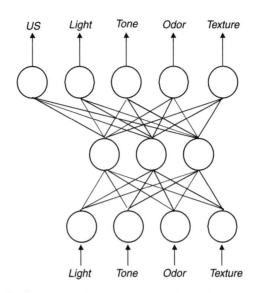

Figure 5.14   A predictive autoencoder is an autoencoder with outputs that reconstruct the inputs *and* predict whether reinforcement (e.g., a US) will occur, given the current inputs. Here, inputs and outputs are labeled to represent four possible sensory stimuli.

For example, suppose that the network is presented with a discrimination paradigm in which one CS (light) predicts the US but the other (tone) does not. The network has one input node corresponding to each possible CS; there are additional input nodes that correspond to the background contextual features (figure 5.15A). For simplicity, the sights, smells, textures, and sounds of the current experimental context are grouped together as context X and represented by a single input node; the sights, smells, textures, and sounds of another experimental chamber might constitute context Y. The network is trained, via error backpropagation, to reconstruct its inputs (whatever CSs and contextual cues are present) and to predict the US on the basis of those inputs.

Initially, presentation of the light in context X will evoke some (random) pattern of activity in the internal-layer nodes (figure 5.15A); presentation of the tone in context X will evoke a different, possibly overlapping representation (figure 5.15B). Presentation of context X alone evokes yet a third representation (figure 5.15C). To master this simple task, the network must adjust the upper-layer weights so that when the internal-layer representation of light is activated, the output nodes corresponding to light, context X, and US are also activated as shown in figure 5.16A. Conversely, when the tone representation is activated, the output nodes for tone and context X—but not

Internal-Layer Representations in the Predictive Autoencoder

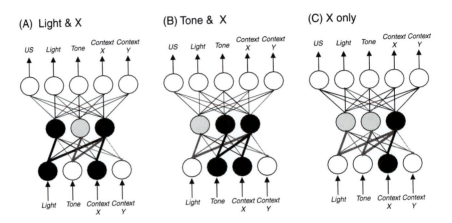

Figure 5.15 Representations in the predictive autoencoder. (A) Presentation of the light in context X activates one pattern of activity in the internal-layer nodes. (B) Presentation of the *tone* in context X activates a second pattern, and (C) presentation of the context X alone—with no explicit CS—generates a third pattern.

Mapping to Outputs in the Predictive Autoencoder

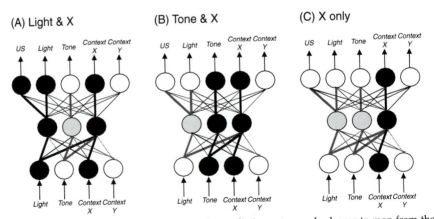

Figure 5.16 The upper layer of weights in the predictive autoencoder learns to map from the internal-layer representations to the correct output. (A) The representation evoked by the light-X input should strongly activate output nodes for light, context X, and the US. (B) The representation evoked by the tone-X input should strongly activate output nodes for tone, context X, and not the US. (C) The representation evoked by the context X alone should strongly activate the output node for X but for no other stimuli.

US—should be activated as seen in figure 5.16B. And, of course, when context X is active but neither light nor tone is present, only the output node for context X should be active, as shown in figure 5.16C.

However, error backpropagation also adjusts the lower-layer weights as well, striving to find a more efficient internal-layer representation. In the case of the current example, the internal-layer representations for light and tone overlap considerably: Both strongly activate the rightmost internal-layer node. Another way of seeing this overlap is shown in figure 5.17A: Light strongly activates the leftmost and rightmost internal-layer nodes, while tone strongly activates the center and rightmost internal-layer nodes. Since light and tone are not redundant (they never co-occur in this example), and

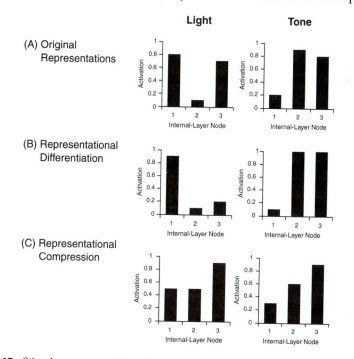

Figure 5.17 Stimulus representations from figure 5.16, encoded as the activity level evoked over a series of nodes. (A) The light stimulus evokes one pattern of internal-layer node activity (strongly activating the leftmost and rightmost nodes), while the tone stimulus activates a different pattern (strongly activating the center and rightmost nodes). (B) If the light and the tone never co-occur, and if they make different predictions about the US, then the autoencoder tends to differentiate their representations, decreasing the overlap. Now, light activates only the leftmost node, and tone activates the other two nodes. In mathematical terms, the difference in representations has increased from D(light, tone) = 1.5 in (A) to D(light, tone) = 2.5 in (B). (C) Conversely, if the light and the tone co-occur and make similar predictions about subsequent US arrival, their representations are compressed or made more similar. Here, D(light, tone) has decreased to only 0.3.

since they make maximally different predictions about the US (light predicts the US, and tone does not), it would be more efficient to **differentiate** their representations. Backpropagation tends to do just this. After many trials pairing light-US and tone-noUS, representations may evolve that are more like those shown in figure 5.17B. Now, there is less overlap, and each internal-layer node is strongly activated by only one cue.

This decreased overlap can be described by subtracting the response of each node to one cue from its own response to the other cues. For example, in figure 5.17A, internal-layer node 1 responds at a rate of 0.8 to light and 0.2 to tone, for a difference of 0.6. The differences in responding to the two cues for the other two nodes are $(0.9 - 0.1) = 0.8$ and $(0.7 - 0.8) = -0.1$. Because we are interested only in the magnitude of the difference, we drop any minus signs, so the differences across the three internal-layer nodes are 0.6, 0.8, and 0.1. Summed across all internal-layer nodes, the difference D in representation of light and tone can be calculated as D(light, tone) $= 0.6 + 0.8 + 0.1 = 1.5$. If the representations are differentiated, as shown in figure 5.17B, D(light, tone) rises to 2.5.

While these representational changes are occurring in the lower layer of weights, the upper layer is learning to generate the desired output: reconstructing the inputs and predicting US arrival. Figure 5.18A shows the activation of the network's US-predicting output node on light and tone trials, as a function of training. Initially, responses to both stimuli are low. For about fifty training trials, there is no difference in the response to light and the response to tone. Then the node begins to respond more strongly to light than to tone; by trial 200, the node gives a near-maximal response to light and almost no response to tone. Meanwhile, the internal-layer representation is changing; figure 5.18B shows how D(light, tone) slowly increases. Initially, there is little difference between the representations of the two CSs, and for the first fifty trials, the network appears to flounder and D(light, tone) actually decreases a bit. At about trial 50, D(light, tone) begins to increase. It is at this point that the network has developed representations that distinguish light and tone: Representational differentiation is occurring. Thereafter, the representations continue to differentiate further until the problem is well learned. Note that only after the representations of light and tone begin to be differentiated (around trial 50) does there begin to be differentiation of responses to light and tone in the output layer (compare figure 5.18A).

The predictive autoencoder doesn't only differentiate representations of stimuli that make different predictions about the US; like the standard autoencoder, it also compresses the representations of redundant (co-occurring) stimuli. Suppose that, instead of a light-versus-tone discrimination, the network is trained that light and tone co-occur and both make the same prediction about US arrival (either a prediction that the US will arrive

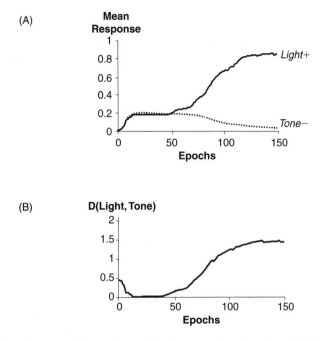

Discrimination Learning in the Predictive Autoencoder

Figure 5.18 Representational differentiation in the predictive autoencoder, trained on light+ and tone−. (A) The activation of the network's US-predicting output node. After about five trials of training, the network begins to predict the US on light+ trials but not on tone− trials. By about trial 150, the responses are strongly differentiated. (B) The differentiation of internal-layer representations, encoded as D(light, tone). Early in training, there is little difference in representations. At about trial 50, the internal-layer representations begin to differentiate the two stimuli, and D(light, tone) rises. Thereafter, the representations become increasingly differentiated. Note that the differentiation in representations in (B) slightly precedes the differentiated responding in (A).

or a prediction that it will not). In this case, the original representations shown in figure 5.17A become more similar, as shown in figure 5.17C. Each internal-layer node comes to respond similarly to light and tone, and this similarity can be quantified by noting the difference D(light, tone) falls from its original value of 1.5 (in figure 5.17A) to only 0.3 (in figure 5.17C).

It is important to note that the degree of compression in a predictive autoencoder does not depend solely on the number of internal-layer nodes. Even with a very large number of internal-layer nodes—enough to devote one internal-layer node to encode every input and output feature—the network still tends to compress the representations of co-occurring inputs (see MathBox 5.1 for further details). This feature of predictive autoencoders has

MathBox 5.1   Hidden Layer Size and Compression

The predictive autoencoder shown in figure 5.16 has an internal layer that contains fewer nodes than either the input layer or the output layer. Thus, if the network is to reconstruct the input, it is forced to compress redundancies in the internal layer, to ensure that nonredundant information makes it through to the output layer. However, even if the number of internal-layer nodes is varied, the same principles of representational compression and differentiation hold.

This is easily shown by example. Suppose that an autoencoder has seven inputs, representing three CSs (A, B, and C) and four contextual cues. The network has eight output nodes, reconstructing the seven inputs and also predicting the US. The network is trained that the stimulus compound AB+ predicts the US but stimulus C− does not.

If the autoencoder has only two internal-layer nodes, then it is necessary to compress the representations of A and B to solve the problem. Then, one internal-layer node can become active when AB is present, and it can activate the output nodes for A, B, and the US; another internal-layer node can become active when C is present and activate the output node for C; when neither internal-layer node is active, only the context output nodes should be active. Thus, as shown in figure A (top), $D(A, B)$ is very low—approximately 0—reflecting compression of the representations of A and B, while $D(A, C)$ and $D(B, C)$ rise, reflecting differentiation of the representation of C from the other two CSs. Within about 2000 training blocks, the network learns to give the correct US prediction to both AB+ and C− (figure A (bottom)).

Two internal-layer nodes is the minimum number with which the predictive autoencoder can solve the problem. If the number of internal-layer nodes is doubled, to four, the network can learn the original problem rather more quickly: Only about 1000 training trials are needed to learn AB+ versus C− (figure B (bottom)). However, the pattern of representational changes is largely the same as it was for the two-node case: Representations of A and B are compressed ($D(A, B)$ is low) while the representation of C is differentiated from A and B (figure B (top)).

As the number of internal-layer nodes is increased still further, to eight (figure C), there is yet more increase in learning speed, but the basic pattern of representational changes remains the same. Note that with eight internal-layer nodes, it would in principle be possible for the network to adopt a "local" representation, with one internal-layer node coding the presence or absence of each input and one coding the expectation of the US. In this case, once the representations are established, there would be little change in representations even when contingencies are switched: All the same information would be encoded in both phases. However, this is not what happens. The representation of stimuli is generally distributed among all the nodes in the network, independent of how many nodes there are.

If the number of internal-layer nodes is increased still further, to 32 (figure D), more than enough to encode all the information in the inputs, the representations still show the same qualitative pattern, compressing and differentiating representations on the basis of stimulus co-occurrence and meaning.

Thus, as long as there are a certain minimum number of internal-layer nodes, adding additional nodes may facilitate learning but may not cause a qualitative effect in the bias to compress and differentiate representations.

MathBox 5.1   (*Continued*)

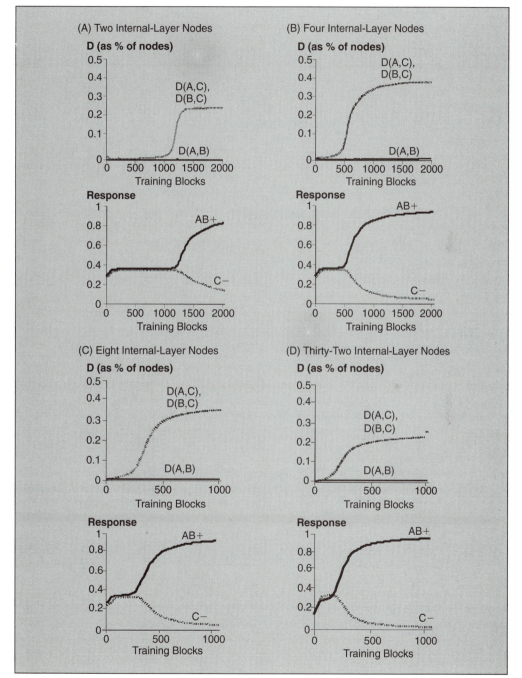

proven useful in many domains in which a neural network is used to pull out the important statistical regularities in a complex data set. (It is thus similar to, though not identical to, the mathematical technique of principal components analysis.[24])

In summary, *a predictive autoencoder forms new representations biased by two constraints: first, a bias to compress (make more similar) the representations of redundant (co-occurring) stimuli and, second, a bias to differentiate (make less similar) the representations of stimuli that make different predictions about the arrival of the US or other reinforcement.*

In the last several chapters, we have repeatedly used the sensory preconditioning paradigm as an example of how learning occurs from mere expo-

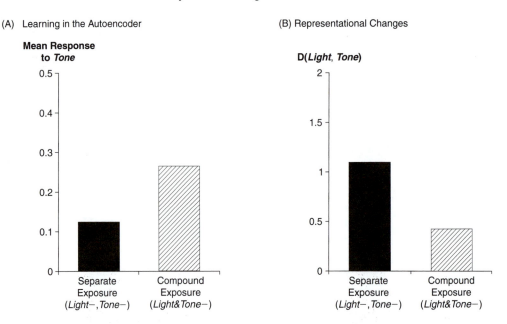

Figure 5.19 Sensory preconditioning in the predictive autoencoder. One group of simulations is given separate exposure to the light and tone stimuli, while the other group is given exposure to the light-and-tone compound. Next, all simulations are given light+ training, pairing the light stimulus and the US. Finally, the tone is presented alone, and the response of the network's US-predicting node is measured. (A) Prior exposure to the light-and-tone compound results in stronger responding to the tone alone than exposure to the light and the tone separately: the sensory preconditioning effect. (B) The representational changes in the autoencoder reflect greater compression (reflected in lower *D*(light, tone)) following compound than separate exposure.

sure to stimulus relationships. To review the paradigm: Unreinforced exposure to a stimulus compound (e.g., light and tone) increases the degree to which subsequent learning about one of the components (light) transfers to the other component (tone).

Animals with hippocampal-region damage do not show sensory preconditioning (refer to figure 2.18); nor does a simple feedforward network such as the ones discussed in chapters 3 and 4. However, a predictive autoencoder can demonstrate sensory preconditioning, as shown in figure 5.19. During phase 1 exposure, the light and the tone are presented together, and neither predicts US arrival; so their representations become compressed. As a result, phase 2 learning about light transfers strongly to tone—more strongly than in a control condition in which there was only separate exposure to the light and tone components in phase 1.

The next chapter will demonstrate that sensory preconditioning is only one of a range of hippocampal-dependent associative learning behaviors that can be demonstrated by a model incorporating a predictive autoencoder.

5.4   INTERIM SUMMARY: WHERE ARE WE NOW?

Chapters 3 through 5 have been largely tutorial, covering the basic principles of error-correction learning, representation, and autoassociation in neural networks. Chapters 6 through 10 will show how these principles can be applied to models of the hippocampus and how it interacts with other brain structures during associative learning.

Before moving on, it seems appropriate to take a few moments to review what has gone before.

Chapter 2 reviewed the kinds of memory impairments that result from hippocampal-region damage in humans and animals. In brief, hippocampal-region damage devastates declarative ("fact") memory but spares many forms of procedural learning. For example, simple CS-US association may be spared, but more complex conditioning involving multiple cues, temporal sensitivity, or latent learning (such as the sensory preconditioning procedure) tend to be disrupted. Electrophysiological studies that record neuronal activity suggest that the hippocampus is intimately involved in all new learning, even the simplest CS-US association, although it may not be necessary for that learning.

Chapter 3 introduced the Rescorla-Wagner model, a powerful model of associative learning from psychology that incorporates an error-correction rule from engineering: the Widrow-Hoff rule. This learning model assumes that there are modifiable weights between nodes representing CSs and USs and that stimuli compete with each other to predict the US. Thus, a CS that predicts the US only some of the time will gain less associative weight as compared to another, co-occurring CS that reliably predicts every occurrence of the US. The error-correction learning embodied in the Rescorla-Wagner model appears compatible with anatomical, neurophysiological, and behavioral data regarding cerebellar circuits. Thus, it is possible that the cerebellum is a circuit-level instantiation of the error-correcting principle of the Rescorla-Wagner model; it is able, on its own, to show just those behaviors accounted for by the model but requiring other brain regions to show more complex behaviors. While the Rescorla-Wagner model can account for many conditioning phenomena, it cannot show configural learning (e.g., negative patterning). It also makes no provision for stimulus representations that encode superficial similarity or allow generalization between stimuli with similar meanings.

Chapter 4 introduced multilayer networks, able to form novel and complex stimulus representations at an internal layer of nodes. One powerful algorithm for training such networks is the error backpropagation algorithm. Multilayer networks can form internal-layer representations that encode arbitrary relationships between stimuli; they can also show configural learning. However, even with this modification, a standard error-correction network fails to show latent learning (e.g., sensory preconditioning). The problem is that error-correction networks learn on the basis of the difference (error) between the US and the network's prediction of the US (measured as the anticipatory conditioned response). In latent learning, in which there is no US, there is no prediction error and hence there is no learning. Interestingly, latent learning is disrupted by hippocampal-region damage.

Chapter 5 began by introducing the concept of an autoassociative network, which learns relationships between co-occurring stimuli. Several features of an autoassociative network—especially high interconnection between nodes—appear in hippocampal subfield CA3. This led many influential modelers to suggest that the hippocampus might operate as an autoassociator. Indeed, an autoassociator is capable of storing arbitrary patterns (memories) and later retrieving them when given partial cues, an ability that seems quite consonant with a hippocampal role in episodic memory. However, autoassociators do not learn explicit CS-US associations, nor are they capable of forming new stimulus representations. The predictive autoencoder is a network that combines some of the most powerful features of all the other networks: It can perform CS-US association and also learn CS-CS associations, and it has an internal node layer, in which new stimulus representations are constructed that compress redundancies while differentiating predictive information—two biases that optimize generalization between stimuli. A predictive autoencoder is capable of latent learning.

Having worked through this material, we are now ready, in the next chapter, to show how such a predictive autoencoder model of the hippocampal region can be used to address a large body of empirical data on the role of the hippocampal-region in associative learning.

II Modeling Memory

6 Cortico-Hippocampal Interaction in Associative Learning

Chapter 4 argued that computational models of learning need to incorporate **stimulus representations** to allow appropriate generalization of learning between stimuli. The appropriate degree of generalization will depend on the particular problem, implying that representations should be adaptable to suit current task demands. However, the computational resources required to create appropriate new stimulus representations on the fly are considerable; neural-network researchers have addressed this problem by developing the error backpropagation algorithm described in chapter 4.

However, it is not clear that the sophisticated neural machinery needed to create the necessary new stimulus representations exists throughout the brain. One possible evolutionary alternative would be to localize some of the mechanisms for representational change in a central location (such as the hippocampus) so that other brain regions (such as cerebral cortex and cerebellum) could make use of these mechanisms as needed for particular tasks. This idea forms the basis for the two models of hippocampal function to be discussed in this chapter.

In both of these models, one network module representing the hippocampal region interacts with other network modules representing other brain regions, as in Marr's model (figure 5.9). *Hippocampal-region damage in these network models is simulated by disabling the hippocampal-region module and observing the behavior of the remaining modules.* These models can implement many aspects of associative learning, particularly classical conditioning, and they are useful for understanding how the hippocampal region may interact with the rest of the brain to facilitate certain kinds of learning.

The first model that we review, called the **cortico-hippocampal model,** is one that we ourselves originally developed to account for the effects of hippocampal-region damage on classical conditioning.[1] The basic idea of this model is that the hippocampal region is simulated as a predictive autoencoder that forms new internal-layer representations to compress redundant information while differentiating predictive information. These adaptive representations are then adopted by long-term storage areas in the cortex and cerebellum.

The second model, called the **Schmajuk-DiCarlo model (or S-D model)** after its originators, takes a very different view of the hippocampal region. It presumes that the hippocampal region is necessary for the kinds of error-correction embodied in the Rescorla-Wagner model. Section 6.2 describes this model and its predictions, with a special emphasis on where it makes predictions that are similar to or divergent from those of our own cortico-hippocampal model.

In addition to these two computational models, there have been many qualitative, or noncomputational, theories of hippocampal-region function that seek to address many of the same behavioral phenomena. Section 6.3 reviews several prominent qualitative theories and shows how they relate to the computational models in sections 6.1 and 6.2.

Finally, section 6.4 describes one avenue of cognitive neuroscience research that has evolved out of the modeling work. As predicted by our cortico-hippocampal model, under some special conditions, individuals with medial temporal lobe (hippocampal-region) damage can actually learn simple associations faster than normal control subjects.

6.1   THE HIPPOCAMPAL REGION AND ADAPTIVE REPRESENTATIONS

Saul Steinberg created a famous cover for the *New Yorker* magazine, caricaturing his view of a typical New Yorker's mental map of the world. Manhattan was drawn in such fine detail that it took up most of the map. The rest of the country, the area between New Jersey and California, was squashed into a small area on the map, marked only by a farm silo and a few scattered rocks.

This painting satirizes many New Yorkers' belief that they are living in the most important place in the world. But it also illustrates an important psychological point. Fine distinctions that are meaningful to New Yorkers, such as the differences between Ninth and Tenth Avenues, are emphasized and highly differentiated in this mental map; these places are physically pulled apart and separated from surrounding areas. Broader distinctions that are irrelevant to the New Yorker, such as the difference between Kansas and Nebraska, are deemphasized or compressed and given less space in the map.

To some extent, we all create similar idiosyncratic worldviews with distorted representations; distinctions that are important to us are enhanced while less relevant ones are deemphasized. For example, students who are asked to sketch a map of the world tend to draw their home region disproportionately large and in the center of the map.[2] Figure 6.1 is such a map drawn by a student from Illinois, who overemphasized Illinois relative

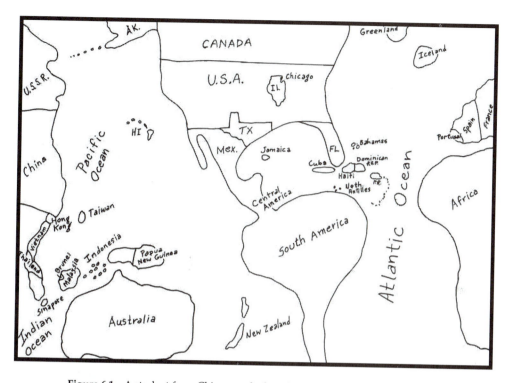

Figure 6.1 A student from Chicago, asked to sketch a map of the world, drew his home state disproportionately large while omitting most of the other states. North America was also disproportionately large in relation to the other continents. (Reproduced from Solso, 1991, Figure 10.11A, p. 289.)

to the rest of the country, omitted most states altogether, and enlarged North America relative to the other continents. Many American students show a similar pattern. In contrast, European students tend to draw Eurocentric maps, while students from Australia often place Australia and Asia in the center.

This kind of representational distortion, although somewhat comic in its egocentricity, is actually very useful. Memory is a limited resource, and individuals need to allocate that resource preferentially to items that are important to them. Thus, an experienced musician may actually devote more area of his brain to the fine control of finger movements than an average person would, while someone who has lost a hand through amputation will show shrinkage of the brain areas associated with finger movement. Chapter 8 will discuss these topics in more detail. For now, though, the chief question is: How can such representational changes come about? Who decides what kind of information is important enough to merit extra space and what is irrelevant enough to be shrunk like the Midwest on Steinberg's map?

Several years ago, we proposed a theory of hippocampal function in associative learning in which we argued that the hippocampal region is presumed to operate as an information gateway during the learning process.[3] Our theory assumes that the hippocampal region selects what information is allowed to enter storage and how it is to be encoded by other brain regions. Specifically, the theory argues that *the representation of redundant or unimportant information is shrunk, or* **compressed,** *while the representation of usefully predictive or otherwise meaningful information is elaborated, or* **differentiated.** According to this theory, the hippocampal region is critical for forming the kind of idiosyncratic maps of the world shown in figure 6.1. It turns out that this theory accounts for a range of behavioral data on representational processing with and without the hippocampus.

The Cortico-Hippocampal Model

Our theory assumes that the hippocampal region monitors statistical regularities in the environment and forms new stimulus representations that reflect these regularities. Specifically, *if two stimuli co-occur or make similar predictions about future reinforcement, their representations will be compressed to increase generalization between the stimuli. Conversely, if two stimuli never co-occur, and if they make different predictions about future reinforcement, their representations will be differentiated to decrease generalization between the stimuli.* The idea that the hippocampus can compress redundant information while differentiating predictive information is also consistent with the anatomy and physiology of the hippocampal region, as other researchers, such as William Levy, have noted previously.[4]

As described in chapter 5, a predictive autoencoder is capable of just this kind of function, compressing and differentiating representations in its internal layer. For this reason, our theory models the hippocampal-region network as a predictive autoencoder, mapping from stimulus inputs, through an internal layer, to outputs that reconstruct those inputs and also predict future reinforcement.

However, the hippocampal region is not the final site of memory storage, as is evidenced by myriad empirical data showing that old, well-established memories can survive hippocampal-region damage. Accordingly, *our model assumes that the representations developed in the hippocampal region are eventually adopted by other long-term storage sites in cortex and cerebellum.* Back in chapter 3, we noted that the cerebellar substrates of classical eyeblink conditioning are well characterized, and therefore we initially chose to apply our theory to this behavioral domain.

A modest elaboration of this cerebellar model introduced in chapter 3 is shown in figure 6.2A: Stimulus inputs (e.g., cues and context information) are processed by various primary cortical areas and then travel to the cerebellum via a structure called the pons. The cerebellum learns to map from these inputs to an output that drives a conditioned motor response. There is also an inhibitory feedback loop, through the inferior olive, that measures the error between the actual response (which is a prediction of unconditioned stimulus (US) arrival) and whether the US actually arrived. This allows the cerebellum to update connection strengths via an error-correcting procedure such as the Widrow-Hoff rule.

This simple cerebellar model does not make provision for any cortical learning, so we extended it into a hybrid cortico/cerebellar network as shown in figure 6.2B. Stimulus inputs (CSs and context information) are

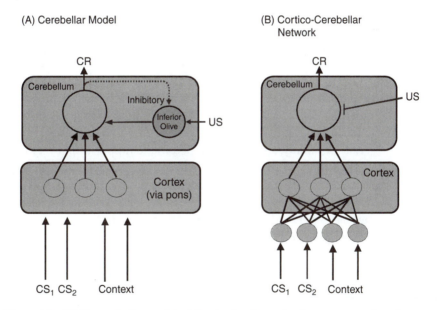

Figure 6.2   (A) The cerebellar model of chapter 3, redrawn to show preprocessing of sensory input by cortex; the cerebellum receives this input as well as direct CS information via a pathway through the pons. According to the model presented in chapter 3, the cerebellum learns to map from this input to a behavioral response (CR); the inferior olive computes the difference between US and CR and returns this error signal to guide learning in the cerebellum via the error-correcting Widrow-Hoff rule. (B) The same network, elaborated to allow an additional level of processing in the cortex. The upper layer of weights in this cortico/cerebellar network can still be trained by error correction to reduce the difference between CR and US; the lower layer of weights needs a training signal before it can use a second application of the error-correction rule.

provided as external input and activate an input node layer. Information travels through modifiable connections to an internal node layer representing cortical processing. In reality, of course, there might be an arbitrary number of successive cortical processing stages; for simplicity, we model only one.

The output of the cortical layer then travels to an output node representing the cerebellum, which integrates its sensory inputs and produces a conditioned response (CR). The difference between the CR and US is used as an error signal to drive learning in the upper layer of weights. The key question in multilayer network models—as discussed in chapter 4—is how one trains the lower layer of weights to alter internal-layer representations to facilitate learning.

This is where we believe that the hippocampal region plays a vital role. As shown in figure 6.3A, new representations formed in the hippocampal network's internal layer can serve as training signals for the cortico/cerebellar network's internal layer. In the simplest case, if each network has the same number of internal-layer nodes, the desired output for each internal-layer node in the cortico/cerebellar network is simply the actual output of the corresponding hippocampal-region network node.

Given this interpretation of the desired output for the cortico/cerebellar network's internal layer, the Widrow-Hoff error-correcting rule (from the Rescorla-Wagner model) can be used to train the lower layer of weights. Over many trials, the cortico/cerebellar network comes to adopt the same representations that were first developed in the hippocampal-region network.*

As figure 6.3B shows, hippocampal-region (HR) damage can be simulated by disabling the hippocampal-region network. In this case, *no new representations are acquired by the cortico/cerebellar network's internal layer. However, any previously acquired representations remain intact.* Thus, the cortico/cerebellar network can still learn new mappings from stimuli to responses based on its existing representations. For this reason, any new learning that does not require new representations (such as simply mapping one CS to a US) is likely to survive HR damage. However, any new learning that does depend

---

*If the total number of internal-layer nodes in the two networks is not equal, then the desired output for each cortico/cerebellar network internal-layer node may be some function of the activations of several nodes in the hippocampal-region network. The result is basically the same: The cortico/cerebellar network comes to adopt a linear transformation of the representations developed in the hippocampal-region network. This means that although there may be superficial differences in the two representations, they will show the same underlying logic: If the representations of two stimuli are compressed (or differentiated) in the hippocampal-region network, they will also be compressed (or differentiated) in the cortico/cerebellar network. See Gluck & Myers, 1993, for additional details.

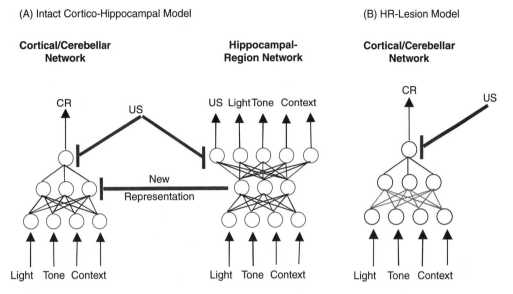

Figure 6.3   The cortico-hippocampal model. (A) The intact model receives inputs representing conditioned stimuli, such as lights and tones, as well as contextual information. One network, representing the processing that is dependent on the hippocampal region, learns to reconstruct these inputs and to predict the arrival of the unconditioned stimulus (US), such as a corneal air-puff. As it does, the hippocampal-region network forms new stimulus representations in its internal layer that compress redundant information and differentiate predictive information. A second network, assumed to represent long-term memory sites in cerebral and cerebellar cortices, adopts the internal representation provided by the hippocampal-region network and then maps from this to an output that represents the strength or probability of a conditioned response (CR), such as a protective eyeblink. (B) The HR-lesion model, in which the hippocampal-region network is disabled. The cortical network is no longer able to acquire new hippocampal-region-dependent internal representations, but it can still learn to map from existing representations to new behavioral responses.

on new representations (such as sensory preconditioning or configural learning) is expected by our model to be disrupted after HR damage. This distinction accounts for a great deal of data regarding HR-lesion effects, as we will describe below.

Representational Differentiation

As we noted earlier, the representations formed in the hippocampal-region network are subject to two biases: a bias to compress the representations of stimuli that are redundant and a bias to differentiate the representations of stimuli that predict different outcomes. Each of these biases can be used to explain data in intact and HR-lesioned animals. First, we give several examples of learning behaviors that appear to involve representational differentiation.

Acquisition.   The most rudimentary eyeblink conditioning task is **acquisition:** learning to respond to a cue that has been paired with the US. The Rescorla-Wagner model and the cerebellar model of figure 6.2 both capture this behavior, suggesting that the cerebellum alone should be sufficient to mediate conditioned acquisition—and hence learning should not be disrupted by HR lesion. Indeed, acquisition of a conditioned eyeblink response is not disrupted by HR lesion in humans (figure 6.4A), rabbits (figure 6.4B), or rats.[5]

Conditioned acquisition is simulated in the intact cortico-hippocampal model by presenting a series of training trials. First, the model is given trials consisting of just the experimental context—call it X—a series of inputs

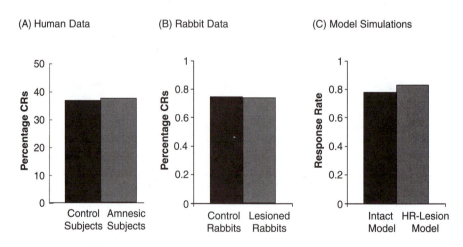

Figure 6.4 Conditioned acquisition, learning that a tone CS predicts an airpuff US, is not disrupted by hippocampal-region damage. (A) Humans with medial temporal lobe damage, including hippocampal-region damage, show normal eyeblink conditioning (Gabrieli et al., 1995). (B) Rabbits with hippocampal-region damage similarly acquire the conditioned eyeblink response as fast as control rabbits (Solomon & Moore, 1975). (C) Similarly, the intact cortico-hippocampal model and HR-lesion model learn at the same speed (Myers et al., 1996). For all graphs, response rate and percentage CRs represent proportion of trials generating CRs after a fixed number of CS-US pairings. (Adapted from Myers, Ermita, et al., 1996, Figure 4.)

Conditioned Acquisition: Model Simulations

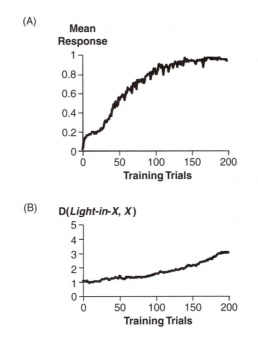

(A)

(B)

Figure 6.5 Conditioned acquisition in the intact cortico-hippocampal model. (A) Learning curve. (B) Representational differentiation of the light CS from the context X alone during training, reflected in increasing D(light-in-X, X).

meant to represent the background sights, smells, and sounds of the experimental setup; the model learns not to give a conditioned response to the context alone. These trials correspond to the time spent acclimating an animal to the experimental chamber, before any explicit training begins, a standard procedure in experimental studies of animal conditioning.

Next comes the actual acquisition training. Because the training takes place in context X, learning to respond to a light CS can be redefined as learning to respond to light-in-X but not to the context alone X−. With enough training, the model learns to respond when the light is present but not to the context alone, as is seen in figure 6.5A.* Figure 6.5B shows the corresponding changes in internal-layer representation in the cortico/cerebellar network, copied from the representations in the hippocampal-region network. The

---

*All figures that show performance of the cortico-hippocampal model are the average of ten simulation runs. Error bars on simulation data reflect variance among multiple simulation runs. Full details of the model presented in section 6.1 are given in Appendix 6.1 at the end of this chapter.

difference in representation between light-in-X and X alone—D(light-in-X, X), as defined in the previous chapter—grows gradually but consistently with increasing training. This representational differentiation facilitates the cortico/cerebellar network's task of mapping the two inputs to different responses.

However, this new differentiated representation is probably not necessary to acquire a conditioned response to a single light CS. The task is so simple that just about any random recoding in the lower layer of cortico/cerebellar network weights is probably sufficient. As long as there is at least one node in the internal layer that gives a different response to light-in-X and X alone, that node can be used to drive the presence or absence of a CR. In fact, the HR-lesioned model can learn the correct response about as quickly as the intact model (figure 6.4C). Thus, the cortico-hippocampal model correctly accounts for the finding that HR lesion does not impair acquisition of a simple CS-US association.

Discrimination and Reversal. Simple **discrimination** involves learning that one CS (light+) predicts the US while a second CS (tone−) does not. This means that conditioned responses should follow light+ but not tone−. In general, discrimination learning in the eyeblink-conditioning paradigm is not disrupted by hippocampal-region damage (figure 6.6A).[6] Similarly, hippocampal-region damage generally does not impair a range of discrimination tasks in animals, including discrimination of odors, objects, textures, and sounds.[7]

In the intact cortico-hippocampal model, the hippocampal-region network constructs new representations that differentiate light+ and tone−, facilitating the mapping of light+ to one response and tone− to another (figure 6.6C,D). However, the discrimination task is so simple that such representational changes are probably not necessary; any random initial representations in the cortico/cerebellar network are probably different enough to allow mapping to different responses. Thus, the HR-lesioned model should be able to learn a conditioned discrimination. As is shown in figure 6.6B, there is indeed no impairment: The HR-lesioned model reaches criterion performance just as quickly as the intact model.

These empirical data have often been interpreted as arguing that conditioned discrimination is hippocampal-independent. Our model offers a different interpretation: *The hippocampal-region may not be strictly necessary for some simple kinds of learning; but when it is present, it normally contributes to all learning.* Even in a simple task such as discrimination (or acquisition), where *a priori* representations probably suffice to allow learning, the hippocampal

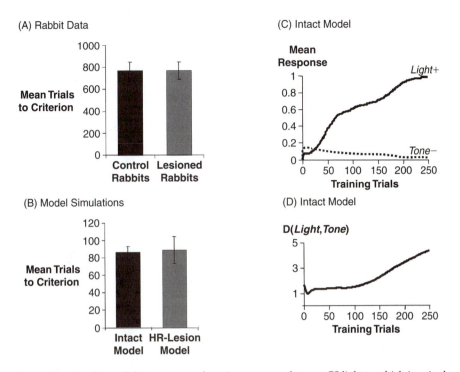

Figure 6.6 Conditioned discrimination: learning to respond to one CS light+, which is paired with the US, but not to CS tone−, which is not paired with the US. (A) Control rabbits learn this task in about 800 trials; rabbits with hippocampal-region lesion learn at the same speed (Berger & Orr, 1983). (B) The intact and HR-lesion cortico-hippocampal model likewise learn at the same speed. (C) In the intact model, there is an initial period when the model responds weakly but equally to both light+ and tone−; then the model begins to discriminate. (D) During learning, the representations of light and tone are differentiated, reflected in increasing D(light, tone).

region is constantly forming new stimulus representations that compress redundant information while differentiating predictive information, whether these new representations are needed or not.

However, the usefulness of this hippocampal participation becomes apparent if task demands change. For example, suppose the discrimination is reversed so that after learning to respond to light+ but not tone−, the contingencies are reversed, so tone+ now begins to predict the US and light− does not. In our intact model, the hippocampal-region network has already done the work of differentiating the representations of light and tone; once the contingencies reverse, all that needs to be done is to map those representations to new responses. In the lesioned model, the situation is quite different: The representations of light and tone are fixed, and so they are not differentiated during the original discrimination. Thus, the reversal

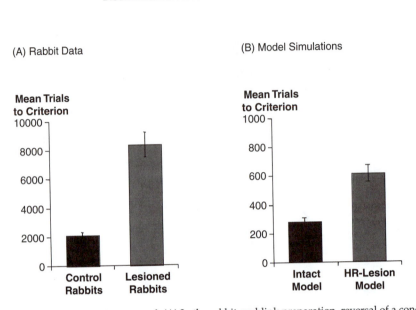

Figure 6.7   Discrimination reversal. (A) In the rabbit eyeblink preparation, reversal of a conditioned discrimination is strongly impaired in animals with hippocampal lesion. (Plotted from data presented in Berger & Orr, 1983.) (B) Similarly, the HR-lesion model is slower to reverse than the intact cortico-hippocampal model.

requires first unlearning the original discrimination and then learning the reversed discrimination. This process may be quite lengthy in comparison to reversal in the intact model (figure 6.7B). In rabbit eyeblink conditioning, several studies show that hippocampal-region damage disrupts discrimination reversal (figure 6.7A).[8]

Other Behaviors Involving Predictive Differentiation.   Our cortico-hippocampal model also predicts that many other paradigms that involve representational differentiation will be disrupted after HR lesion.[9] These tasks include **easy-hard transfer** (the finding that learning a hard discrimination is facilitated by prior training on an easier version of the task), the **overtraining reversal effect** (the finding that reversal is speeded if the original discrimination is trained for many days beyond criterion performance), and **nonmonotonic development of the stimulus generalization gradient** (the finding that learning about one stimulus early in training generalizes strongly to other stimuli, while generalization is reduced when similar learning takes place later in training).

These are novel predictions: no data currently exist documenting the behavior of HR-lesioned animals on these tasks. However, experiments in our lab at Rutgers-Newark are under way to test some of these predictions. The results of such experiments will provide a critical test of the model, either confirming its predictions or showing that the model requires revision.

Representational Compression

Just as the hippocampal region is assumed to differentiate the representations of stimuli that should be mapped to different responses, the hippocampal region is assumed to compress the representations of stimuli that co-occur and should be mapped to similar responses. Behaviors that reflect representational compression should be disrupted after hippocampal-region damage.

Sensory Preconditioning.   One simple example is **sensory preconditioning,** which was discussed in several earlier chapters. Recall that sensory preconditioning involves unreinforced exposure to a compound of two stimuli (tone&light− exposure), followed by light-US pairings (light+ training). The associations learned to the light should partially transfer to tone, as a result of the paired exposure. Hippocampal-region damage (specifically fimbrial lesion) abolishes sensory preconditioning in the rabbit eyeblink preparation, as shown in figure 6.8A.*[10] Because the predictive autoencoder in chapter 5 was sufficient to mediate this effect (refer to figure 5.19), it should come as no surprise that our intact cortico-hippocampal model shows the same effect (figure 6.8B).[11] In the intact model, tone&light− exposure results in compression of the representations of tone and light, since both stimuli co-occur and neither predicts the US or any other salient event. Subsequent associations to light partially activate the representation of tone, and the learning transfers. In the lesioned model, there are no representational changes during the exposure phase, and as long as light and tone are distinct stimuli that activate different (fixed) representations, there is little chance that associations made to light will transfer to tone.

---

*Fimbrial lesion does not involve removal of the hippocampus but instead cuts an important input and output pathway by which subcortical structures communicate with the hippocampus. As such, the effects of fimbrial lesion may not be identical to hippocampal lesion. The implications of damage or disruption to this pathway will be further discussed in chapter 9.

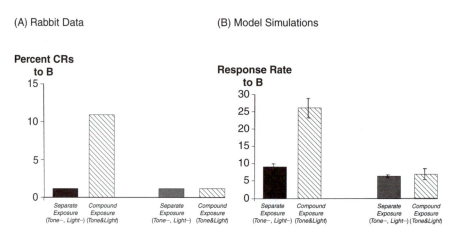

Figure 6.8 Sensory preconditioning. (A) In rabbit eyeblink conditioning, phase 1 exposure to the compound tone&light−, followed by light+ training, results in stronger phase 3 responding to tone than in animals that are given separate exposure to the components (tone−, light−) in phase 1; this effect is eliminated in animals with damage to the hippocampal region (fornix lesion). (Adapted from data presented in Port and Patterson, 1984.) (B) Similarly, the intact but not HR-lesioned cortico-hippocampal model shows sensory preconditioning.

Learned Irrelevance. Another behavior involving representational compression is **learned irrelevance.**[12] The paradigm is schematized in table 6.1. In phase 1, subjects in the exposed group are given presentations of a CS (e.g., light) and a US, uncorrelated with each other. Subjects in the nonexposed group are given equivalent time in the experimental context but receive no presentations of light or the US. In phase 2, all subjects receive light-US pairings. As shown in figure 6.9A, subjects in the exposed group are much slower to learn the light-US association.

In the intact cortico-hippocampal model, phase 1 exposure to a CS (e.g., light) and a US causes representational changes. The representation of the light becomes compressed, together with the representations of the background contextual cues, since neither predicts the US well. In effect, the light is treated as a sometimes-occurring aspect of the context, one that is of no use in predicting US arrival. This representational compression of light and context will hinder phase 2 learning to respond to the light but not the context alone. Thus, as shown in figure 6.9B, there is a learned irrelevance effect in the intact cortico-hippocampal model. Since learned irrelevance is interpreted in terms of representational compression, it is not shown in the HR-lesion model (figure 6.10B).

Table 6.1   The Learned Irrelevance Paradigm

Group	Phase 1	Phase 2
CS/US exposure	Light and airpuff (uncorrelated)	Light → airpuff . . . . *SLOW!*
Sit exposure	(Animal sits in experimental chamber)	Light → airpuff . . . . *normal speed*

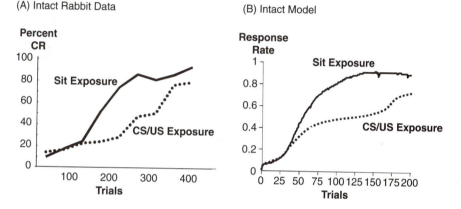

(A) Intact Rabbit Data

(B) Intact Model

Figure 6.9   Learned irrelevance. Both intact rabbits (A) and the intact cortico-hippocampal model (B) show slower learning of a CS-US association following exposure to the CS and US uncorrelated with each other. (A is drawn from data presented in Allen, Chelius, & Gluck, 1998.)

At the time we first published this prediction, it was a novel implication of the cortico-hippocampal model. Since then, we have shown in our lab that learned irrelevance is severely disrupted by HR lesion in the rabbit eyeblink-conditioning preparation (figure 6.10A).[13] These results provide further evidence that the representational compression contributing to learned irrelevance depends on the hippocampal region. Our empirical data further demonstrate that the exact lesion extent is critical in determining whether or not learned irrelevance is disrupted, suggesting that different hippocampal-region structures contribute differently to the effect. We will return to this issue, and the actual empirical data, in chapter 9.

Our cortico-hippocampal model predicts that other behaviors that reflect representational compression will also be disrupted by HR lesion. These include **latent inhibition** and **contextual effects,** which will be discussed more fully in chapter 7. Some of these predictions have also been confirmed by recent experimental studies.

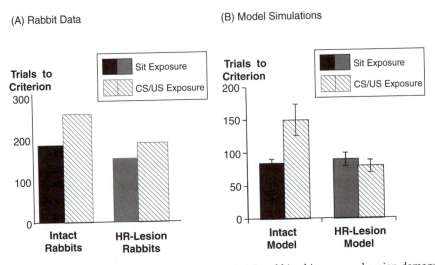

(A) Rabbit Data   (B) Model Simulations

Figure 6.10   Learned irrelevance and HR-lesion. (A) In rabbits, hippocampal-region damage (specifically, entorhinal lesion that also cuts off the major information pathways into and out of hippocampus) eliminates learned irrelevance: Animals that are given prior exposure to the CS and US uncorrelated learn at about the same rate as animals that are given exposure to the context only (Sit Exposure). (B) Likewise, the HR-lesion model does not show learned irrelevance. (A is drawn from data presented in Allen, Chelius, & Gluck, 1998.)

Limitations of the Cortico-Hippocampal Model

Although our cortico-hippocampal model accounts for a considerable range of data on intact and hippocampal-lesioned animals, there are several effects that it does not address. The model is specifically limited to model classical conditioning. This limited domain was chosen specifically because it is possible to construct a model of the cerebellar substrates of eyeblink conditioning with some assurance that the model accurately reflects the brain substrates. However, this approach means that the model does not apply easily to other domains. Recently, we have shown that the model can be extended to address **instrumental conditioning,** a form of learning in which reinforcement is contingent on the subject's response, and **category learning,** in which people learn to classify objects into predefined classes.[14] However, there are other domains that lie well outside the model's ability; these include spatial learning, declarative memory, and delayed nonmatch to sample (DNMS), three behaviors that were mentioned in chapter 2 as important areas of research into hippocampal function. These are limitations of the current computational model but not necessarily of the basic underlying theory. An important direction for future research will be to see how well the fundamental information-processing principles of representational compression and differentiation can account for hippocampal function in more complex behaviors such as spatial learning and recognition learning.

Extinction.   There are, however, phenomena within the model's domain of classical conditioning for which the model fails to accurately account for all relevant empirical data. One example is **extinction.** After learning a response to one CS (light+ training), if an animal is given CS-alone trials (light− training), the conditioned response gradually weakens, or extinguishes. Extinction is problematic as a psychological phenomenon because there is considerable evidence that the process is more complicated than simply undoing a CS-US association; instead, subjects appear to learn a CS-noUS association that competes with the earlier CS-US association.[15] The idea that the earlier CS-US association is not destroyed, but merely suppressed, is consistent with the finding that an extinguished association can be reacquired more quickly than it was originally acquired.[16]

The cortico-hippocampal model does not contain any explicit mechanism for the simultaneous maintenance of CS-US and CS-noUS associations. During extinction, all that occurs is that the mapping between the representation of CS and the US is replaced by a mapping to noUS. No representational changes are involved, and so extinction occurs at the same speed in the intact and lesioned models (figure 6.11B). This behavior is superficially correct—hippocampal-region damage does not affect extinction in animals (figure 6.11A)[17]—but is nonetheless an oversimplification. Extinction also occurs much more quickly in the model than in experimental subjects.

To account for these data, additional mechanisms would have to be postulated in the model to account for all these aspects of extinction. At the present time, sufficient controversy surrounds the true nature of extinction that it seems premature to try to add such a mechanism to the model. However, it would be a fruitful exercise to try to implement some of the possible mechanisms in a model of extinction and see which accounts for the greatest array of empirical data. It has been suggested that extinction does not erase CS-US learning but, rather, makes this learning more sensitive to context.[18] Thus, the correct response in the old context was to produce a CR, but in the new context, no CR should occur. We will return to contextual issues in chapter 7.

Timing Effects.   A second major class of data for which our original cortico-hippocampal model does not account is stimulus interval effects such as **trace conditioning.** Trace conditioning is defined by introducing a short interval between CS offset and US onset (refer to figure 2.17). Trace

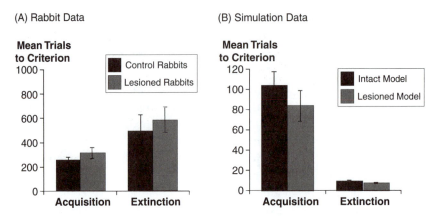

Figure 6.11   Acquisition and extinction. (A) In the rabbit eyeblink preparation, extinction of a trained response is not significantly slowed by hippocampal-region damage. In both cases, extinction typically takes longer than acquisition of the original response. (Plotted from data presented in Berger & Orr, 1983.) (B) In the cortico-hippocampal model, extinction is not slowed in the HR-lesion model; however, in contrast to the animal data, both intact and HR-lesioned models show extremely rapid extinction. The model probably does not adequately capture the complexities of extinction in animals.

conditioning is disrupted by hippocampal-region damage—if the trace interval is long enough.[19] The version of the cortico-hippocampal model described here does not incorporate temporal information such as the number of milliseconds between CS and US onset. Therefore, it cannot directly model stimulus interval effects. Recently, we have developed a generalized version of our model that includes recurrent connections within the network, thereby allowing it to demonstrate some aspects of temporal and sequential processing, including trace conditioning.[20]

However, introducing temporal information into the cortico-hippocampal model does not solve a more fundamental problem. The cortico-hippocampal model assumes that the hippocampal region is critical when new stimulus representations are required that involve redundancy compression or predictive differentiation. There is no obvious way to relate this assumption to the finding of a hippocampal role in trace conditioning; trace conditioning does not seem to require new stimulus representations—only the formation of an association between CS and US. Thus, our theory does not provide a good understanding of why trace conditioning should depend on the hippocampal region. At present, the best that can be done is to note that the model does not rule out additional possible hippocampal-region functions such as a role in short-term memory that might help to maintain a representation of the CS during a trace interval. Interestingly, trace conditioning is not universally reported to depend on the hippocampal region.[21] One possible reason for this discrepancy between studies is variance in exact lesion extent;[22] this would be consistent with a suggestion that different hippocampal-region subareas perform different functions and that some are more involved in trace conditioning than others.

Many other computational models do address a role for the hippocampus in timing (including trace conditioning).[23] Future work remains to determine whether a single model can capture both the representational and temporal aspects of hippocampal-region function (and also spatial learning, DNMS, and episodic memory).

Neurophysiological Support for the Cortico-Hippocampal Model

If the hippocampal region does adapt stimulus representations to minimize redundancy while preserving predictive information, it should be possible to observe the results of this process via neurophysiological recordings of cell firing in the hippocampal region. It is now possible to simultaneously record the activation of dozens of neurons within a small area of brain. The set of firing activity across a set of neurons is a pattern analogous to the activities across a set of nodes in a network model and can be viewed as the brain's representation of the current inputs. The difference between the brain's representation of one input A as a pattern of neuronal firing and a second input B can be quantified by using a $D(A, B)$ metric just like that defined for the network model. Thus, it is possible to measure $D(A, B)$ in a specific region of the brain both before and after training and then calculate whether the neural representations have become more or less similar. This approach has obvious limitations: It is possible to simultaneously record only a small sample of the vast number of neurons in any brain region, and—as with any sampling method—it is possible that the small sample may not accurately reflect the larger population. However, if the predicted changes in $D(A, B)$ are visible among even a small sample of neurons, it is a reasonable inference that similar changes occur throughout the population.

By using this method, it is possible to observe changes in hippocampal firing patterns as a result of learning. For example, during rabbit eyeblink conditioning, some neurons in the hippocampus that do not respond strongly to a CS will gradually increase responding to that CS if it is repeatedly paired with a US.[24] In a discrimination task, some neurons will respond to the CS (light+) but not to the CS (tone−).[25] Averaged over many neurons, these changes will result in increased $D(\text{light}, \text{tone})$ much like that shown in figure 6.6D. Importantly, these changes in hippocampal neuronal activity *precede* the development of the behavioral CR,[26] just as representational changes precede development of the response in the predictive autoencoder of our hippocampal model (refer to figure 5.18).

Rabbits are not the only animals to show these kinds of changes predicted by our cortico–hippocampal model. In one experiment, monkeys were trained on a visual discrimination, in which they had to make an arm movement when they saw one stimulus A+ but not when they saw a second stimulus B−. Figure 6.12A shows how a single neuron in the hippocampus responded during this task.[27] Initially (trials 1 through 20), there is a similar response to both stimuli A and B. With further training, these neurons begin to become more active when stimulus A was presented than when stimulus B was presented. These changes preceded the behavioral evidence of learning, evidenced by correct arm movements. Of all the hippocampal neurons

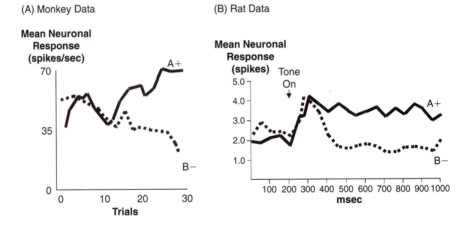

Figure 6.12 Representational changes during discrimination learning. Neurophysiological recordings of neuronal activity suggest representational differentiation during learning. (A) Recordings from monkey hippocampus during learning to make a motor response to one stimulus (A+) but not a second (B−). Initially (trials 1–10), there is little difference in responding to the two stimuli; with further training (trials 20–30), there is significantly greater neuronal activity to the rewarded stimulus A+. (Adapted from Cahusec et al., 1993, Figure 2.) (B) Recordings from rat dentate gyrus during training to respond to tone A+ but not tone B−. The graph shows the pattern of responding on a single presentation of the tones, averaged across several trials, in an animal that had learned the appropriate responses. When either tone comes on (200 msec into the trial), there is initially a response. However, only for the rewarded stimulus A+ is this response maintained for the duration of the trial. (Adapted from Deadwyler, West, & Lynch, 1979, Figure 4.)

that showed task-related activity, about 22% altered their activity patterns to discriminate the two stimuli; most of these maintained these new response patterns across the experiment. However, many did not maintain their new activity patterns once the behavior was fully acquired. As the authors of this study note, this would be consistent with the idea that the hippocampus has a limited capacity for pattern storage, and at some point, old learning is transferred elsewhere (e.g., cortex) and new learning overwrites the old in hippocampus.[28]

In another study, Deadwyler and colleagues recorded neuronal activity in the dentate gyrus of rats that were being trained to make a motor response to one tone A and not to another tone B.[29] Initially, neuronal activity (in the form of extracellular unit discharge patterns) looked similar after presentation of either tone. By the time the conditioned response had been acquired, neuronal discharge in the dentate gyrus differentiated the two stimuli; specifically, neurons might respond to both stimuli, but only the rewarded stimulus (A) elicited sustained activity (figure 6.12B). Although these tone-evoked responses occur slightly before the initiation of the behavioral response, Deadwyler et al. argue that the dentate activity is probably not directly related to the production of a motor movement. Instead, the dentate gyrus may contribute to learning which of two or more competing responses is appropriate to a given stimulus and may encode information about expected reward by means of differential discharge patterns. A related study has also shown that hippocampal cells in the rat that encode place information change as a result of learning, differentiating the representations of landmarks.[30]

Taken together, *the neurophysiological evidence currently available is remarkably consistent with the implications of our cortico-hippocampal model, suggesting that hippocampal neuronal representations can and do change to reflect associations between stimuli and rewards.* The results do not prove that the hippocampus itself creates these representational changes; it is possible that another brain region develops appropriate representations and merely passes this information to hippocampus. However, these neurophysiological findings are clearly consistent with the idea that the hippocampus creates new stimulus representations, much like the internal-layer nodes in a predictive autoencoder.

6.2 SCHMAJUK AND DICARLO (S-D) MODEL

Nestor Schmajuk and his colleagues have presented in several papers an evolving series of computational models of cortico-hippocampal interaction in conditioned learning.[31] These models are similar in spirit and aim to our cortico-hippocampal model in that these models are concerned with

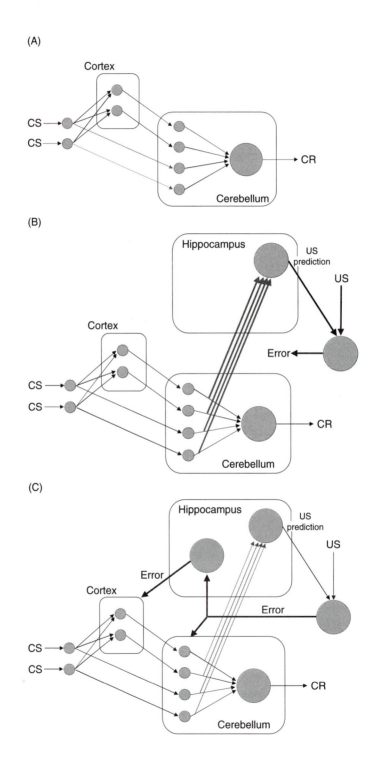

information-processing roles for different brain subregions and how these subregions exchange information. Moreover, Schmajuk's models are also meant to address much of the same body of empirical data as our cortico-hippocampal model. However, the particular function that Schmajuk and his collaborators assign to the hippocampus differs from that supposed by our model, leading to some predictions that may differentiate the two models.

Schmajuk and DiCarlo have presented a computational model of the hippocampal-system processing in classical eyeblink conditioning, often referred to as the **S-D model.**[32] *The S-D model assumes that CS information reaches the cerebellum via two routes: a direct path and an indirect path involving association cortex (figure 6.13A).* This dual-pathway assumption seems anatomically valid.[33] Schmajuk and DiCarlo suggest that CS information is combined in the cortex to allow configural learning. Then, they argue, the cerebellum integrates information from both the direct and indirect pathways to produce a CR.

The S-D model assumes that the hippocampal system has two roles in conditioned learning. The first is shown in 6.13B. According to the Rescorla-Wagner learning rule (refer to MathBox 3.1), learning is proportional to an error measure, which is the difference between the actual and predicted US. The S-D model assumes that the hippocampus is critical in computing this error. Specifically, *the hippocampus in their model is presumed to calculate the US prediction; other brain areas compare this predicted US against the actual US and calculate the total error.* This error signal is then used to guide learning.

Figure 6.13   (A) The S-D model of classical eyeblink conditioning (Schmajuk & DiCarlo, 1992) assumes that CS information reaches the cerebellum by two pathways: a direct CS-cerebellum pathway and an indirect pathway via neocortex. This assumption is consistent with known anatomy. The S-D model assumes that the neocortex recombines CS information to allow configural learning. Finally, the cerebellum integrates information from both the direct and indirect CS pathways to produce a CR. (B) The S-D model assumes that the hippocampus has two roles in conditioned learning. First, it calculates the strength of the US prediction by summing the activations from cerebellum. The hippocampal output is a measure of how strongly the US is predicted. This US prediction measure is passed to other brain regions, which compare it against the actual US and compute a prediction error. This prediction error is similar to the error measure in the Rescorla-Wagner rule, and the learning rate is proportional to the magnitude of this error. (C) The second function of the hippocampus in the S-D model is to broadcast the error signal to the neocortex. According to this model, hippocampal-region damage should impair both the computation of the aggregate error signal as well as the ability of the neocortex to develop new configural nodes.

Figure 6.13C illustrates the second role for the hippocampal region in the S-D model: *The cerebellar units can update weights directly on the basis of the error signal, whereas the cortical units require specialized error signals broadcast by the hippocampus.* In neural network terms, the cortical units are hidden units between the input and output layers, and the hippocampal circuitry is specialized to compute error signals for these hidden units—by implementing a version of error backpropagation.

Hippocampal-system damage is simulated in the S-D model by disabling *both* of the putative hippocampal functions. First, there is no longer any way to calculate the predicted US. Most of the power of the Rescorla-Wagner model (and the Widrow-Hoff learning rule) comes from the ability to predict the US on the basis of *all* available cues. The lesioned S-D model cannot form such an **aggregate prediction** of the US and is reduced to simple learning about individual CSs. Thus, the S-D model predicts that hippocampal damage will impair behavioral phenomena such as blocking that require this error signal based on an aggregate prediction of the US.

Second, the lesioned S-D model cannot form new configural nodes in the cortex, and it is restricted to simpler CS-US learning in the cerebellum. Thus, the S-D model correctly produces unimpaired CS-US learning after hippocampal lesion: The indirect CS-cortex-cerebellum pathway is dysfunctional because the cortical units cannot update without hippocampal error signals, but the direct CS-cerebellum pathway is operational and allows learning. Other forms of learning, such as sensory preconditioning, that depend on CS-CS associations, are disrupted by damage either to the cortical system or to the hippocampal system that provides its error signals.

There are numerous additional complexities to the S-D model that are not discussed here,[34] but the description given above is sufficient to illustrate the basic principles by which the model operates. Applied to classical conditioning, the S-D model can account for a sizable range of empirical findings. These include the sparing of discrimination learning, but impairment of reversal, after hippocampal lesion; the broadening of the generalization gradient in lesioned animals; and the loss of latent inhibition after hippocampal lesion.[35] In addition, because it is a real-time model, it can successfully account for such temporal effects as trace conditioning and phasic cue occasion setting, which are beyond the scope of our own cortico-hippocampal model.[36]

In later work, the S-D model has been extended to include attentional processing and novelty detection.[37] The basic idea behind these subsequent models is that when a mismatch occurs between prediction and reality, attention to the current stimuli is increased and the prediction generator is updated. Thus, during the first CS-US pairing, the unfamiliar CS generates high attention, facilitating its association with the US; during latent inhibition, the CS becomes familiar, reducing attention and impairing the ability of that CS to enter into subsequent associations. More recently, Schmajuk has suggested that the two hippocampal-system functions proposed in the S-D model can be subdivided and mapped to various hippocampal-region substructures.[38] Chapter 9 will discuss these elaborations in more detail.

Comparison with Gluck and Myers's Cortico-Hippocampal Model

Because the S-D model and our cortico-hippocampal model both address the same domain (classical eyeblink conditioning), there is a great deal of overlap in their predictions. However, there are several important points on which the two models differ. The most basic of these concerns the ability to predict the US based on all available CSs. The S-D model sites this aggregate prediction in the hippocampus and assumes that hippocampal lesion abolishes it. Our cortico-hippocampal model, by contrast, follows Thompson's cerebellar theory[39] in assuming that this (and all other aspects of the Rescorla-Wagner model) are implemented in the cerebellum. The HR-lesioned cortico-hippocampal model does continue to compute a prediction of the US based on all available cues and to use this information to guide error-correction learning. Thus, the S-D model and cortico-hippocampal model make different predictions about the effects of hippocampal-region damage on behavioral effects that, in the intact animal, reflect aggregate prediction of the US. While there are behavioral data testing these predictions, the data are unfortunately mixed in many cases.

Conditioned Inhibition.   One example of such an effect is **conditioned inhibition:** learning to respond to one cue (e.g., light+) when presented alone but not when paired with another cue (e.g., tone&light−).

The Rescorla-Wagner model can solve this task by setting a positive weight on light and a negative weight on tone so that light alone produces a response but tone and light together cancel each other out and produce no response. Both the Rescorla-Wagner model and the cerebellar model of chapter 3 show this effect. This implies that the cerebellum should be sufficient to mediate conditioned inhibition, and therefore hippocampal-region damage should not disrupt performance. Paul Solomon tested this idea in rabbit eyeblink conditioning and found that rabbits with hippocampal-region damage could learn the task just as well as control rabbits, as shown in figure 6.14A.[40]

Because the cortico/cerebellar network of figure 6.2B incorporates the error-correcting learning procedure from the Rescorla-Wagner model, both

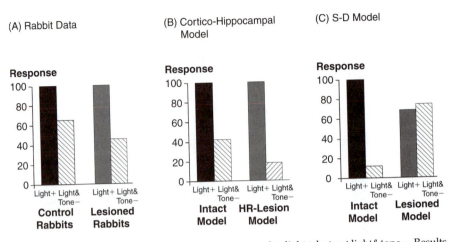

Figure 6.14   Conditioned inhibition: learning to respond to light+ but not light&tone−. Results are expressed as a percent of response to light+ in intact animals or model. (A) Rabbit eyeblink conditioning data: Both intact and hippocampal-lesioned animals can learn a strong response to light+ and a weak response to light&tone− after about 700 blocks of training; the lesioned animals are slightly better at withholding responses to light&tone−. (From data presented in Solomon, 1977, Figure 2.) (B) The cortico-hippocampal model: After 1000 blocks of training, both the intact and HR-lesion models give strong responses to light+ and weaker responses to light&tone−; again, the HR-lesion model learns slightly faster. (C) The S-D model makes the opposite prediction: Although the intact model can learn the task, the lesioned model is unable to discriminate light+ and light&tone− and gives intermediate responses to both. This is because the S-D model assumes that the hippocampus is necessary for cue competition effects. (From data presented in Schmajuk & DiCarlo, 1992, Figure 11.)

our intact and HR-lesioned models show conditioned inhibition, as is seen in figure 6.14B.

The intact S-D model can also produce conditioned inhibition. However, the lesioned S-D model cannot, as is shown in figure 6.14C. This is because the S-D model assumes that hippocampal-region damage disrupts the ability to compute the output error that is needed to learn competing responses to light depending on whether tone is present or absent. Therefore, the lesioned S-D model cannot learn different responses to light and to tone and light and cannot produce conditioned inhibition.[41]

Thus, the data from Solomon and colleagues study of conditioned inhibition are consistent with our cortico-hippocampal model but conflict with the predictions of the S-D model.

Blocking.   Another behavioral paradigm in which our cortico-hippocampal model and the S-D model make differing predictions is **blocking.** The basic

Table 6.2   The Blocking Paradigm

Group	Phase 1	Phase 2	Phase 3: Test
Pretrained	Tone → airpuff	Tone&light → airpuff	Tone → ?
			⇒ *no blink*
Sit exposure	(Animal sits in experimental chamber)	Tone&light → airpuff	Tone → ?
			⇒ *partial blink*

paradigm is schematized in table 6.2. Animals in the Pretrained group receive tone+ training followed by tone&light+ training; when later tested with the light alone, they show no response. By comparison, control animals in the Sit-exposure group, which receive only tone&light training, show at least partial responding to the light stimulus.

Figure 6.15A shows that blocking is unaffected in the HR-lesioned cortico-hippocampal model; by contrast, the lesioned S-D model predicts that the light CS will acquire strong associative strength (figure 6.15B). Unfortunately, the empirical data are ambiguous here; blocking has been reported to be both impaired and spared following hippocampal-region damage in different studies.[42] It is not clear what conclusions to draw from these conflicting results. Perhaps future data will clear up this controversy and provide strong support for one model or the other. Another possibility is that the brain has multiple sites that subserve stimulus competition effects—in the hippocampus and cerebellum and elsewhere—and the particular effects of hippocampal-region damage will depend critically on details of the procedural parameters used in each study. This is especially relevant given that the empirical studies of blocking cited above employed a variety of lesion techniques that produce different degrees of HR damage.

Configural Learning (Negative Patterning).   The notion that a task may be either impaired or spared after hippocampal lesion, depending on a variety of procedural details, has implications for a wide range of tasks. One significant task for studies of hippocampal function in recent years has been configural learning, such as the **negative patterning** task. Recall from chapter 3 that this task involves learning to respond to two stimuli (e.g., light+ and tone+) but not to their compound (light&tone−).

Many animal studies have found that hippocampal lesion disrupts the ability to learn negative patterning (e.g., figure 6.16A), but a few studies also showed that negative patterning was spared.[43] Both the cortico-hippocampal

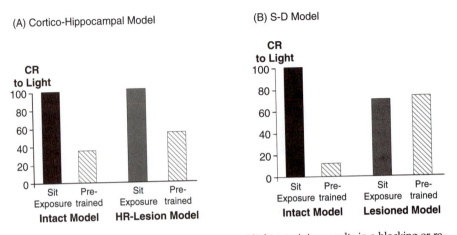

Figure 6.15 Blocking: Tone+ training before tone&light+ training results in a blocking or re-duction of associative strength to light. Results are response to light, expressed as a percent of response intact animal or model control condition. (A) The cortico-hippocampal intact and HR-lesion models both show blocking: Responding to light is reduced following tone+ and tone&light+ pretraining relative to a naive condition that just received training to tone&light+. (B) The S-D model predicts that blocking should be eliminated by hippocampal lesion. (Redrawn from data presented in Schmajuk & DiCarlo, 1992, Figure 7.)

and S-D models predict that negative patterning should, in general, be dis-rupted by hippocampal-region damage, as figures 6.16B and C show. The two computational models make similar predictions here because both assume that the hippocampal region is necessary to form new representa-tions that encode cue configurations (though the two models assume that somewhat different mechanisms underlie this process).

However, both models also assume that hippocampal-region damage will not affect the cue configurations that are already learned and stored outside the hippocampal region (e.g., in cortex). This leads to a subtle prediction of both models: For some configural tasks, preexisting configural representa-tions may exist and suffice to allow the problem to be solved—even without the benefit of hippocampal processing.

Figure 6.17 shows an example from the cortico-hippocampal model:* 100 simulation runs with the intact and HR-lesioned model were trained on the

*Note that the simulations shown in figure 6.17 were not generated from the standard cortico-hippocampal model used elsewhere in chapters 5 and 6 but were instead a version that had fewer internal-layer nodes (four each in the hippocampal region and cortico/cerebellar net-works) and also stronger initial weights in the lower layer of the cortico/cerebellar network. This increased the probability that some HR-lesioned networks would reach criterion perfor-mance, for demonstration purposes.

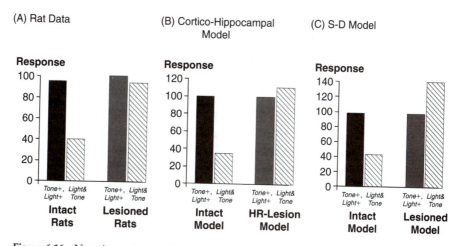

Figure 6.16   Negative patterning involves learning to respond to two cues, light+ and tone+, but to withhold responding to their compound light&tone−. (A) Normal rats can learn to respond to the components but not the compound; hippocampal-lesioned rats are generally found to be unable to withhold responding to the compound light&tone−. Both the cortico-hippocampal model (B) and the S-D model (C) predict that, on average, this and other configural tasks will be greatly disrupted after HR-damage. (A is plotted from data presented in Sutherland & Rudy, 1989, Figure 2. B is plotted from data presented in Schmajuk & DiCarlo, 1992, Figure 14.)

negative patterning task. Solving the task was defined as reaching a criterion performance level, defined as ten consecutive trials on which the simulation generated a CR greater than 0.8 to the components light+ and tone+ but less than 0.2 to the compound light&tone−. By this definition, 80% of the intact simulations did solve the task, reaching criterion performance on discriminating the light+ and tone+ trials from the light&tone− trials. Of the remaining 20%, most simulations still responded somewhat more strongly to the components than to the compound.

The results were very different for the HR-lesion model: 80% of HR-lesion simulations failed to solve the task. Interestingly, the 20% of HR-lesion simulations that did master the task reached criterion performance just as quickly as the intact simulations; in fact, the fastest learners were HR-lesioned, not intact, simulations. This seemingly paradoxical result arises because the intact model is slowed down in learning because it has to construct new stimulus representations to differentiate components light+ and tone+ from the compound light&tone−; in the HR-lesioned model, these representations rarely exist (and hence 80% of the simulations fail), but if by chance the representations do already exist, then learning is very rapid because all that needs to be done to reach criterion performance is to map from these preexisting representations to the correct responses.

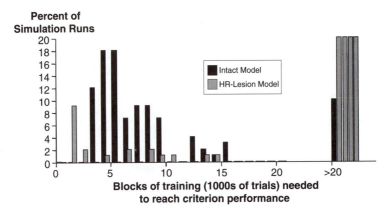

Figure 6.17 Individual performance on negative patterning in the cortico-hippocampal model. The cortico-hippocampal model and S-D model both predict that, while HR lesion will disrupt negative patterning on average, occasionally and seemingly at random an animal's preexisting representations may suffice to solve the problem. Out of 100 simulation runs with both the intact and HR-lesion cortico-hippocampal model, 80% of intact and 20% of HR-lesioned simulations solved the negative patterning problem within 20,000 training blocks. Those HR-lesioned simulations that solved the problem did so as fast as or faster than the intact simulations.

Thus, under certain (possibly rare) conditions, learning in the HR-lesioned model may be faster than in the intact model. Certain kinds of experimental procedures may be especially likely to tap into preexisting, hippocampal-independent systems, in which case configural learning may be reliably faster after hippocampal-region damage. Such results have occasionally been reported in the literature,[*44] lending support to this model prediction.

---

*Gallagher & Holland, 1992, showed that rats with hippocampal lesions were slightly faster than normal to acquire feature-neutral association (AC+, A−, BC−, B+). Han, Gallagher, & Holland (1998) showed that this effect was strengthened if the time between trials was reduced. Bussey et al., 1998, showed that rats with fornix lesions learned faster than normal on a transverse patterning task (prefer A over B, B over C, and C over A). Eichenbaum & Bunsey, 1995, reported that rats with hippocampal lesions were better than control animals in a paired-associate task (AB+, CD+, AC−, BD−). Each of these tasks embeds configural components. It is very much an open question which precise features of these experiments (including animal species, stimulus modalities, procedural variations, and precise lesion techniques) contribute most to the finding of impaired, spared, or facilitated configural learning after hippocampal-region damage.

6.3   RELATIONSHIP OF MODELS TO QUALITATIVE THEORIES

The previous sections reviewed two computational models that were meant to address information processing in the hippocampal region and how that information might be used by other brain structures during learning. One advantage of computational models is that they provide a reality check: A researcher might propose a mechanism for learning that sounds plausible as a verbal argument, but would not work in practice. If the mechanism can be implemented in a computational model, that suggests that the mechanism would indeed operate as expected. A computational model does not *prove* that the brain operates in a certain way, but if the model successfully accounts for a large portion of existing data and makes predictions that are later confirmed by experimental testing, then that suggests that the model is on the right track.

A second use of computational models is that they can often provide possible explanations for issues that were not obvious before. For example, the cortico-hippocampal and S-D models provide one interpretation for the paradoxical finding that, although configural learning may often be devastated following hippocampal-region damage, in some rare cases it is spared or even facilitated. *Thus, it may not be particularly useful to attempt to dichotomize tasks according to whether they can or cannot survive hippocampal-region damage. The computational-modeling approach suggests that it is more useful to consider what kinds of information the hippocampal region normally processes and which tasks may be expected generally to depend on this information.*

Other researchers have also taken information-processing approaches to understanding the hippocampal region and have developed qualitative theories about the hippocampal region's role that are often very useful as heuristics to predict behavior in the lesioned animal or human. In many cases, these qualitative theories are consistent with the computational models described above. This section reviews several prominent qualitative theories of hippocampal-region function, and notes how they relate to the computational models described in sections 6.1 and 6.2.

Stimulus Configuration

Several prominent theories of hippocampal-region function have assumed that the hippocampal region is involved in **stimulus configuration** (or **"chunking"**), whereby a set of co-occurring stimuli come to be treated as a unary whole (or configuration) that can accrue associations.[45] For example, the negative patterning task requires subjects to learn to respond to two stimuli (light+ and tone+) but not their compound (light&tone−). This is easily solved if it is assumed that light and tone can enter into direct excitatory associations with the US but that the compound light&tone is a separate entity that can enter into direct inhibitory associations with the US. In fact, early studies demonstrated that such configural tasks were especially sensitive to hippocampal-region damage.[46] However, later studies suggested that hippocampal-lesioned animals could indeed solve some configural problems.[47] While configuration may be especially sensitive to hippocampal-region damage, it is clearly not universally abolished by such damage.

An alternative interpretation of configuration is embodied by the cortico-hippocampal model. The model assumes that the hippocampal region forms new stimulus representations that may compress (or chunk or configure) co-occurring stimuli. This will facilitate learning of such tasks as negative patterning that depend on stimulus configuration. In the lesioned model, the cortico/cerebellar network is left with a set of fixed lower-layer weights, which do perform a recoding of stimulus inputs. Depending on the initial state of these weights, there is always some probability that a random configuration may be encoded by those weights. In such a case, a configural task may well be solved by the lesioned model. Thus, the cortico-hippocampal model expects only a general tendency toward a lesion deficit in configural learning, not an absolute deficit. This interpretation is consistent with the finding in a few studies that, although lesioned animals are generally impaired at a configural task, they may occasionally solve a configural task as quickly as—or faster than—control animals.[48] It is also consistent with the observation, in many studies, of wide individual variance in how animals solve configural tasks. For example, near the end of a study of negative patterning in normal rabbits, most animals were reliably giving eyeblink CRs to the components light+ and tone+ but not to the configuration light&tone−.[49] However, about one-fourth of the rabbits were showing a different pattern: responding strongly to one component and weakly to the configuration—but also failing to respond to at least one of the components. An additional rabbit was showing the opposite failure: responding reliably to both components and also responding strongly to the compound.[50] Thus, as in the model in figure 6.17, some individual rabbits learn quickly and some learn slowly or not at all. The variation can be even more pronounced in lesioned animals.

Thus, the computational models implement much of the spirit of the configural theory while also demonstrating how and why exceptions to the rule might exist.

Contextual Learning

A related class of theory implicates the hippocampal region in contextual processing. Specifically, the hippocampus has been proposed as the source for *contextual tags* to memories, which identify the spatial and temporal settings in which events occur.[51] **Context** is usually defined as the set of background cues that are present during a learning experience but distinct from the experimentally manipulated CS and US; example contextual stimuli include visual features of the room, background noises, temperature, and time of day. Contextual processing is often disrupted after hippocampal-region damage. For example, humans with medial temporal lobe amnesia can often acquire new information but not recall the spatial and temporal context in which it occurred.[52] Conversely, the nondeclarative (or incremental or procedural) learning that is often preserved in amnesia tends to be acquired slowly, over many trials, and therefore is less strongly associated with any particular context.

Chapter 7 will consider the role of the hippocampal region in contextual processing in more detail; for now, it is sufficient to note that *the cortico-hippocampal model assumes that all co-occurring stimuli (CS, US, and context) influence the development of hippocampal-mediated stimulus representations.* Thus, if CS-US learning occurs in one context, the representation of CS will include contextual information. In contrast, the lesioned model does not develop new stimulus representations but only forms direct CS-US associations; in most cases, the context will not be sufficiently predictive of the US to enter into any associations. Thus, in many cases, there are differences between the context-sensitivity of the intact and lesioned model, and these differences parallel the behavior of intact and lesioned animals.

Stimulus Selection

Some early theories of hippocampal function viewed the hippocampal region as an attentional control mechanism, responsible for reducing attention to stimuli that are not significant, are not correlated with reinforcement, or are irrelevant with respect to predicting reinforcement.[53] These theories are concerned with **stimulus selection**: how individual stimuli are "tuned in" or "tuned out" of attention.

Traditionally, psychological theories of stimulus selection have fallen into two broad classes: **reinforcement modulation theories** and **sensory modulation theories.** Reinforcement modulation theories consider the effectiveness of the reinforcer (e.g., the US) to be modulated by the degree to which the US is unexpected, given all the cues (e.g., the CS) present. So a reinforcer that is predicted by a CS would not support new learning, while one that is unexpected would support new learning. The Rescorla-Wagner model described in chapter 3 is an example of a reinforcement modulation theory.

In contrast, sensory modulation theories of stimulus selection focus on the ability of CSs to enter into new associations, on the basis of how much they add to the overall ability to predict reinforcement.[54] Thus, a CS that predicted an otherwise unpredictable US would be very likely to enter into associations; a CS that did not add to the ability to predict the US would not enter into new associations. Both reinforcement and sensory modulation theories can account for some—but not all—learning behaviors.

Interestingly, a few behaviors, such as blocking, can be explained in terms of either (or both) approaches: At the end of phase 1, the trained CS (e.g. tone+) perfectly predicts the US. When the second light+ CS is added, reinforcement modulation theories expect that the well-predicted US should not enter into new associations with the light. At the same time, sensory modulation theories expect that the light, which adds no new information, should not enter into new associations with the US. Thus, both sensory modulation and reinforcement modulation may normally contribute to a strong blocking effect.

The cortico-hippocampal model and the S-D model of hippocampal-region function incorporate both sensory and reinforcement modulation. The cortico-hippocampal model assumes that the cortico/cerebellar regions (which are capable of error-correction) can perform reinforcement modulation, while the hippocampal region is needed for sensory modulation. Thus, our model predicts that some—but not all—stimulus selection effects will be disrupted after hippocampal-region damage. Specifically, reinforcement modulation should survive HR lesion, while sensory modulation should not.

More generally, because stimulus selection depends on two substrates (cortico/cerebellar and hippocampal), our model expects that many behaviors that reflect stimulus selection may be reduced but not eliminated by HR lesion, because removing one of two sources of stimulus selection may leave the other intact. This may explain why some stimulus selection behaviors, such as blocking, sometimes survive hippocampal lesion and sometimes are eliminated.

Intermediate-Term and Working Memory

The fact that HR-lesioned monkeys are impaired at delayed nonmatch to sample—but only if there is a long enough delay between sample and choice—suggests that the hippocampal region has a role in maintaining information over the course of a few minutes. This kind of memory is often called **intermediate-term memory** (as distinct from the short-term memory that we use to remember a telephone number by constant rehearsal or long-term memory, which can last years). A related concept is **working memory:** intermediate-term memories that contain information relevant to the current task at hand. For example, in the monkey delayed nonmatch to sample (DNMS) paradigm, working memory allows the monkey to remember the sample item across a short delay; however, on each new trial, the sample item is different, and working memory updates to reflect this. A working-memory task in rats might involve a maze in which there is food in a number of locations at the start of each trial; to obtain all the food in the shortest possible time, the rat must use working memory to remember which locations it has visited (and depleted) so far on the current trial. Performance on this kind of task is disrupted by hippocampal-region damage.[55] Trace conditioning also requires the ability to maintain CS information during the short interval until the US arrives and is likewise disrupted by hippocampal-region damage.

Several researchers have suggested that a critical component of these tasks is the ability to represent information over short periods of time, and some have suggested that the hippocampus functions as a buffer, holding critical bits of information for a short time.[56] In fact, there are some neurophysiological data suggesting that neuronal activity in the hippocampus may temporarily encode recent stimuli.[57] More recently, researchers have suggested that the hippocampus is critical when the task has a temporal discontinuity, meaning that the items to be associated do not overlap in time.[58]

Howard Eichenbaum, Tim Otto, and Neal Cohen have suggested that the intermediate-term memory buffer can be specifically localized within the **parahippocampal region,** including entorhinal, perirhinal, and parahippocampal cortices.[59] One function of this buffer would be to compress or "fuse" individual stimuli into compound percepts.[60] We will return to the possible selective role of entorhinal cortex and other parahippocampal structures in chapter 9; for now, we note that the stimulus fusion that Eichenbaum and colleagues attribute to the entorhinal cortex is perfectly consistent with the stimulus compression that the cortico-hippocampal model views as one aspect of hippocampal-region function.[61] The hippocampal region may be involved in constructing new representations that compress together stimuli that co-occur or are similar in meaning; this compression could apply equally to stimuli that are superficially dissimilar, and to those that are separated in time or in space.[62]

Cognitive Mapping

Perhaps the most devastating effect of hippocampal-region damage in rats is on spatial learning. The strong spatial impairment in hippocampal-lesioned rats has led to theories suggesting that the hippocampus (or hippocampal region) is specialized as a spatial mapping system.[63] Partial support for these theories comes from neurophysiological studies showing that individual cells in hippocampal subfields CA3 and CA1 respond preferentially when the animal is in a particular region of space. A variety of computational models have shown that the known anatomy and physiology of these subfields is sufficient to give rise to place field behavior and allow various kinds of spatial learning.[64]

Perhaps the primary problem with the simplest spatial theories is that hippocampal-region damage can result in a broad range of deficits that have no obvious spatial component; examples include conditioning tasks such as disrupted sensory preconditioning in HR-lesioned animals and disrupted recognition in humans with medial temporal damage (refer to chapter 1). The spatial theory has since been extended to assume that the hippocampus is only disproportionately, but not exclusively, involved in spatial processing[65] or that the hippocampal region is involved in **cognitive mapping,** which ties spatial as well as contextual, semantic, and other information into unified memories.[66] This, then, would lead to the impairment in episodic learning observed in human amnesia.

An alternative interpretation of the lesion impairment in spatial learning suggests that the hippocampus is not specialized for spatial learning per se, but rather that a "place" is simply a configuration of local views of space.[67] Thus, since configural processes seem to be especially sensitive to hippocampal-region damage, spatial learning is also susceptible to hippocampal-region impairment. This interpretation is consistent with the fact that some hippocampal cells that show spatially determined responses during a spatial task can have other behavioral correlates during a nonspatial task.[68]

"Flexible" Memory

In contrast to theories that implicate the hippocampal region specifically in one kind of memory—be it configural, contextual, spatial, or even declarative—some researchers have suggested that the hippocampal region of an intact animal is involved in learning even the most elementary associations. For example, in the cortico-hippocampal model, the hippocampal region is not *necessary* for learning a CS-US association; however, in the intact model, the hippocampal region constructs new representations even during such a simple task and thereby influences the way in which CS-US associations are formed. This may not be evident during learning, and so there may be little or no difference in the CR development of an intact or hippocampal region-lesioned animal (or model). But the hippocampal-mediated representations will become very evident if the animal (or model) is later challenged to use that learning in a generalization or transfer task.

Eichenbaum, Cohen, and colleagues have advanced a qualitatively similar view.[69] They propose that the hippocampus is involved in forming stimulus representations that are sensitive to the relationships between stimuli.[70] Hippocampal-independent memories are assumed to be inflexible, in the sense that they can be accessed only through reactivation of the original stimuli and situations in which the learning took place. For example, rats can be trained to prefer odor A+ over odor B− and to prefer odor C+ over D−. Later, when presented with odors A and D, normal rats reliably choose A but hippocampal-lesioned rats may choose randomly—as if they had never been exposed to either odor before.[71] In chapter 8, we will discuss this kind of task in more detail and show how the cortico-hippocampal model can be extended to address some of its features. For now, though, we simply note a surface similarity between Eichenbaum and Cohen's theory and the cortico-hippocampal model. A central feature of Eichenbaum and Cohen's flexible learning is the creation of stimulus representations that emphasize the relationships between stimuli. This is consistent with the cortico-hippocampal model, in which hippocampal-region representations emphasize predictive features and deemphasize irrelevant features; such representations may be used flexibly in new contexts whose irrelevant features differ from those of the learning context.

6.4   IMPLICATIONS FOR HUMAN MEMORY AND MEMORY DISORDERS

The first and most important implication of the computational models discussed in this chapter is that hippocampal-region damage does not indiscriminately abolish the ability to learn. Animals with HR lesion can acquire some kinds of new information, including simple acquisition of conditioned eyeblink responses and other stimulus-response associations.

It is now well established that humans with anterograde amnesia from medial temporal (including hippocampal-region) damage can also learn motor-reflex responses.[72] Similarly, by focusing on what amnesic subjects can do rather than on their impairments, it may be possible to accomplish significant and subtle learning in these individuals. Amnesic subjects are able to acquire and retain new motor skills such as mirror-tracing and cognitive skills such as grammatical rules if the learning takes place incrementally, over many trials, and does not require episodic memory of individual learning sessions.[73] Similarly, amnesic subjects can learn to categorize objects on a computer screen into arbitrary classes by repeated exposure to members of the categories.[74] Amnesic subjects have even been taught rudimentary computer programming skills using methods that take advantage of spared learning abilities.[75]

The animal and model data also suggest that some kinds of conditioning should be disrupted by HR lesion. For example, discrimination reversal may be greatly slowed in relation to controls, although HR-lesioned animals may master the reversal given enough trials. One question is whether humans with medial temporal (HR) damage will show a similar pattern of impaired and spared learning. At this point, it is still very much an open question whether amnesic individuals can reverse a learned discrimination as well as control subjects do.[76]

In other kinds of paradigm, in which control animals are slowed by prior exposure, HR-lesioned animals can outperform control animals. For example, controls but not HR-lesioned animals are slow to learn a CS-US association following uncorrelated exposure (learned irrelevance) to the CS and US. Recently, we developed in our laboratory a computerized task that embeds some features of learned irrelevance into a video game task.[77] The task involved learning that some screen events (like CSs) predict other screen events (like USs). Subjects were seated at a computer screen and told that they would see a magician trying to make a rabbit appear under his hat (figure 6.18). On each trial, the subjects were to guess whether or not the magician succeeded. The appearance of the rabbit was conceptually analogous to the to-be-predicted US, and the subjects' predictions were equivalent to an anticipatory CR.

Subjects in our study were divided into two groups: Exposed and Nonexposed. In phase 1, for all subjects, the appearance of the rabbit US was contingent on a particular "magic word" in the magician's cartoon word balloon. For subjects in the Nonexposed group, the cartoon balloon was always uncolored (gray). For subjects in the Exposed group, the cartoon balloon was colored red or green, and the color was not correlated with the rabbit US. Later, in phase 2, the balloon color perfectly predicted the rabbit US. Thus, balloon color was the CS that predicted US arrival. Subjects who had previously been exposed to this color CS, uncorrelated with the US, were slower to learn the association between CS and US in phase 2 than were

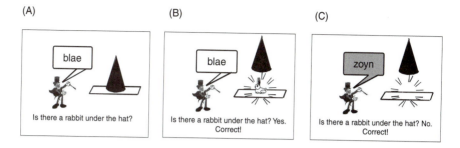

Figure 6.18 A computerized task that embeds some aspects of learned irrelevance. Subjects watch a computer screen that shows a magician trying to produce a rabbit under his hat (A). Conceptually, the appearance of the rabbit is the to-be-predicted event (US). Subjects guess whether the rabbit will appear on each trial. The hat is then raised to show whether the rabbit is present (B, C), and corrective feedback is given. In phase 1, the rabbit is predicted by a particular magic word in the magician's cartoon word balloon. In phase 2, the rabbit is predicted by a particular color (red or green) in the word balloon. (Adapted from Myers, McGlinchey-Berroth, et al., 2000, Figure 1.)

subjects who had not been exposed. Thus, normal subjects showed learned irrelevance.[78]

Recently, we tested a group of individuals with amnesia resulting from medial temporal (HR) damage and a group of matched control subjects on this task.[79] In phase 1 (in which the "magic word" predicted the rabbit), amnesic and control subjects all learned quickly, regardless of exposure condition (figure 6.19A). In phase 2, the control subjects showed a strong learned irrelevance effect: The Exposed group learned more slowly than the Nonexposed group. However, among amnesic subjects, the learned irrelevance effect was eliminated: Exposed and Nonexposed groups learned at the same rate (figure 6.19B).

One implication of these findings in animals and humans is that *under certain conditions that slow CS-US learning in normal subjects, the amnesic subjects learn more quickly than controls!* Of course, the normal subjects learn more slowly because they are learning more: They are learning about environmental regularities during exposure, and this same learning is what disrupts later association.

A second implication of these findings is that *although both controls and amnesic subjects appear to learn similarly in phase 1, they are actually learning differently.* This difference shows up during phase 2, when subjects are challenged to apply their learning in new ways. Thus, transfer tasks may be a more useful way to demonstrate differences between these groups than the initial learning. This in turn has potential implications for diagnosing syndromes,

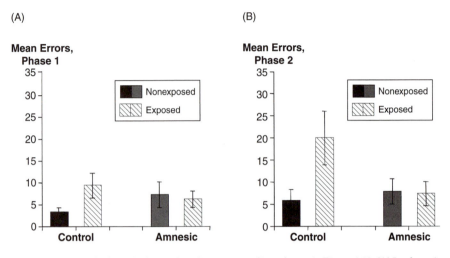

Figure 6.19   Results from the learned irrelevance paradigm shown in Figure 6.19. (A) In phase 1, subjects learned to predict the rabbit US on the basis of a neutral cue (a particular magic word). Subjects in the exposed condition were also given uncorrelated exposure to a color CS; subjects in the nonexposed condition never saw this CS in phase 1. Among normal subjects, there was no significant difference in total errors between the two conditions; amnesic subjects in both conditions also performed the same as controls. (B) In phase 2, the color CS predicted the rabbit US. Normal subjects who had been exposed to the CS in phase 1 took longer to learn this CS-US association than did nonexposed subjects. Thus, normal subjects showed learned irrelevance. By contrast, amnesic subjects did not show learned irrelevance: Exposed and nonexposed amnesic subjects learned the phase 2 task at the same speed—and much faster than exposed control subjects. (Adapted from Myers, McGlinchey-Berroth, et al., 2000, Figure 2.)

such as Alzheimer's disease, that involve hippocampal-region damage. We will consider the application of related human experiments to the prediction of the early stages of Alzheimer's in chapter 9.

SUMMARY

• Hippocampal-region damage in network models is simulated by disabling a hippocampal-region module and observing the behavior of the remaining modules.

• Gluck and Myers's cortico-hippocampal theory argues that the hippocampal region plays a crucial role in the recoding or rerepresentation of stimulus representations during learning. Specifically, if two stimuli co-occur or make similar predictions about future reinforcement, their representations will be compressed to increase generalization between the stimuli. Conversely, if two stimuli never co-occur and make different predictions about future reinforcement, their representations will be differentiated to decrease generalization between the stimuli.

• The cortico-hippocampal model assumes that the representations developed in the hippocampal region are eventually adopted by other long-term storage sites in cortex and cerebellum.

• The hippocampal region may not be strictly *necessary* for some simple kinds of learning; but when it is present, it normally contributes to *all* learning.

• The cortico-hippocampal model has limitations in accounting for data on extinction and response timing.

• Taken together, the neurophysiological evidence that is currently available is remarkably consistent with the implications of our cortico-hippocampal model, suggesting that hippocampal neuronal representations can and do change to reflect associations between stimuli and rewards, much like the internal-layer nodes in a predictive autoencoder.

• The Schmajuk-DiCarlo (S-D) model assumes that CS information reaches the cerebellum via two routes: a direct path and an indirect path involving association cortex. Specifically, the hippocampus in this model is presumed to calculate the predicted US, while other brain areas compare this predicted US against the actual US and calculate the total error. This error signal is then used to guide learning. In addition, cerebellar units can update weights directly on the basis of the error signal, whereas the cortical units require specialized error signals broadcast by the hippocampus.

• It may not be particularly useful to attempt to dichotomize tasks according to whether they can or cannot survive hippocampal-region damage. Computational modeling suggests that it is more useful to consider what kinds of information the hippocampal region normally processes and which tasks may be expected generally to depend on this information.

• In many cases, qualitative theories of the hippocampal region are very consistent with a subset of the implications of computational models when the models are applied to specific domains or tasks.

• Because selective attention depends on both cortico/cerebellar and hippocampal substrates in the cortico-hippocampal model, the model expects that many behaviors that reflect selective attention may be reduced but not eliminated by HR lesion.

• In studies of associative learning in cognitive analogs of conditioning tasks, both control and amnesic subjects appear to learn similarly during an initial phase of training, but transfer task performance suggests that they are actually using different strategies to learn.

APPENDIX 6.1   SIMULATION DETAILS

The cortico-hippocampal model of section 6.1 was described at a very general level, without reference to mathematical details such as number of nodes or learning rates. In fact, over the years, we have implemented the model with a wide number of parameter choices; the qualitative behavior of the model is usually independent of these choices, although the absolute speed or accuracy of learning may vary. All of the cortico-hippocampal model simulations presented in section 6.1 were based on a single implementation (the same one used in Myers & Gluck, 1994), and each figure represents the average of ten simulation runs with that implementation, except as otherwise noted in the text.

The external inputs consisted of four CSs and fourteen contextual stimuli, each of which could be either present or absent. The contextual stimuli were initialized randomly but thereafter held constant for the remainder of the experiment. (A different set of randomly initialized contextual stimuli was used if there was to be a contextual shift in the experiment.) At any given moment, one or more CSs could be present along with the US. A **trial** consisted of one presentation of each stimulus combination to be trained, interspersed with context-alone trials in a 1:19 ratio. Thus, for discrimination learning (CS A predicts the US, but CS B does not), one trial would include a presentation of A (with the US), nineteen context-alone presentations, a presentation of B (with no US), and nineteen more context-alone presentations.

The hippocampal-region network contained eighteen input nodes, ten internal-layer nodes, and nineteen output nodes. The output nodes learned to reconstruct the eighteen inputs as well as predicting whether the US was present. The network was trained by error backpropagation, as described in MathBox 4.1 and Rumelhart, Hinton, and Williams (1986). The learning rate was set at 0.05 when the US was present and 0.005 otherwise; the momentum was set at 0.9.*

The cortico/cerebellar network also contained eighteen input nodes, along with sixty internal-layer nodes and one output node. The activity of the output node was interpreted as the strength or probability of a CR in response to the current inputs. The upper layer of weights was trained according to the Widrow-Hoff rule (MathBox 3.1); desired output was the same as the US. The

---

*Note that there is a wide range of parameters for the model that would produce similar rates of learning; for example, setting the learning rates to be equivalent on US-present and US-absent trials but greatly increasing the ratio of context-alone versus CS+ trials would produce generally similar, though not necessarily identical, behavioral properties.

learning rate was set at 0.5 when the US was present and 0.05 otherwise. For each internal-layer node c, the desired output was defined as the sum over all hippocampal-region network internal-layer nodes h of the activity of h times the weight from h to c. These weights were initialized according to the random distribution $U(-0.3\ldots+0.3)$ and were held constant throughout the experiment.

All nodes in the system used a sigmoidal output function as defined in Math-Box 4.1, Equation 4.3. All weights and biases in the hippocampal-region network were initialized according to the random distribution $U(-0.3\ldots+0.3)$. Upper-layer weights and output bias in the cortico/cerebellar network were initialized in the same way. Lower-layer weights and internal-layer node biases in the cortico/cerebellar network were initialized according to the random distribution $U(-15\ldots+15)$. This, in combination with the large number of internal-layer nodes in the cortico/cerebellar network, maximized the chance of useful representations existing in the HR-lesioned model.

Before any training, the entire system was initialized with 500 context-alone presentations, simulating the time spent acclimatizing an animal to the experimental chamber before any conditioning begins. The model was assumed to have "learned" a task when it reached **criterion** performance, defined as ten consecutive trials correctly generating a CR of at least 0.8 whenever the US was present and at most 0.2 when the US was absent.

7 Cortico-Hippocampal Interaction and Contextual Processing

Chapter 6 presented some examples of computational models of cortico-hippocampal interaction in classical conditioning. These models considered how conditioned stimuli were associated with responses and what role the hippocampal region might play in this association. But any conditioning experiment—indeed, any form of learning—takes place against a background, or **context,** including the sights, sounds, and smells of the environment. There are also internal contextual cues such as motivation and drives. Typically, researchers try to minimize contextual cues or control for them by making sure that all subjects experience similar context. Nevertheless, it has long been recognized that contextual cues can and do affect what is learned.[1]

From the early days of hippocampal research, it has been apparent that the hippocampal region plays an important role in contextual processing. Indeed, two early influential theories of hippocampal-region function suggested that the region's chief function is contextual processing in general[2] or processing spatial contexts in specific locations.[3] This chapter reviews several different approaches to interpreting the role of the hippocampus for learning about context.

7.1 OVERVIEW OF CONTEXTUAL PROCESSING

One of the difficulties in developing a theory of contextual processing is that context can be interpreted in several distinct manners. Context can be thought of as a set of unchanging, or **tonic,** cues. This contrasts with the more familiar, experimentally manipulated **phasic** cues, such as tones and lights, which have well-defined and limited duration and presentation rate. The CS is presented against a background of other tonic stimuli, such as the overhead lighting, the noises of the ventilation system, and the subject's knowledge of the time of day. Normally, the very nature of these background tonic cues means that they are not particularly useful as predictors of exactly when the US will appear. By contrast, a phasic cue, such as a light or tone, that always occurs just before the US will be a much better warning signal.

However, if no phasic cues are present, or if they are not good predictors of the US, then tonic contextual cues may be the only available predictors of reinforcement. For example, suppose food reinforcement is occasionally available in one experimental chamber X but never in a second chamber Y and there are no phasic cues, as schematized in figures 7.1A and 7.1B. In this case, animals will tend to approach the food cup in context X but not in context Y, as shown in figure 7.1C. Apparently, the animals have learned an association between context X and reinforcement, as if context were not fundamentally different from any other kind of CS. This kind of learning is not dependent on the hippocampal region: Animals with hippocampal damage can still learn to respond in context X but not in context Y.[4]

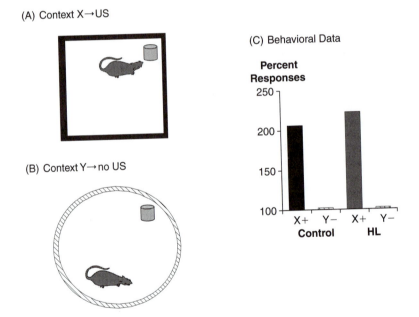

Context = "Just Another CS"

(A) Context X→US

(B) Context Y→ no US

(C) Behavioral Data

Percent Responses

Figure 7.1   In an experimental paradigm, there may be both phasic cues, with explicit temporal duration, and tonic or contextual cues, which are present throughout the experiment. If no phasic cues reliably predict the US, then contextual cues may be the best available predictors. For example, if food is available in context X (A) but not in context Y (B), then animals will learn to make a response (e.g., approach the food cup) in context X but not Y. In this case, the context may enter into direct associations with the food US, just like any other CS. (C) Hippocampal-lesioned (HL) rats learn this distinction just as well as controls. Data are presented as percentage of baseline responding in unrewarded context (Y–). (Plotted from data presented in Good & Honey, 1991.)

However, context can also function as something more than just a collection of tonic cues. *Context can provide a framework against which other learning occurs.*[5] For example, suppose an animal is placed in a particular experimental chamber (context X) and trained that a cue, such as a light, predicts a US, as shown in figure 7.2A. The animal will learn to respond to the light. Once this light-US association is well learned, the animal is then tested in a new context Y that is dramatically different from X, as illustrated by figure 7.2B.

Under many conditions, if the light is presented in this new context Y, normal (control) animals will give a significantly reduced response, compared to the responding in the old context X, as shown in figure 7.2C.[6] This reduced responding in the new context implies that the animal learned not only about the light, but also about the context X in which the light originally occurred. In this case, the context appears to modulate responding to the light, helping to determine what kind of response is appropriate on the current occasion.

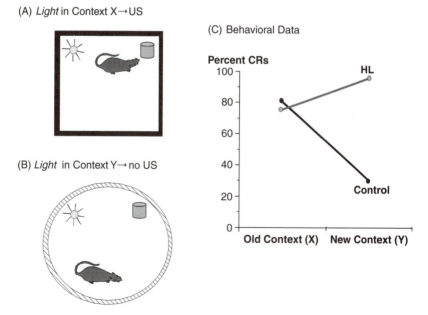

Figure 7.2   Context can also provide a framework for interpreting the meaning of phasic CSs. (A) For example, an animal is trained that a light cue predicts a US (e.g., food) in one context X. (B) If the light cue is then presented in a novel context Y, there may be a decreased level of responding. (C) In rabbit eyeblink conditioning, hippocampal-lesion (HL) eliminates the context shift effect. (Plotted from results presented in Penick & Solomon, 1991.)

This kind of contextual processing—sometimes called **occasion setting**—does appear to be dependent on the hippocampus, since hippocampal-lesioned animals show responding at the same level when a familiar cue is presented in a novel context (figure 7.2C).[7] Note that this different behavior for hippocampal-lesioned animals is not necessarily more or less desirable than that seen in intact controls; what is clear is that the hippocampal-lesioned animals generalize differently than the intact controls to novel contexts.

The use of context to disambiguate the meaning of a stimulus is not limited to classical conditioning experiments. Most of us will react differently to a snake, depending on whether we encounter it in the context of a barefoot walk through the woods or in the context of a visit to the zoo. Context is also not limited to external cues such as physical setting. Context can include internal states such as motivation. For example, a rat can be placed in the base of a T-shaped maze and trained to run into the left or right arm of the maze to obtain a reward. If the left maze arm contains food and the right maze arm contains water, then the correct response (run left or run right) depends on whether the animal is hungry or thirsty. After a few trials, the rat will learn to run toward the water when it is thirsty and toward the food when it is hungry.[8] In this example, the maze itself is the conditioned stimulus that elicits responding, and the animal's internal state is the context that determines which of two competing responses is appropriate. Hippocampal-region damage greatly disrupts an animal's ability to learn the correct response, indicating that the hippocampal region is also involved in using internal contextual cues to guide responding.[9]

In summary, depending on the situation, context sometimes can act just like any other kind of conditioned stimulus cue, thereby entering into direct associations with the US. The first part of section 7.2 describes a computational model of this kind of contextual processing. On the other hand, context also stands in a special, superordinate relationship to the cues that it contains simply by virtue of its tonic nature throughout a conditioning experiment; as such, context appears to be able to mediate responding to cues, without itself entering into direct associations with the US. The second part of section 7.2 describes a computational model that includes this kind of contextual mediation. Animal data suggest that the former, associative properties of context are not dependent on the hippocampal region, while the latter, mediating properties of context do depend on the hippocampal region. Richard Hirsh extrapolated from these and similar results and proposed that contextual processing is a chief role of the hippocampus. Specifically, Hirsh argued that, *while the hippocampus is not needed to mediate the associative properties of context (the ability of context to enter into direct associations with the US), the hippocampus is critical for contextual occasion-setting (using context to mediate choice between competing responses to a stimulus).*[10] The last part of section 7.2 shows how computational models of hippocampus can incorporate both these kinds of contextual processing without requiring any special representational status for contextual cues.

7.2   COMPUTATIONAL MODELS

Context as "Just Another CS"

In the original description of the Rescorla-Wagner model, the authors noted that contextual cues (such as the odor and texture of the experimental chamber) could acquire associative strength just like the experimentally manipulated cues, such as tones and lights.[11] Rescorla and Wagner proposed that if the set of contextual cues is collapsed into a single compound cue X, then X could be associated with the US just like any other CS. Training to respond to a light in context X could be thought of as mixing presentations of the light&X compound with presentations of X alone (figure 7.3A); light&X would be paired with the US, while X alone would not. In this case, the light is a perfect predictor of the US and will accrue strong associative strength. Context X, by contrast, is only sometimes paired with the US; it will accrue little or no associative strength. Thus, there will be little responding to X alone in the absence of the light.

Alternatively, the experimenter may arrange things so that the context is a better predictor of the US than any other available cue. For example, suppose that the US sometimes appears in context X but never appears in context Y. Under these conditions, context X will accrue some positive associative strength (figure 7.3B). If the US appears only occasionally, context X will accrue associative strength proportional to the rate of US presentation compared to the total time spent in context X. On the other hand, since the US never appears in context Y, Y will not accrue any associative strength. In fact, this appears to be what actually happens: Animals show a higher rate of CRs in context X than in context Y.[12] This behavior is also shown in rats with hippocampal-region damage,[13] a result suggesting that the hippocampal region is not necessary for learning to condition to tonic contextual cues.

The convention that context can be viewed as just a collection of tonic cues that compete with phasic CSs for associative strength has been adopted by several other computational models.[14] This seemingly simple idea does, however, lead to surprisingly subtle and important implications.

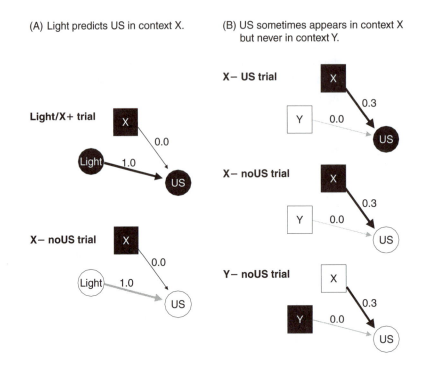

(A) Light predicts US in context X.

(B) US sometimes appears in context X but never in context Y.

Figure 7.3   If context is treated as just another kind of cue, it can accrue direct association with the US if it is the best predictor of the US. (A) Learning that light predicts the US in a particular context X can be interpreted as mixing light-X+ trials with X− trials. In this case, light is a good predictor of the US and will accrue strong associative strength; X is only occasionally paired with the US and will acquire little or no associative strength. (B) Alternatively, the context may be the best available predictor of the US. If the US always occurs in context X but never in context Y, this is equivalent to intermixing X+, X−, and Y− trials. Context X will acquire associative strength, and the amount of associative strength will be related to how often the US appears in context X as a function of total time spent in context X. Context Y will acquire no associative strength, since it is never paired with the US.

For example, several models of spatial navigation adopt this same general framework.[15] Figure 7.4A shows an example of a canonical network that learns to map from a set of contextual cues (representing current location) to generate the next appropriate move. At each time step, the current location is provided as input to the network. Initially, the network generates a random output, representing a movement direction; some external process may then compute the resulting location and distance from the goal. If the goal is now closer than it was at the start of the trial, the network weights are updated to increase the likelihood that, next time the network is in the same initial position, it will make the same move. If the goal is farther away, then the weights

(A)

(B)

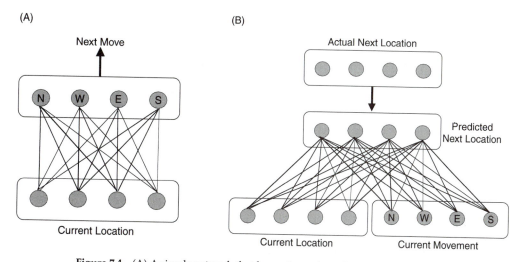

Figure 7.4   (A) A simple network that learns to navigate. Inputs represent the contextual cues that are available at the current location. Outputs represent possible next moves (typically, a movement of one step in the north, west, south, or east direction). Only one output may be active at a time. If a reward is encountered, the weights are adapted to increase the probability of making the same movement the next time that location is encountered. This general format can be made more sophisticated in a number of ways: The inputs can be extended to include additional information about head direction and egocentric coordinates, the implementation can be mapped onto various brain regions, and so on. The basic principle still remains that responses are made by allowing contextual information about spatial location to accrue direct associative strength. (B) A slightly more sophisticated network that learns to predict the next location in a spatial navigation task. Inputs represent the current location and the current movement; outputs represent the predicted next location. This is compared to the actual next location, and weights are updated accordingly. If the network is allowed to "imagine" the expected results of each possible movement, another module can choose between possible movements on the basis of which generates the most desirable next expected location (e.g., closest to goal). This network can also act as a sequence generator if the predicted next location is fed back into the inputs to generate further predicted next locations. With enough iterations, the network may generate an entire path from the current location to the goal location.

are updated to increase the chances that the network will choose a different move next time. When the network is fully trained, it can accept a single location as input and generate a movement trajectory leading to the goal.

Figure 7.4B shows a related spatial navigation network, which takes inputs coding both the current location and the current move and learns to predict the next location.[16] If the network is allowed to experiment with different moves, it can "imagine" the effects of each possible movement and determine which results in an expected next location that is closest to the goal. This kind of network is not limited to spatial learning, but can also perform general sequence learning, mapping from one state to output that predicts the next state.*[17]

Networks such as those shown in figures 7.4A and 7.4B allow tonic contextual cues representing place to enter into direct associations with outputs that can be used to guide behavioral responses—either directly (figure 7.4A) or indirectly (figure 7.4B). Such networks largely ignore the occasion-setting properties of context, by which context can influence stimulus-response learning without itself accruing associative strength.

Combining the Associative and Occasion-Setting Properties of Context

Section 7.2A reviewed some computational models that focus on the *associative* properties of context: namely, the ability of tonic contextual cues to enter into associations if they are reliable predictors of reinforcement. This is distinct from the *occasion-setting* properties of context, whereby context is used to disambiguate competing responses to a stimulus. The associational processes appear to survive hippocampal-region damage, while the occasion-setting properties of context may depend on the hippocampal region. Apparently, these two contextual processes are separable and may be instantiated in different locations within the brain.

Our cortico-hippocampal model (figure 7.5) is also a two-process model, which proposes that *associational* CS-US learning is mediated by extrahippocampal substrates, while some kinds of *representational* CS-CS learning may require the involvement of the hippocampal region. To the extent that tonic contextual cues enter into associative learning, they are no different from any other CS, and so this kind of learning is based in the cortico/cerebellar network within the model.

For example, the background contextual cues are present not only when the US arrives, but also during long intertrial intervals when the US is *not* present. In contrast, a phasic cue that is present only just before US arrival is a much better predictor of the US. Because all cues (phasic and tonic) compete for associative strength, phasic CSs usually accrue associations at the expense of tonic contextual cues.

---

*These spatial navigation networks are interesting as computational devices that can be used to guide robot movements, but there is also a neurobiological tie-in. There are neurons in the hippocampus that respond when an animal is in a particular region of space. These neurons, called place cells, may provide the kind of information needed as input to the networks shown in figure 7.4. Thus these networks provide one possible interpretation of how place cells might be exploited in the brain. For a fuller discussion of place cells in the brain, see O'Keefe, 1979, Kubie & Ranck, 1983; Taube, 1991; Redish, 1999.

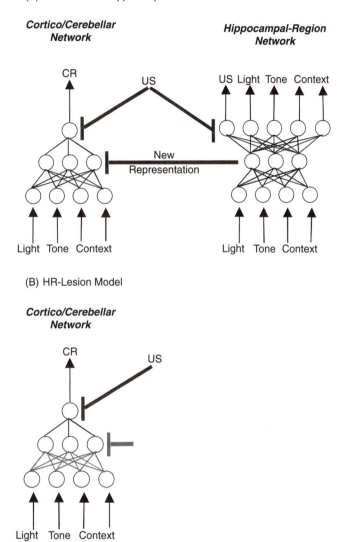

Figure 7.5 The cortico-hippocampal model, as introduced in section 5.2D, instantiates two kinds of contextual processing. In the intact model (A), the hippocampal-region network forms new stimulus representations that include information about all co-occurring cues, including the context in which a phasic CS occurs. Thus, it can implement contextual occasion-setting. At the same time, contextual cues are free to enter into associations with the US if they are the best available predictors of that US. This ability of the context to enter into direct associations with the US can occur in both the hippocampal-region and cortico/cerebellar networks. In the HR-lesion model (B), the occasion-setting properties of context are lost, but context can still enter into direct associations with the US.

However, in the absence of phasic CSs that reliably predict the US, contextual cues will compete for associative strength (refer to figure 7.1). If the US occasionally occurs in context X but never in context Y, both the intact and HR-lesion models will show stronger responding in X than in Y (figure 7.6A).[18] Similarly, both intact and hippocampal-lesioned rats can learn to make a conditioned response more often in context X than context Y (figure 7.6B).[19]

On the other hand, the hippocampal-region network contains representational processes in which the representation of any cue is affected by all the other cues—phasic and tonic—with which it co-occurs. Because of this, tonic contextual cues can develop occasion-setting properties and be used to disambiguate the meaning of phasic CSs. *Thus, our cortico-hippocampal model provides a way to reconcile the associational and occasion-setting properties of context without requiring any special treatment of context.*[20] Because the contextual occasion-setting processes are localized within the hippocampal-region

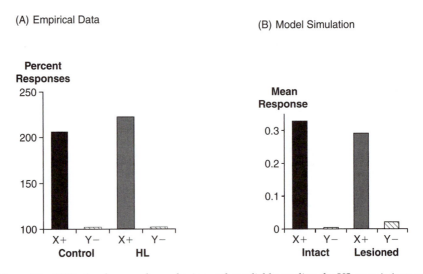

Figure 7.6   (A) In the absence of any phasic cue that reliably predicts the US, associations can be formed directly between context and US. One example is a situation in which a food US often arrives in context X but never in context Y. Normal rats will learn to approach the food cup more often in context X than in context Y. Hippocampal-lesioned (HL) rats show the same discrimination. Responses are plotted as a percentage of mean responding in context Y: typically about 2.5 to 3.5 responses per minute. (Plotted from mean response rate data reported in Honey & Good, 1993.) (B) The cortico-hippocampal model shows similar behavior, with both the intact and HR-lesion models giving a stronger response in context X than in context Y. After extended training, the strength of the response in X will be related to the frequency of US arrival in X compared to the total time spent in X. (Taken from Myers & Gluck, 1994, figure 5C.)

network, they do not occur in the HR-lesion model. This is consistent with animal data demonstrating that hippocampal-lesioned animals are generally less sensitive to the effects of context on learned CS-US associations. Two examples of this effect occur in the behavioral paradigms of context shift and latent inhibition, which will be discussed in the next section.

Context Shift Effects.   As we noted in section 7.1, an intact animal that is trained to give a strong response to a cue in one experimental context X will often show a decrement in responding when that cue is presented in a different experimental context Y, as is illustrated in figure 7.7A.[21] Our intact cortico-hippocampal model shows a similar response decrement after context shift (figure 7.7B).[22] Initially, the presentation of a tone cue in context X (tone&X+) and X-alone (X−) may evoke a very similar internal-layer representation in the hippocampal-region network, since the inputs overlap a great deal.

However, since tone&X+ and X− are to be associated with very different responses, the hippocampal-region network generates representations that are very distinct and overlap little (figure 7.8A,B). Once this is done, it is fairly trivial for the upper layer of weights to be set so that the representation

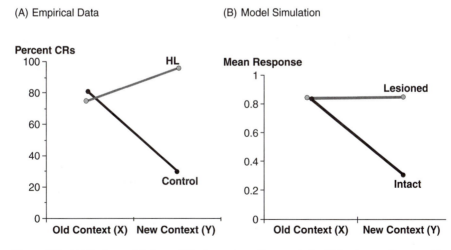

Figure 7.7   (A) In the eyeblink conditioning preparation, control rabbits show a decrement in responding when the trained cue is presented in a novel context X. Hippocampal lesion (HL) eliminates this response decrement after context shift. (Data plotted from results in Penick & Solomon, 1991.) (B) The cortico-hippocampal model shows similar behavior: The intact model but not the HR-lesion model shows decreased responding in the novel context. (Adapted from Gluck & Myers, 1994, figure 3A.)

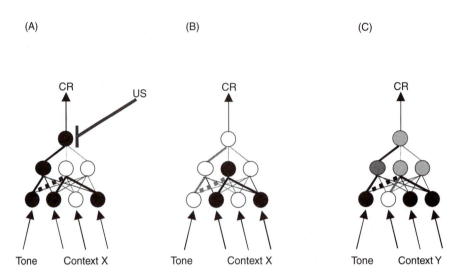

Figure 7.8 Contextual learning in the intact cortico-hippocampal model. (For simplicity, only the cortico/cerebellar network is shown.) Dark circles represent active nodes, lighter circles are more weakly activated nodes, and white circles represent inactive nodes. The network has been trained that a phasic cue, a tone, in context X predicts the US but context X alone does not. Internal-layer representations evolve that differentiate the tone&X inputs and X-alone inputs. (A) Tone&X activates a particular representation (strongly activating the leftmost internal-layer node but inhibiting the center one), and this representation is in turn mapped to a conditioned response. (B) When context X is presented alone, a different representation is activated. (C) The tone is presented in a new context Y, which shares some features with X. Elements of the representation of tone&X are weakly activated, and other nodes may be partially activated too, depending on their preexisting (fixed) connections with the input nodes encoding Y. The resulting representation may cause some output activity, but this is typically weaker than the robust conditioned response produced by tone&X.

of tone&X+, when activated, causes a strong response, while the representation of X− does not.

Now suppose that the tone is presented in a different context Y (figure 7.8C). The new stimulus tone&Y will activate a different subset of internal-layer nodes than tone&X; this in turn will mean that tone&Y will evoke a weaker response than tone&X. Thus, the intact model shows decreased responding when a trained cue is presented in a novel context. In this case, context modulates the response to a cue without itself accruing associative strength: Context X-alone does not evoke any kind of behavioral response in the absence of the tone cue.

The situation is quite different for the HR-lesion model. Recall that the HR-lesion model has only a cortico/cerebellar network and the internal-layer representations are not adapted. Thus, initially, tone&X and X-alone generate some random activity patterns in the internal layer nodes, and these representations are not adapted. Since there is high overlap between the inputs encoding tone&X and X-alone, there will generally be high overlap between their internal-layer representations too (figure 7.9A,B). The network must learn to ignore those common elements and strongly weight associations to the output node from the internal-layer nodes that are activated by tone&X but not by X-alone. In this way, tone&X generates a CR, but X-alone does not. In effect, the network learns to completely ignore context and respond on the basis of whether the tone is present. When the tone is presented in a new context Y (figure 7.9C), context is still ignored, and the usual CR is generated. Thus, the HR-lesion model shows little decrement in responding after a context shift (figure 7.7B).[23] Consistent with this account, there is no decrement in responding after a context shift in hippocampal-lesioned animals (figure 7.7A).[24]

Latent Inhibition.   Latent inhibition is a behavioral paradigm in which unreinforced exposure to a stimulus, such as a tone, can retard later learning

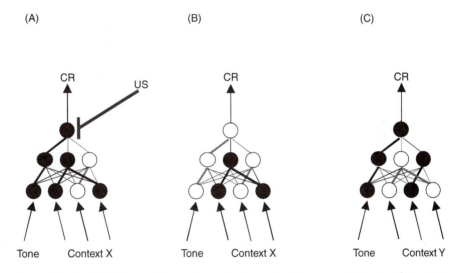

Figure 7.9   The HR-lesion model cannot construct new stimulus representations to differentiate tone&X from X alone. Whatever (fixed) representation is evoked by tone&X (A) will be partially activated by X alone too (B). To solve the task of responding only when A is present, the network must learn to strengthen weights from exactly those elements of the representation that are activated by tone&X but not by X alone. In effect, the system learns to ignore the context and focus only on whether the CS is present. Then, if the tone is presented in a new context Y (C), the network is relatively oblivious to this change, since the context has already been largely ignored. The result is that the lesioned system shows little or no decrement in responding when a trained cue is presented in a novel context.

about that stimulus. One way of interpreting latent inhibition is in terms of context exposure whereby exposure to a tone in context X (tone&X−, X−) retards subsequent acquisition of a response to that stimulus (tone&X+, X−).

Latent inhibition has been extensively studied in animals and humans with various forms of brain lesion and under various pharmacological agents. There are probably several substrates in the brain, all of which may contribute to the effect. One important contribution to latent inhibition appears to be attention: During the exposure phase, subjects learn to "tune out" the cue, which makes it harder to later acquire associations involving that cue. This attentional effect is beyond the scope of the cortico-hippocampal model. However, it is an important issue, given that latent inhibition is indeed disrupted in subjects who have attentional disorders (such as schizophrenia) or have been given attention-altering drugs (such as amphetamine).[25]

The cortico-hippocampal model provides an alternative, representational account of latent inhibition. During the first exposure phase (tone&X−, X−), neither the tone nor the context X predicts any salient future events. As the hippocampal-region network forms new representations, it tends to compress the tone and X, since they frequently co-occur and do not predict different outcomes. In effect, the network treats the tone as an occasionally occurring feature of the context X. In the second acquisition phase (tone&X+, X−), the network must differentiate the representations of tone&X and X if it is to learn to map one to a conditioned response and the other to no response.

This differentiation takes time, retarding learning relative to a condition in which there was no prior exposure to the tone and hence no compression of the tone and X to undo. Thus, in the intact model, after 100 trials of tone&X+ and X−, simulations that received exposure only to the context are already giving strong (0.8) responses to tone&X; in contrast, simulations that received exposure to tone&X− and X− are giving much weaker responses to tone&X (figure 7.10B).[26]

Because these representational processes depend on the hippocampal-region network, no latent inhibition is produced by the lesioned model (figure 7.10B). This is consistent with data showing attenuation or elimination of latent inhibition in animals with hippocampal-region damage (figure 7.10A).[27] More recent data have shown that various substructures of the hippocampal region may contribute differentially to latent inhibition; we will return to this issue in chapter 9.

Our cortico-hippocampal model also has several implications for latent inhibition in intact systems. For example, since latent inhibition is assumed to reflect representational compression of the tone and context X during the exposure phase, our model expects that the effect should be context

Latent Inhibition

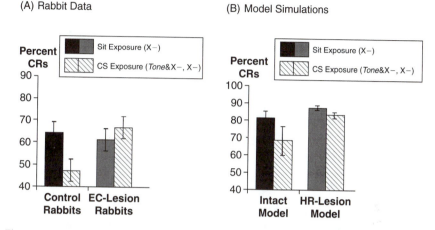

Figure 7.10 (A) In the rabbit eyeblink preparation, control rabbits show latent inhibition: Animals are slower to learn a response to a cue A following unreinforced exposure to a tone, relative to a Sit Exposure group that received equivalent exposure to the context X alone. Hippocampal-region damage can attenuate or eliminate latent inhibition, so exposure does not retard subsequent learning. (Plotted from data presented in Shohamy, Allen, & Gluck, 1999.) (B) The model shows a similar latent inhibition effect: In the intact model, unreinforced exposure to the tone slows subsequent learning compared to simulations that received equivalent amounts of exposure to the context alone; the lesioned model does not show the latent inhibition effect (Myers & Gluck, 1994). Note that the hippocampal region is only one of several substrates implicated in latent inhibition, which may be one reason why latent inhibition is more robust in the intact animal than in the intact model.

sensitive.[28] Thus, if exposure takes place in context X but acquisition takes place in context Y, there should be a release from latent inhibition, as is seen in figure 7.11. There is now good evidence that latent inhibition is similarly reduced by a context shift in rats and in humans.[29]

In a similar fashion, the cortico-hippocampal model shows disrupted latent inhibition if there is an intervening exposure to the context alone between exposure and acquisition phases (figure 7.11).[30] During the context-exposure period, the hippocampal-region network continues to update its representations. Since the context continues to appear without the tone, the tone gradually disappears from the representation of context. Given enough time, the representations of the tone and context will be redifferentiated, eliminating the compression that gives rise to latent inhibition. Empirical

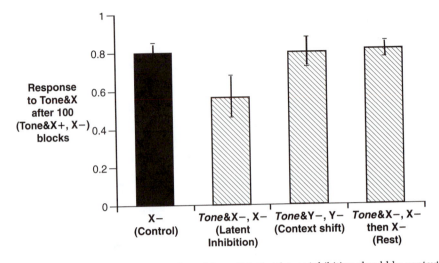

Figure 7.11   The cortico-hippocampal model predicts that latent inhibition should be context sensitive. Prior exposure to the stimulus (tone&X−, X−) results in slower learning to respond to tone&X+ than a control condition that received exposure to the context alone: the latent inhibition effect. However, if there is a context shift between phases, the latent inhibition effect disappears: tone&Y−, Y− exposure does not slow tone&X+, X− learning relative to the control condition. Normal animals do show such a release from latent inhibition following context shift (Lubow, Rifkin, & Alek, 1976; Hall & Honey, 1989). Similarly, exposure to the context alone between exposure and training phases eliminates the latent inhibition effect. A similar effect may also occur in animal conditioning, though further studies are indicated to test this prediction. (Adapted from Myers & Gluck, 1994, figure 4.)

data on this question are mixed: Many animal studies found that adding context-alone trials between exposure and acquisition can reduce latent inhibition, but another careful study found no such effect.[31] One study in humans found that a delay between exposure and training phases did not affect latent inhibition, but here the delay between training phases lasted only 120 seconds; possibly, a longer duration delay would be needed to show the effect.[32]

Finally, the cortico-hippocampal model predicts that overexposure to a cue may eliminate latent inhibition. For example, during ordinary exposure, the tone and the context X are equally unpredictive of any future salient event, and so their representations are compressed together. However, the hippocampal-region network is not only learning to predict the US; it is also learning to reconstruct its inputs including cue and contextual information. This means that on tone&X− trials, the hippocampal-region network should reconstruct the tone and X, while on X− trials, it should reconstruct X alone. Therefore, although the presence of the tone may not signal the US, it does signal that tone should appear in the hippocampal-region network's outputs. For this reason, although there is a bias to compress the tone and X on the basis of their nonprediction of the US, there is a competing bias to differentiate the representations of the tone and X. With enough exposure, the hippocampal-region network will develop representations that do indeed differentiate the tone and X somewhat. At this point, latent inhibition will be abolished. We are aware of one study directly addressing this issue in rabbit eyeblink conditioning; the results showed that overexposure to the CS could reduce the latent inhibition effect, just as predicted.[33]

Thus, the representational processes in Gluck and Myers's cortico-hippocampal model appear sufficient to address a broad range of latent inhibition data. Like the other contextual effects, this is accomplished without giving context any special status: All cues, including context and phasic CSs, color the representation of all co-occurring cues. The model does not address the attentional explanation of latent inhibition. However, the representational and attentional explanations of latent inhibition are in no way mutually exclusive. Both may operate in parallel in the normal brain, producing similar latent inhibition effects for different reasons. More likely, the two mechanisms may cooperate.

The brain substrates that are believed to underlie the attentional component of latent inhibition—particularly the nucleus accumbens[34]—have reciprocal connections with the hippocampal region. In fact, it makes a certain amount of intuitive sense that the two systems would cooperate: Attention may be important in deciding which cues are emphasized or deemphasized within the hippocampal representation, while the hippocampus can help to detect novel cue configurations that are worthy of engaging attention.[35]

Occasion-Setting Properties of Phasic Cues

Occasion-setting is the ability to modulate responding without directly entering into associations with a US. Context is not the only kind of stimulus that can function as an occasion-setter. Peter Holland and others have documented the circumstances under which phasic cues can become occasion-setters.[36] For example, in ordinary **conditioned inhibition,** a cue (light+) predicts the US, while the compound (tone&light−) predicts no US (figure 7.12A). Normally, on light&tone trials, light and tone co-occur. However, if tone precedes light (figure 7.12B), then the presence or absence of tone determines the correct response to light. This kind of task is sometimes called a **feature-negative discrimination.** Similarly, in a **feature-positive discrimination,** light preceded by a cue (odor) predicts the US, while light alone predicts no US (figure 7.12C). In these cases, the tone and odor cues are

(A) Conditioned Inhibition

Light+ Trials

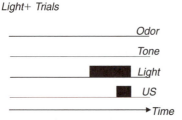

Tone&Light− Trials

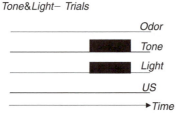

(C) Feature Positive (FP)

Light− Trials

Odor

Tone

Light

US

Time

Odor → Light+ Trials

Odor

Tone

Light

US

Time

(B) Feature Negative (FN)

Light+ Trials

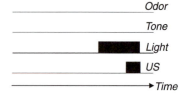

Tone→Light− Trials

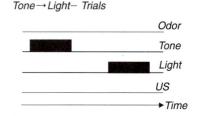

(D) Simultaneous FN/FP

Tone→Light− Trials

Odor

Tone

Light

US

Time

Odor → Light+ Trials

Odor

Tone

Light

US

Time

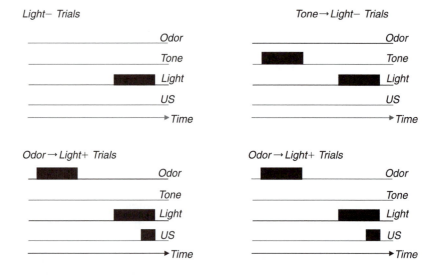

Figure 7.12 Occasion-setting with phasic cues. (A) In a conditioned inhibition paradigm, a CS (light) is reinforced when it occurs alone but not when it co-occurs with a second CS (tone). (B) In the feature-negative (FN) paradigm, light is reinforced when alone but not when preceded by tone. (C) In the feature-positive (FP) paradigm, light is reinforced when preceded by a cue (odor) but not when presented alone. (D) The FN and FP discriminations can be presented simultaneously so that light is reinforced when preceded by one cue (odor) but not by a second cue (tone). Unreinforced presentations of the individual cues (light, tone, and odor) may also be interspersed to ensure that the subject is not learning simple associations between tone or odor and reinforcement.

occasion-setters, which determine the correct response to light, although they themselves do not enter into direct association with the US.[37]

In at least one study, animals with hippocampal lesions could learn simultaneous feature-positive and feature-negative discriminations as well as controls; in fact, under some circumstances, the lesioned animals even showed facilitated learning.[38] This particular study used a lesion technique that destroys hippocampus and dentate gyrus but not nearby structures such as entorhinal cortex; it may be the case that broader hippocampal-region damage would indeed disrupt learning. Another study found that, while a selective lesion of the hippocampus did not disrupt feature-positive learning, a broader lesion that included nearby brain structures did indeed disrupt learning.[39] Clearly, further study is needed to resolve this issue. However, on the basis of the limited existing data, it appears that the hippocampus is not always needed for occasion-setting using phasic cues.

This in turn suggests that what is disrupted following hippocampal damage is specifically the ability to use context as an occasion-setter; this again points to a critical dependence of contextual processing on hippocampal-region mediation.

7.3   RELATIONSHIP OF COMPUTATIONAL MODELS TO QUALITATIVE THEORIES

Several prominent theories of hippocampal-region function focus on contextual processing. Hirsh and others have suggested that contextual processing is the hippocampus's chief role.[40] Our cortico-hippocampal model suggests a way in which the hippocampal region could contribute to contextual occasion-setting without having to define this as the region's special purpose. Context acts to mediate between competing responses to a cue by virtue of its inclusion in stimulus representations. This is no different from the way in which all (tonic and phasic) cues mediate the representations of all cues with which they co-occur.

Thus, there is no special treatment of context in our model; nevertheless, the model can account for a wide range of contextual phenomena. A similar argument can be made for spatial mapping: Place is simply one specialized form of context, consisting of a configuration of local views of space.[41] Thus, the devastating spatial impairment seen after hippocampal-region damage is really only a task-specific effect of disrupted contextual processes. Of course, in an animal such as the rat that depends heavily on spatial navigation, it is an especially visible effect.

A somewhat different view of contextual occasion-setting has been set forth by Mark Bouton and colleagues after years of elegant empirical studies examining the nature of contextual processing.[42] One of the most telling results to emerge from Bouton's lab is the contextual sensitivity of extinction. In one example, a CS is paired with shock in one context (context X) and then extinguished in another context (context Y); when the CS is again presented in context X, the response is renewed.[43] Various manipulations have shown that this effect cannot be ascribed simply to direct excitatory associations between context X and the US (or direct inhibitory associations between context Y and the US). The most parsimonious explanation seems to be that there are two associations: CS-US and CS-noUS; the context determines which response is retrieved.[44] During initial training, a CS-US association is created in context X (figure 7.13A); subsequently, during extinction, a CS-noUS association is created in context Y (figure 7.13B). At this point, the

(A) CS-US learning in context X

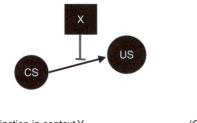

(B) Extinction in context Y   (C) Renewal in context X

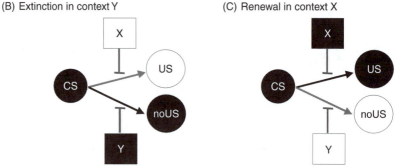

Figure 7.13 An account of extinction and renewal that involves contextual occasion-setting (Bouton, 1991). (A) Original learning that a CS predicts the US occurs in one context X. That context modulates the CS-US association but does not itself become associated with the US. (B) Subsequent extinction in context Y involves the development of a new association between CS and noUS. That association is retrieved during extinction training in context Y, making it appear as if the earlier CS-US learning has been extinguished. (C) However, if the CS is presented back in context X, the original association is retrieved, and the responding to CS is renewed. Thus, the context modulates which of the competing associations to CS is retrieved.

CS-US association learned in X has not disappeared, even though there is no responding to the CS in context Y. When the animal is returned to context X, the original CS-US association is retrieved, and the response "spontaneously" reappears (figure 7.13C).

We noted in chapter 6 that the cortico-hippocampal model does not adequately address extinction. When trained to give a response to a CS (tone+), this response can be eliminated by extinction trials (tone−). However, what the model does in this case is simply unlearn the response to the tone, setting the weights from the internal representation to the output nodes to zero. The model does not adequately learn a second, CS-noUS association, as is shown in figure 7.13.

It is possible that simple addition of multiple output nodes in the cortico/cerebellar and hippocampal-region networks would alleviate this problem, allowing internal representations to activate either a US or a noUS output. The particular representation that is activated on a current trial would depend not only on the CS, but also on the context, and thus context would affect the response retrieved in much the way Bouton and colleagues have suggested. If this is the case, there may be little theoretical difference between Bouton's theory of contextual occasion-setting and that embodied in our cortico-hippocampal model. Importantly, in Bouton's theory, as in the model, there is no qualitative difference in the ability of contextual cues and phasic CSs to operate as occasion-setters.[45]

There is some evidence that this kind of contextual modulation of extinction is dependent on the hippocampus and that various conditions that lead to renewal of an extinguished response in normal animals do not cause renewal in animals with hippocampal-region damage.[46] However, the data are mixed, and further study is needed to tease out the conditions under which hippocampal-lesioned animals may or may not show renewal of extinguished responding.

Another interesting aspect of the body of empirical studies amassed by Bouton and colleagues is their finding that, generally, there is no response decrement after context shift.[47] This is in contrast to the findings reported in the above section (refer to figure 7.7), but occasionally, other researchers have similarly failed to find a context shift effect.[48]

One factor that contributes to these conflicting results may simply be differential sensitivity to different kinds of contextual cues among different animals;[49] thus, some animal paradigms might be more likely than others to show context effects. Another possibility is that contextual dependence is increased when phasic CSs are poor predictors of the US.[50] Thus, if a CS only sometimes predicts US arrival, animals are more likely to respond to the context alone;[51] interestingly, this effect is disrupted by hippocampal lesion.[52]

Our cortico-hippocampal model suggests a third factor that may contribute to contextual sensitivity of learned associations; as usual, this possibility may operate in parallel with the other factors suggested above. In the model, contextual sensitivity is a function of training time. It was mentioned above that latent inhibition in the model can be reduced by overexposure; it turns out that contextual sensitivity can be similarly affected by overtraining. Early in training, the hippocampal-region network is constrained to compress co-occurring cues; if a CS is always presented in a particular context X, then the features of X become part of the representation of the CS. However, *compression* is not the only bias constraining representations; there is also a constraint to *differentiate* the representations of stimuli that are useful predictors of future reinforcement. If the CS is the best predictor of US arrival, its representation should be differentiated from that of all other stimuli—including contextual stimuli. As a result, with extensive training, the representation of the CS may actually include less information about context. As a result, overtraining of a response to a CS will gradually decrease the amount of response decrement after context shift (figure 7.14).

In animal paradigms, different kinds of discrimination are learned at widely varying rates; an animal may acquire a conditioned fear response within a single trial, an odor discrimination within a few dozen trials, and a conditioned eyeblink response within a few hundred trials. If, as the model suggests, context sensitivity is reduced with overtraining, the exact number of trials required to eliminate contextual sensitivity may depend on the exact paradigm. However, there should still be a general trend to less context sensitivity with more training.

In 1994, we conducted a literature review and found this principle to hold across studies.[53] For example, rat conditioned suppression involves a hungry rat that is engaged in pressing a lever to obtain food; when a shock US appears, the animal briefly freezes, reducing (or suppressing) its normal fast rate of lever pressing. If a tone or light CS is paired with the US, the animal will come to suppress responding in the presence of the CS, anticipating US arrival. The degree of suppression to the CS is one measure of how well the CS-US association is learned. Conditioned suppression tends to be learned fairly quickly; most rats learn to suppress responding in the presence of the CS after only a few trials.[54] In this preparation, the response decrement effect occurs if the context is shifted after a single training trial[55] but not after 15–23 training trials.[56] In a slower preparation, rabbit eyeblink conditioning, the response decrement effect is seen even if the context is shifted after more

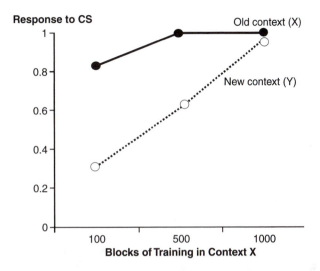

Figure 7.14 The cortico-hippocampal model predicts that contextual sensitivity may be reduced or eliminated by overtraining. After training to respond to a CS in one context X for 100 trials, the intact model develops a strong CR; if that CS is then presented in a novel context Y, the response drops dramatically. However, after 500 training trials in context X, there is less of a decrement in responding when the CS is presented in Y. After overtraining (1000 trials), there is no decrement in responding when the CS is presented in Y: The learned response is no longer context-sensitive. The model thus predicts that overtraining may similarly eliminate the response decrement with context shift in animal preparations. However, the precise amount of training that constitutes overtraining may vary, especially given that different kinds of learning are acquired at different speeds (e.g., it may take 40–70 trials to acquire a conditioned response but only one trial to acquire a fear response). (Adapted from Myers & Gluck, 1994, figure 3B.)

than 600 training trials;[57] the cortico-hippocampal model suggests that with enough overtraining, even this effect should disappear. Currently, our prediction of parametric sensitivity remains to be explicitly tested; however, we are aware of no data that contradict the prediction that a context shift will affect responding early in training but not after overtraining.

7.4 IMPLICATIONS FOR HUMAN MEMORY AND MEMORY DISORDERS

Just as Eichenbaum and colleagues describe their hippocampal-lesioned rats as "inflexible,"[58] Daniel Schacter has noted that humans with MT amnesia often seem inflexible or "hyperspecific" in their learning.[59] Although amnesic subjects may be able to acquire new information, they are often unable to express that learning if test conditions differ significantly from learning conditions. For example, in one paper, Schacter and colleagues recount a study of an amnesic individual who was first read a list of little-known facts.[60] A few minutes later, he retained a few of them but generally forgot where he had heard them. He claimed that he guessed the answers or read about them in a magazine. By contrast, control subjects recall most of the facts—and also that they learned them in the course of the experiment. Thus, one important aspect of learning in amnesic individuals is an inability to remember the context in which information was acquired, a condition that is sometimes called **source amnesia.**[61]

The idea of contextual occasion-setting schematized in figure 7.13 also has implications for how to improve learning in amnesic subjects. Figure 7.13B suggests that a single CS can be associated with multiple outcomes (US or noUS) and multiple responses (CR or noCR) and that context helps to disambiguate which of these is appropriate at the present time. If an amnesic individual cannot use context in this way, then a single CS will be associated with multiple outcomes and responses, and there is no easy way to determine which is currently appropriate. The default may simply be to choose the most recent or most often-repeated response rather than the one that is appropriate in the current context.

This may account for the finding that amnesic subjects are often disproportionately impaired at reversing a trained discrimination.[62] Typically, amnesic subjects (and hippocampal-lesioned animals) can learn to respond to one stimulus A+ but not a second stimulus B− as well as controls; the problem comes when it is time to acquire responses to A and B that compete with the old ones: An old association between A and the US conflicts with a newer one in which A predicts noUS. Control subjects may be able to interpret the two phases of the experiment as different "contexts": The response that was appropriate in the old context is no longer appropriate now. Without this contextual occasion-setting, amnesic subjects have a hard time favoring the newly developing A-noUS association in preference to the older, well-established A-US one. The result is that reversal may be very hard indeed.

This kind of interference may be a very general phenomenon. During most discrimination learning, there is a period of trial and error in which there are some correct responses and some incorrect responses. In normal subjects, the correct responses eventually win out, and the incorrect responses are suppressed; but in amnesic subjects, the incorrect responses may be much more able to compete, hindering learning. An amnesic subject's impairment in learning may therefore not only reflect absolute task difficulty, but also how many errors were made during learning—and thus how much interference was generated.[63]

One way to ameliorate the interference may be to reduce the likelihood that competing responses develop in the first place. One way to do this is through a technique, developed by Herb Terrace, called **errorless learning.**[64] In errorless learning, the subject is prevented from making incorrect responses (or is guided toward making correct ones). For example, Terrace used errorless learning techniques to train pigeons to peck at a red light but not a green light to obtain food reward (for pigeons, this is a very difficult task to learn).[65] First, the experimenter turned on the red light and waited for the pigeons to randomly peck in the vicinity of the light; when they did, they obtained a food reward. The procedure was repeated many times, until the pigeons came to peck at the red light fairly reliably. Next, the experimenter would wait until the pigeons were not in a good position to peck and then briefly darken the red key. Slowly, the experimenter lengthened the amount of time the key was darkened and also gradually changed the color from red to green. The pigeons came to associate the red light with food and the green light with no food. Eventually, after many such trials, the experimenter could flick the light from red to green no matter where in the cage the birds were; the pigeons would peck only while the key was red. In this way, the pigeons were trained to discriminate red from green—all without ever having made a single erroneous response to the green key.

The same basic errorless learning strategy can be applied to humans.[66] One application is in the stem completion task. In the learning phase, subjects are shown a list of stems (e.g., "TH___") that can each be completed in a variety of ways to form common five-letter English words. Subjects are asked to guess the correct completion for each stem (e.g., "THUMB"). Often, of course, the subject will guess incorrectly (e.g., "THINK," "THING," "THANK"). If the subject does not guess correctly within four tries, the experimenter gives the correct answer. The process is repeated several times with the same list of word stems until the subject reliably generates the correct completion for each word stem. Next comes a testing phase, containing questions of the form: "One of the words you saw before began with TH. Can you remember what the word was?" Under these conditions, normal control subjects can correctly recall 60–80% of the studied words. Amnesic subjects achieve only some 30% correct, even if the testing phase comes immediately after the end of the learning phase.[67]

However, given an errorless version of the same task, amnesic performance improves considerably. In this version, subjects do not have to guess the word stem completions but are told that the correct completion for "TH___" is "THUMB." This prevents subjects from making any mistakes (incorrect guesses) during the learning phase. This errorless learning improves control subjects' performance on the testing phase: They now get 80–100% correct. Performance of amnesic subjects reaches as high as 70% correct—almost as good as control subjects.[68] Apparently, preventing the amnesic subjects from making mistakes during learning somehow improves their ability to retain that information.

The same technique of errorless learning may be fruitful in more realistic situations. For example, a similar method was used to help a man with profound anterograde amnesia learn to program an electronic memory aid, even though he had completely failed to master this skill using normal (trial-and-error) learning techniques.[69]

SUMMARY

• Context—the tonic environmental stimuli, both external and internal—can and does affect what is learned.

• Some contextual learning involves direct associations between contextual cues and reinforcement (US). This kind of contextual processing can be described by the Rescorla-Wagner model and appears to be hippocampal-independent.

• Some contextual learning appears to involve contextual occasion-setting, in which context determines which of several competing responses to a stimulus should be retrieved. This kind of contextual processing appears to depend on the hippocampal region. It can be modeled by allowing context to influence CS-US associations but not itself enter into associations with the US.

• The cortico-hippocampal model assumes that all cues (including context) are part of the representation of all other cues with which they co-occur. In this way, context can affect the representations of CSs without itself requiring special representational status. The cortico-hippocampal model can show both context-US learning and contextual occasion-setting and assumes that the latter depends on hippocampal-region representational changes.

• Phasic cues (CSs) can also operate as occasion-setters; it appears that this kind of occasion-setting may survive hippocampal-region damage, meaning that contextual occasion-setting is selectively dependent on the hippocampal region.

• Hippocampal-region damage may eliminate the ability to use context to discriminate between competing responses to a stimulus. This in turn may imply that amnesic individuals are especially susceptible to interference from trials in which they made erroneous responses, as these errors will compete with memories of the correct response. Errorless learning may be a useful technique for reducing this interference.

8   Stimulus Representation in Cortex

The computational models of hippocampus discussed in previous chapters have considered the role of the hippocampal region in stimulus representation and memory. However, most of these models acknowledge that the hippocampus does not operate as an isolated structure. Any information processed by the hippocampus must eventually be transferred to other brain areas for long-term storage. Models of hippocampal consolidation make this point explicitly, but our cortico-hippocampal model[1] also assumes that representations developed in the hippocampal region are eventually adopted by other brain areas such as the cortex and cerebellum.

Most of the models that we have discussed so far assume that the hippocampal region operates directly on sensory input (such as CSs). This is also an oversimplification. The hippocampal region is the culmination of a long and intricate processing chain. Sensory inputs from receptors such as retinal transducers and taste buds travel through the thalamus and into areas of cerebral cortex that are specifically devoted to processing different kinds of sensory information. From there, information travels to higher cortical areas, which combine and integrate across sensory modalities, before finally reaching the hippocampal region.

Thus, among its other functions, cerebral cortex preprocesses hippocampal-region inputs. To fully understand what the hippocampal region is doing, it is therefore necessary to have some understanding of its inputs—and hence what the cerebral cortex is doing.

In this chapter, we review some basics of cortical representation. We show how certain types of network models can be related to cortical architecture and physiology. We then present a specific model that combines a cortical module with a hippocampal-region module; with this model, we then explore how these brain systems might interact. Finally, we present an example of how research into cortical representation is leading to a real-world application to help children who are language learning–impaired.

8.1   CORTICAL REPRESENTATION AND PLASTICITY

The cerebral cortex is a grayish sheet covering most of the mammalian brain and containing the cell bodies of neurons. The output processes of these cells, **axons,** form the underlying "white matter" that makes up much of the bulk of the brain in higher species. Most mammalian cortex is only a few millimeters thick but has six distinct layers, each characterized by the presence or absence of various cell types (figure 8.1A). Only mammals have six-layered cortex; reptiles and birds have a simpler kind of cortex—sometimes called **paleocortex** or **allocortex**—with only two layers (figure 8.1B). Six-layer cortex is often called **neocortex** or **isocortex,** reflecting the assumption that it developed later in evolution. However, there are a few places in the mammalian brain that are also two-layered paleocortex, and these may be evolutionary remnants from which neocortex developed.

Although overall brain weight is related to an animal's body size, the cerebral cortex is disproportionately elaborated in higher species. For example, if a rat's brain were enlarged to be the same size as a human brain, many parts would be similar in the two species (figure 8.2). However, the rat's olfactory

(A)   (B)

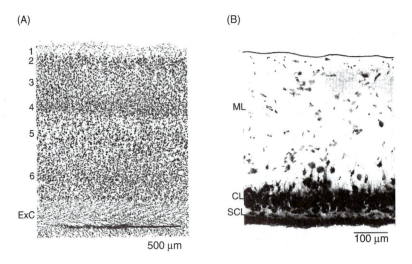

500 μm   100 μm

Figure 8.1   (A) High-power photomicrograph of a slice through mammalian neocortex (rat), showing complex cellular and laminar structure. Cortical layers 1 through 6 are labeled. The top of the figure corresponds to the outer layer of cortex; ExC = external capsule lies below the cortex. The scale bar near the bottom of the picture equals 500 μm. (B) High-power photomicrograph of a slice through reptilian cortex (turtle), showing much simpler two-layered structure. The ridge near the top of the picture is the outer layer of the brain. CL = cellular layer; ML = molecular layer; SCL = subcellular layer (sometimes considered a third layer). The scale bar at the bottom of the picture equals 100 μm. (Reprinted from Zigmond et al., 1999, p. 1289, figure 50.3C,E.)

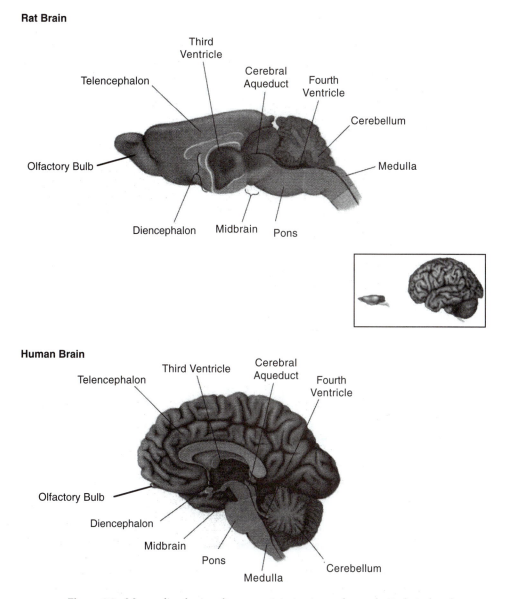

Figure 8.2 Mammalian brains show a variety in size and complexity but also share many features, including the presence of six-layered neocortex. For example, the rat brain (top) and human brain (bottom), drawn to be equivalent in size, show many of the same structures (a few are labeled for comparison). However, different structures are elaborated in different species. The rat's olfactory bulb is disproportionately large relative to the human's, presumably reflecting the importance of olfactory stimuli to the rat. Conversely, neocortex reaches its highest elaboration in humans, resulting in the characteristic wrinkled surface, which allows the large cortical sheet to fit in the confines of the skull. (Adapted from Bear et al., 1996, p. 176, figure 7.21.)

system would be proportionately larger than the human's, while the rat's neocortex would still only be a fraction the size of the human's. The cortex of an adult human would measure about 1.5 square feet if spread out into a flat sheet; the characteristic wrinkled appearance of the human brain reflects the fact that the cortex has to fold to fit inside the confines of the skull. The rat cortex, by contrast, fits quite comfortably inside the rat skull without wrinkles.

Most areas of neocortex share the same basic organizational structure: Tissue from different areas of neocortex looks very similar to that shown in figure 8.1A. However, different areas of neocortex process different kinds of information, and this differentiation arises from the different inputs they receive.[2]

For each sensory modality, the first cortical processing occurs in a specific region: **primary visual cortex** (or **V1**) for vision, **primary auditory cortex** (or **A1**) for sounds, and so on. From there, sensory information progresses to higher sensory areas, which integrate information further, first within and then across modalities. One of the most interesting features of primary sensory cortex is that it is organized **topographically.** That is, *each region of cortex responds preferentially to a particular type of stimulus, and neighboring cortical regions respond to similar stimuli. Thus, it is possible to draw a "map" of sensory space on the cortical surface.*

For example, **primary sensory cortex** (or **S1**) is a thin strip of cortex running down each side of the brain in humans (figure 8.3A). By recording the activity of individual neurons in S1 while touching various areas of the skin, it was found that different neurons respond maximally when different body regions are stimulated. Thus, some cells respond to touch stimulation on a particular finger, some on a region of the face, and so on. If this recording is done for a large number of S1 neurons, it is possible to draw a "map" of the body on S1 so that each body part lies over the cortical region that responds to it (figure 8.3A).

Moreover, adjoining areas of S1 contain cells that tend to respond to adjoining areas of body surface. Parts of the body that are especially sensitive to touch, such as fingers and lips, activate larger areas of S1. The result is a distorted neural representation of the human figure, often called a **homunculus,** with exaggerated hands and lips but a greatly shrunken torso. Primary somatosensory cortex in animals shows similar organization except that the homunculus is replaced by a distorted figure of the species in question, and this figure will be distorted to reflect body areas that are more or less critical for that animal. Thus, primates receive a great deal of touch information through their fingers, so these are disproportionately elaborated in the cortical map, while rats receive a great deal of information from the displacement of their whiskers, so that area is disproportionately represented in a rat's cortical map.

Primary auditory cortex (A1) lies near the top of the temporal lobe in humans and is organized as a topographic map, as shown in figure 8.3B. In A1, however, neurons respond to sound instead of touch stimulation. Adjoining areas of A1 respond to similar tone frequencies in an orderly fashion. Similar maps could be drawn for other primary sensory areas; neighboring areas tend to respond preferentially to similar stimuli. This neat topographic organization of primary sensory cortex seems to be a consistent feature

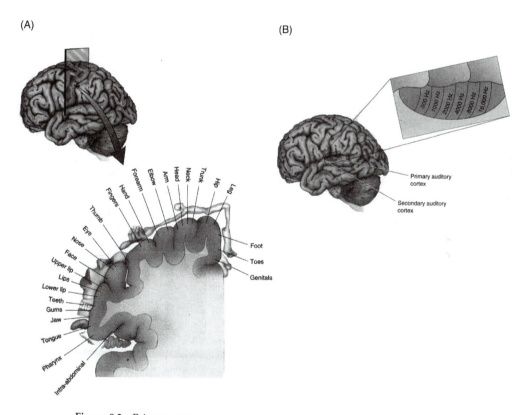

Figure 8.3 Primary sensory areas in mammalian neocortex are organized into topographic maps, meaning that neighboring regions of cortex tend to respond to neighboring stimuli. (A) In primary somatosensory cortex (S1), cells respond to touch stimuli on different parts of the body surface. Neurons in each area are most responsive to the body parts shown above them. These areas are organized into a distorted map of the body, often termed a homunculus. (B) In primary auditory cortex, cells respond to auditory stimuli of different frequencies; adjoining areas respond to similar frequencies. (Reprinted from Bear et al., 1996, figures 12.20 and 11.28.)

across modalities and across mammalian species. The output from primary sensory cortex travels to higher-order cortical areas, where it appears that the obvious topographic ordering may be lost, or else information may simply be coded in a topographic manner that researchers don't yet fully understand.

For many years it was believed that cortical topographic maps were fixed—predominantly hard-wired from birth and subject to fine-tuning only during a **critical period** that extended through the first few months of life. Certainly, the maps are especially plastic at that early period. For instance, in a normal cat, primary visual cortex (V1) contains alternating patches of cells that respond to input from either the left eye or the right eye. If a kitten is reared from birth with its left eye sealed shut, V1 will reorganize accordingly: Proportionally more area will respond to input from the active right eye than from the inactive left eye. Another way of saying this is that the representation of the active eye expands, and the representation of the inactive eye is compressed. If the kitten matures into a cat and the sealed eye is then opened, the visual map in V1 cannot reorganize enough to accommodate the drastic change. The result is that the visual cortex cannot process information from the left eye; the animal will be functionally blind in the left eye, even though that left eye is now fully operational.[3]

However, more recent experimental findings have demonstrated that cortical plasticity can and does occur in adult animals. For example, when a limb is amputated, the part of S1 representing the lost limb is deafferented, meaning that it receives no more sensory input. Rather than allowing that region of cortex to remain idle, nearby areas on the homunculus may "spread" into the vacated space.[4] If two or more fingers are always stimulated together, so that the different fingers always experience exactly the same sensory inputs, the parts of S1 representing those fingers may fuse, so that a single area comes to represent the input from both fingers.[5]

One of the most important findings in this area of research in recent years is that cortical reorganization can occur as a function of learning. In one study, Michael Merzenich and colleagues first mapped out the topographic representations in the area of S1 of the monkey that encodes stimulation to the hand (figure 8.4A).[6] This was done by inserting recording electrodes into various sites in S1 (figure 8.4C) and then stimulating various regions of the hand (figure 8.4B) to see how skin surface mapped to cortical area. The resulting map, shown in figure 8.4D, revealed a neat topography, in which different strips of cortex responded to stimulation of each of the five fingers and within each strip there was an orderly progression from distal sites (fingertips) to proximal sites (near the base of the finger).

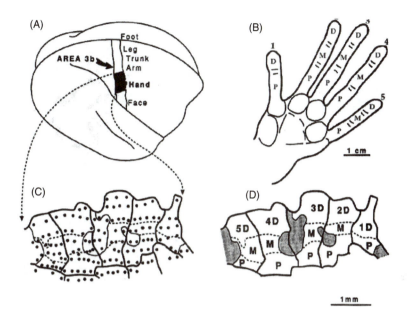

Figure 8.4   (A) The somatosensory cortex of the owl monkey brain contains a small area containing a topographic representation of the hand. (B) The palm of the monkey hand can be divided into areas according to finger (1−5) and site (P = proximal, M = middle, D = distal). (C) Recording electrodes are lowered into S1 at various sites (dots) to record neural activity while different areas of the hand are stimulated. (D) The recordings reveal a topographic map: The five fingers are represented in roughly parallel strips (shown here running from left to right). Within each strip, there is an orderly progression from distal to proximal sites. Dark patches responded to stimulation on the back (hairy side) of the associated finger. The boundary lines in C are drawn to match those discovered in D. (Adapted from Jenkins et al., 1990, figure 1.)

Next, Merzenich and colleagues trained the monkeys for several weeks on a task that required touching a textured spinning disk with the tips of fingers 2 and 3. During training, these fingertips received extensive stimulation in a meaningful context, since the stimulation was associated with obtaining reward. After several weeks, the areas of S1 representing these two fingertips expanded (figure 8.5)—sometimes by a factor of 3.[7] The representations of the other, unstimulated fingers shifted and even shrank to make room for the expanded fingertip representations.

In another study, Merzenich and colleagues considered changes to primary motor cortex (M1), a strip of cerebral cortex that lies just forward of primary sensory cortex (S1). Like S1, M1 is laid out in the form of a homunculus with exaggerated lips and hands. Stimulation of a region in M1 can result in motor movements in the corresponding part of the body. When monkeys

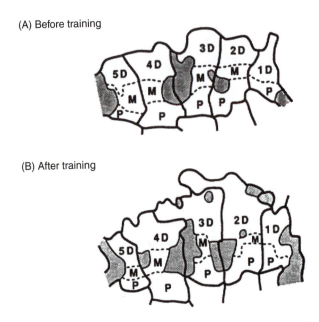

(A) Before training

(B) After training

Figure 8.5 Cortical map reorganization following behavioral training (Jenkins et al., 1990). (A) Hand representation within somatosensory cortex S1 of a normal adult owl monkey shows a regular topographic layout, with two rough axes encoding finger (1–5) and position (P = proximal, M = medial, D = distal). The fields encoding distal portions of each finger are approximately equal in size. (B) After several weeks of training on a behavioral task that involved fine sensory stimulation of the tips of fingers 2 and 3 (and occasionally 4), the map changes. The area encoding the stimulated skin surfaces (2D and 3D) are expanded relative to the other fingers and relative to their own original size (A). The representation of 2D has expanded from 0.32 mm^2 to 0.92 mm^2—nearly a threefold increase; the representations of 3D and 4D increase by about 33% and 25%, respectively. The areas encoding nonstimulated areas have shifted to accommodate these expansions, and the area encoding the nonstimulated finger 5 has shrunk to about 80% of its original size. (Adapted from Jenkins et al., 1990, figure 3B,D.)

were trained on a task requiring skilled use of digits, the M1 representation of those digits expanded, while the amount of space devoted to representation of other, nontrained areas (such as wrist and forearm) shrank.[8]

These and related studies suggest an important principle of cortical plasticity: *The representations of stimuli compete for space in the cortical map.* Stimuli that are important, such as those required to execute a task or those that predict reward, increase their areas of cortical representation, and this expansion occurs at the expense of other, nonpredictive stimuli. The topographic nature of the map in primary sensory cortices is generally preserved during these changes, as is shown in figure 8.5B.

The idea that cortical representations are differentiated and compressed on the basis of the predictive nature of stimuli and whether they co-occur is clearly reminiscent of the representational ideas discussed in chapters 6 and 7 in the context of hippocampal-region function and our own cortico-hippocampal model. One important unresolved question is: To what degree do these representational changes in cortex reflect hippocampal-mediated learning, or is this kind of cortical plasticity—observed by Merzenich and others through electrophysiological studies—independent of hippocampus? The answer awaits further experimental studies.

Computational models of cortex have been developed that are consistent with features of cortical anatomy and physiology and that can be used to explore cortical plasticity and the development of topographic maps.[9] In the next section, we first describe the general principles of these models (often called **competitive** or **self-organizing** networks) and then show how they can be applied to model specific regions of cortex. Next, we show how such a cortical model can be integrated with our existing model of hippocampal-region function, to examine how the two systems might interact to adapt stimulus representations during learning.

8.2   COMPUTATIONAL MODELS

Competitive Learning and Topographic Maps

The error-correcting networks that were described in earlier chapters are **supervised** learning systems, meaning that they learn on the basis of the error between network response and some target. Supervised learning works well in many domains in which the desired response is known or can be inferred. For example, in classical conditioning, the response (such as an eye-blink) should predict reinforcement (such as an airpuff US). A network that performs error correction on the basis of the difference between its response and the US is performing supervised learning.

An **unsupervised** learning system, however, does not learn to produce any predefined desired output. Instead, the network discovers underlying regularities—statistically salient features—of the inputs it is given. For this reason, these networks are also called self-organizing networks, since they do not depend on external reinforcement (such as a US). The autoassociative network discussed in chapter 5 was one kind of unsupervised network. Another class of unsupervised network is a competitive network, meaning that the nodes in the network compete with one another for the right to respond to stimuli. Competitive networks (or networks that embed competitive learning principles) have been considered by a variety of researchers.[10]

An example of a competitive network is shown in figure 8.6A. It consists of a single layer of nodes, each of which has weighted connections with every input element. The nodes are organized into nonoverlapping clusters. Within a cluster, only one node can become active at a time. Thus, nodes within a cluster compete with one another for the right to respond. The winner will be the node that is most strongly activated by the current input pattern; it will become maximally active and will inhibit the activity of the other nodes in the cluster. For example, the input pattern in figure 8.6B activates one node in

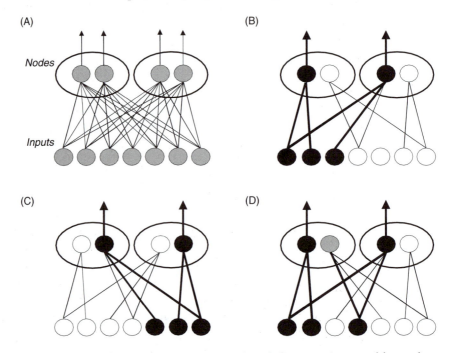

Figure 8.6   (A) Schematic of a competitive network, including seven inputs and four nodes organized into two two-node clusters. Nodes within a cluster compete with each other, meaning that only one can be active to a particular input. The winning node responds to the input; other nodes in the cluster are silenced. The winning node also undergoes plasticity to make it more likely to respond to similar inputs in the future. Over many training trials, the network discovers underlying regularities in the input patterns, so similar inputs generate similar activity patterns over the nodes. (B) Example of a network that has been trained on two input patterns. Here, one input pattern activates one node in the left cluster and one node in the right cluster; other nodes are suppressed. (C) A different input pattern generates a very different activity pattern. (D) A novel input pattern, which shares some features with the pattern in (B), generates an intermediate response. In the left cluster, only one node is activated; it wins the competition by default. In the right cluster, two nodes are partially activated; the stronger one wins and suppresses the other. The result is that the network will respond to this novel input in the same way as it responded to the input in (B); hence, the network will classify the novel input as belonging to the same category as the input in (B).

each cluster; the other nodes are silenced. Within each cluster, the weights from active inputs to the winning node are strengthened to make that node even more likely to win the competition next time the same input pattern is presented. A very different input pattern may generate a very different pattern of activity over the clusters (figure 8.6C).

If there are N nodes in a cluster, each node in the cluster can be considered to represent one of N categories. Each input pattern will be categorized depending on which node in the cluster is activated. For example, if input stimuli range in color along a red-green axis, then one node in a two-node cluster might respond maximally to red stimuli while the other might respond maximally to green stimuli; the color of an arbitrary input can be classified as "red" or "green" by observing which node in the cluster responds to it. Thus, without any external teaching signal, the network learns to classify the inputs. If a novel input is shown that shares some features with one of the trained input patterns (figure 8.6D), it will tend to activate the nodes that are activated by similar inputs. Thus, the novel input will be classified according to the same rules as the trained inputs.

This simple idea can be elaborated in many ways. One possibility is a network with a single, large cluster of nodes arranged in a two-dimensional array (figure 8.7). Each node receives weighted connections from all the inputs; initially, these weights are random. When an input is presented, one of the nodes is maximally activated and wins the competition (e.g., node X in the figure). The weights from active inputs to X are then increased a bit, so that next time the same input is presented, X is even more likely to win the competition again. Then, the immediate neighbors of X (e.g., nodes labeled Y in the figure) undergo similar but smaller weight increases. More distant neighbors (e.g., nodes labeled Z in the figure) may have increasingly smaller weight increases. MathBox 8.1 gives additional details of this learning rule.

One effect of this weight change is that if the same pattern is presented again and again, over many trials, it will come to evoke a "bubble" of activation centered on X. The fact that nearby nodes are encouraged to respond to similar patterns means that a topographic map eventually develops in which similar inputs are represented by nearby nodes in the network. In this case, the network may be termed a **self-organizing feature map,** since it forms a topographic representation based on some features of the input. Although such a map may be similar to the cortical maps shown in figures 8.3 and 8.5, it is important to note that the network topography depends purely on the frequency and overlap of different input patterns rather than any predefined idea of similarity that may make sense to a human observer.

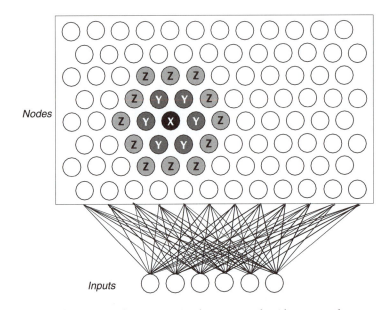

Figure 8.7   A self-organizing feature map is often a network with many nodes arranged in a two-dimensional array. Each node receives weighted connections from all of the input, and these weights are initialized randomly. When an input pattern is presented, one node (X) will become maximally active; it wins the competition. The weights from active inputs to X are strengthened, which means that next time this input pattern is presented, X will respond even more strongly and will be even more likely to win the competition. The weights of X's neighbors are also strengthened, the magnitude of weight change decreasing with distance. Thus, immediate neighbors (Y) will receive a moderate weight increase, more distant neighbors (Z) may receive a mild weight increase, and beyond some neighborhood, there will be no weight changes—or there will even be a mild weight decrease. Over many trials, the input that most strongly activates X will also partially activate immediate neighbors (Y) and mildly activate distant neighbors (Z)—so that a bubble of activation is evoked. Depending on the number of nodes and the size of the neighborhood used, a topographic map will develop in which nearby nodes tend to respond to similar input patterns.

To better understand how these sort of networks function, it is instructive to describe in detail one example from the work of Teuvo Kohonen and his colleagues, who have made extensive study of self-organizing feature maps. They have proposed a "neural phonetic typewriter"[11] that learns to transcribe spoken words into output and could be used to generate typewritten text. (For the interested reader, MathBox 8.2 gives some specifics of speech analysis.)

Because Kohonen and many of his collaborators are from Finland, they considered the Finnish language. Finnish has the convenient property of being orthographically regular, which means that words are spelled

MathBox 8.1   Self-Organizing Feature Maps

A self-organizing network learns to represent input patterns on the basis of their structure and frequency, rather than according to any external classification, such as whether they predict reinforcement (e.g., a US). The canonical form of a self-organizing network consists of a single layer of nodes, often arranged as a two-dimensional array (see figure 8.7). Each node has a weighted connection from every element in the input pattern. The weights are initialized to small random numbers in the range 0…1 and may be normalized, meaning that the sum of all the weights coming into each node is the same for all nodes in the network.

When an input pattern is presented, each node j calculates its activation V_j as a weighted sum over the n inputs:

$$V_j = \frac{\sum_i o_i\, w_{ij}}{n} \tag{8.1}$$

where o_i represents the activation of the ith input and w_{ij} is the weight from that input to j. Since the inputs take on values from 0 to 1, V_j can range from 0 to 1. V_j will be maximized if the n weights coming into j have the same values as the n elements of the input pattern.

Once activation is calculated for all nodes, the winning node w is chosen as the node with maximal activation. (If two or more nodes tie with maximal activation, some probabilistic rule is used to choose between them.) The weights coming into winning node w are updated to increase the correlation between them and the current input pattern, which in turn increases the probability that w will win the competition next time that input pattern is presented. At the same time, nodes that are close to w in the array are updated, and the magnitude of weight change decreases with increasing distance from w. This is done by

calculating the distance from w for each node, d_{wj} (with $d_{ww} = 0$), and then making the magnitude of weight change decrease as d_{wj} increases. A simple learning rule to accomplish this is:

$$\Delta w_{ij} = \beta(o_i - w_{ij})f(d_{wj}) \tag{8.2}$$

where $f(x) \rightarrow 0$ as x gets sufficiently large. β is a learning rate, set to a small positive value. In some cases, β is initially set to a larger value, to allow the net to quickly map out rough organization, and is then slowly decreased to allow progressively finer-grained changes.

Over many training trials, this learning rule has the effect that nearby nodes will tend to respond maximally to similar input patterns, while distant nodes will tend to different kinds of input patterns. This will lead to a rough topography of the kind shown in figure 8.8. Different initial conditions (i.e., different numbers of nodes, different initial weights, and different learning rules) will lead to different topographic maps.

If the number of input patterns is not equal to the number of nodes, then some sharing will occur. In the example of speech recognition (figure 8.8), phonemes that occur most often (e.g., /a/ in Finnish) tend to be represented over several nodes, each of which responds maximally to one variant of the phoneme; infrequent phonemes (e.g., /d/) may be represented by a few nodes, each of which responds to many variants of one phoneme—or even to several similar phonemes.

The learning rules presented here are only examples; many other variations of self-organizing networks have been studied.[12] Self-organizing feature maps have been used in a wide variety of applications in which it is useful to use a computer algorithm to discover underlying order in a large database.[13]

MathBox 8.2   A Brief Introduction to Speech

Speech consists of a continuous stream of acoustic signal. Within any language, this signal can be broken down into meaningful sounds called **phonemes.** For example, the spoken word *cat* is composed of three phonemes: /k/, /æ/, /t/. The phonemic representation of a spoken word often bears no close relationship to the written spelling, especially in a language such as English; for example, the spoken word *knight* would be represented as /nayt/. Different languages recognize different phonemes as significant; for example, /l/ and /r/ are not distinguished in Japanese, while the German /x/ (the guttural final sound in *Bach*) does not occur in English. English uses 38 phonemes; all the languages in the world use a total of about 200.

Phonemes can be defined by their manner of production. Thus, both /t/ and /d/ are generated by forcing through the vocal tract while pushing the tongue against the roof of the mouth just behind the teeth; the difference between /t/ and /d/ is that the vocal cords vibrate during production of a /d/ but not a /t/. (You can feel this by putting a finger against your throat while uttering each phoneme.) The phonemes /k/ and /g/ stand in a similar relationship, except that the tongue is pressed against the roof of the mouth nearer the back. Phonemes that involve briefly blocking off the passage of air (usually by the tongue or lips) are called consonants; phonemes for which the vocal tract is unobstructed are called vowels.

Each phoneme in a language is associated with a cluster of sound events called **phones;** thus, in English, the first sound in the word "took" and the last sound in the word "out" are both phonemic /t/, even though the actual acoustic sounds (phones) are somewhat different. A native speaker of English will recognize both as the same meaningful unit: "t".

Each phone generates acoustic energy patterns at different frequencies. This can be plotted as a **speech spectrogram** (see figure 8.A). The vertical

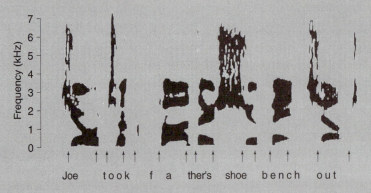

Figure 8.A   A speech spectrogram of an English sentence. The vertical axis plots sound frequency, and the degree of darkness indicates amount of acoustic energy at that frequency. The horizontal axis plots time; the sentence being uttered is spelled out below the axis. Most vowels (e.g., /o/, /a/, /e/) consist of several bands of energy that are relatively steady across time, while consonants contain variable onset times and rapid transitions of frequencies. There are also often brief periods of silence (indicated by arrows) during transitions between consonants such as /b/, /p/, /t/, /d/, /k/, /g/, and so these phonemes are often called stop consonants. Although voice, intonation, and speed can vary across and even within speakers, the relative patterns of energy are constant enough that phonemes can be reliably recognized. (Reprinted from Zigmond et al., 1999, p. 1494, figure 57.6.)

MathBox 8.2   (*Continued*)

axis represents different sound frequencies, and the horizontal axis represents time; the degree of darkness represents the amount of energy present at a given frequency at a given time. Notice that there is no obvious break in energy between words or even between syllables. Instead, there is often a brief period of silence during transitions involving **stop consonants** such as /t/ and /f/, indicated by arrows in the figure. The lack of obvious segmentation between words is one reason why it is so difficult for computers to recognize speech; yet most native speakers of a language perform this task easily.

The precise pattern of acoustic energy generated by a phone will differ with variations in speaker voice; even within a single speaker, changes in intonation and even nearby phones can affect the spectrogram. Thus, in figure A, the /t/ in *took* generates a somewhat different pattern than the /t/ in *out*, because nearby phones affect pronunciation. Nonetheless, phones—and associated phonemes—can be consistently identified on the basis of the relative combinations of active frequencies of energy. Figure 8.B shows speech spectrograms for the vowels /a/ and /æ/ and for the consonant-vowel syllables /ba/ and /da/.

Vowels such as /a/ and /æ/ tend to produce long-lasting, relatively stable energy at several frequencies. Consonants show rapid transitions. For example, the consonant-vowel combinations

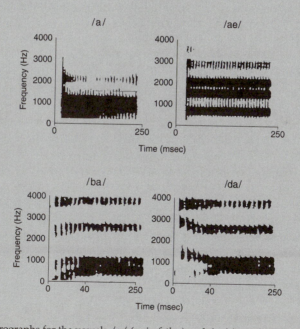

Figure 8.B   Spectrographs for the vowels /a/ (as in *father*) and /æ/ (as in *bad*) and for the consonant-vowel syllables /ba/ and /da/. The vowels consist of relatively steady-state activation across a range of frequencies that may last hundreds of milliseconds. Consonants, by contrast, contain variable onset times and rapid transitions of frequencies that may last only a few tens of milliseconds. Distinguishing the /ba/ and /da/ syllables therefore requires discriminating the very rapid transitions that differ between /b/ and /d/. (Reprinted from Fitch, Miller, & Tallal, 1997, figures 1 and 2.)

MathBox 8.2   (*Concluded*)

/da/ and /ba/ differ only in the initial 40-msec segment. This can make them very difficult to discriminate, yet most native speakers of a language make similar discriminations with little conscious effort.

A continuous stream of speech can be converted into a spectrogram, and the spectrogram can then be divided up into short sequences, each of which represents the pronunciation of a single phone, similar to the vowel spectrograms above. Each phone can then be represented as a string of numbers representing the amount of acoustic energy at each frequency. The result is a pattern representing the phone. Changes in speaker inflection and other variations mean that different instances of the same phone may generate different patterns.

A neural network can be trained to take these input patterns and generate output classifying them as phonemes they represent.[14] The output of such a network could then be translated into typewritten text.

In practice, there may be a considerable degree of additional preprocessing before raw speech signals are translated into input patterns; discussion of such preprocessing strategies is beyond the scope of this book, but the interested reader may refer to specialized publications such as Ramachandran & Mammone, 1995.

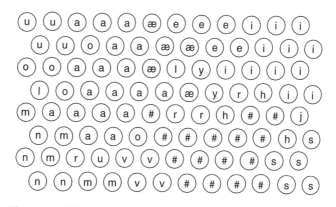

Figure 8.8   The nodes of the phonetic typewriter, labeled with the symbols of the phonemes for which they give best responses. Kohonen and Hari (1999) give the pronunciation guide as follows: /a/ as in *cut*, /æ/ as in *cat*, /e/ as in *bet*, /i/ as in *bit*, /o/ as in *pot*, /u/ as in *put*, and /y/ as in the French word *duc*; /#/ means /k/, /p/, or /t/. (Note that these mappings vary slightly from formal linguistic definitions of phonemes.) To a large extent, similar phonemes are represented by nearby nodes, Therefore, the vowels are grouped together: /m/ and /n/—both involving nasal resonance—are nearby, and so on. Additionally, the amount of space devoted to a phoneme generally reflects frequency; the phoneme /a/, which is the most common in the Finnish language, maps to fully 18 of the 96 nodes. (Adapted from Kohonen & Hari, 1999, figure 2.)

approximately the way they sound. In contrast, English, with its changeable vowels (e.g., the "i" sound differs in "fin" and "fine") and its strange consonant clusters (e.g., "knight"), has many orthographic irregularities.

Kohonen and colleagues started with recordings of natural speech, which they converted into 15-element input patterns, each representing one speech sound or **phoneme.** These patterns were provided as input to a self-organizing feature map that had 96 nodes arranged in a two-dimensional array. Each node in the network competed to respond to every input, with the winning nodes strengthening their own weights as well as those of their immediate neighbors. After much training, each node in the network came to respond maximally to a preferred phoneme. Figure 8.8 shows the nodes in the network, with each node labeled according to its preferred phoneme.* Several characteristics are evident. First, nodes responding to a particular sound tend to be clustered together. Second, clusters responding to similar sounds tend to

*Note that since this network was trained on examples of Finnish speech, the set of phonemes is not quite the same as a set of phonemes from English speech (Finnish has relatively few fricatives such as sh-, ch-, and th-). Also, note that the node labels shown in the example of figure 8.8 do not map exactly to formal phoneme definitions: The /o/ phoneme is usually take to be more like the "oh" sound in "hotel" than the "ah" sound in "pot." The labels are for illustration only.

be close together: The nodes responding to /æ/ (as in "cat") and /e/ (as in "bet") are nearby, reflecting the high similarity in sounds; the nodes responding to /m/ and /n/—two consonants that involve nasal resonance—are neighbors; and so on. More generally, vowels are gathered near the top half of the map, while consonants are gathered in the bottom half. The topography is not perfect; for example, the nodes responding to /l/ are quite widely distributed across the network, while the highly similar consonants /p/, /t/, and /k/ are not well distinguished (represented as /#/ in figure 8.8). Nevertheless, considering that the network was given no supervision on how to encode phonemes, the map does quite a good job of representing the acoustic similarities between sounds. Finally, there is rough correspondence between the importance of phonemes and the amount of total area representing them: /a/, which is the most common Finnish phoneme, activates fully 18 of the 96 nodes, while the less common /j/ activates only one node maximally.

These emergent properties of the self-organizing map are quite reminiscent of the topographic maps that are encountered in primary sensory cortex (refer to figures 8.3 and 8.5): In each case, cells evolve that preferentially respond to particular types of input, and neighboring cells tend to respond to similar inputs. Thus, this class of network is a possible model for how topographic maps could develop in the brain during early exposure to a set of stimuli. Of course, there may be many ways such maps could emerge, and self-organizing networks instantiate only one of these possibilities. However, many of the assumptions inherent in such a network are consistent with features of cortical anatomy and physiology, a topic to which we turn next.

Piriform Cortex

Most parts of cerebral cortex in mammals are six-layered neocortex (figure 8.1A). However, there exist a few places in the brain where the cortex begins to change, gradually becoming two-layer paleocortex similar to the reptile cortex shown in figure 8.1B. One such area is the olfactory cortex (also known as **piriform cortex**). The hippocampus itself is also a two-layered sheet of paleocortex, although it is folded in on itself to create its characteristic "C" shape. The piriform cortex abuts the hippocampal region; in some species such as the rat, the piriform cortex actually merges into nearby cortical areas, and it is therefore difficult to make a precise division between the two regions. One theory is that hippocampus and piriform cortex are remnants of the "primitive brain" from which more complex neocortex evolved.

Whatever its history, the relatively simple organization of the piriform cortex suggests that it is a logical place to begin exploring how cortical anatomy could give rise to computational function. Additionally, although human olfactory cortex is relatively small, the olfactory cortex of most mammals is much larger, reflecting the importance of odor information to those species. Dogs, for example, have almost fifty times as many olfactory neurons as humans do. Therefore, the olfactory cortex is especially convenient for animal studies.

Olfaction (the sense of smell) begins with a thin sheet of olfactory receptor cells, high up in the nasal cavity shown in figure 8.9, called the olfactory epithelium. It contains olfactory receptor cells that transduce chemical stimuli (odors) into nerve impulses by processes that are still incompletely understood.

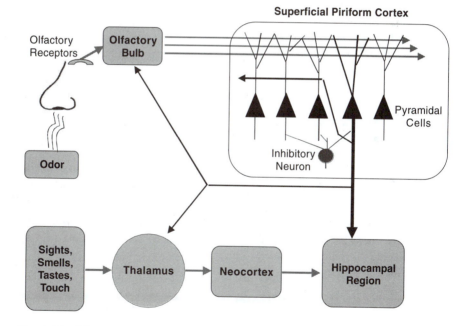

Figure 8.9 Schematic of olfaction. Odors enter the nose and reach olfactory receptors in the olfactory epithelium, which in turn transmit information to the olfactory bulb and thence to the olfactory cortex. Piriform cortex is one subarea of olfactory cortex. Pyramidal cells in the piriform cortex in turn project to other pyramidal cells as well as to local inhibitory neurons, which inhibit activity in nearby pyramidal cells. Pyramidal cells also project out of piriform cortex to thalamus, hippocampal region, and back to olfactory bulb. Olfaction is unique in that it is the only sensory modality in which sensory inputs project directly to cortex; most other sensory information travels through thalamus before reaching neocortex. Piriform cortex is also the only primary sensory cortical area with substantial direct projections to the hippocampal region.

The axons of the olfactory receptor cells form the olfactory nerve and travel to the **olfactory bulb;** from there, information projects to the olfactory or piriform cortex. This arrangement is special: No other sensory information has direct access to cortex. Most other sensory information travels first to thalamus and then to primary sensory areas in neocortex. The direct access of odors to cortex means that it should be possible to model the function of piriform cortex in some detail without first requiring a full understanding of thalamic preprocessing.

A final special characteristic of piriform cortex is that it is the only sensory cortex with a sizable direct connection to the hippocampal region; all other sensory information passes through several layers of unimodal and polymodal association cortex before reaching the hippocampal region.[15]

Several researchers have presented computational models of olfaction;[16] Richard Granger, Gary Lynch, and colleagues proposed a competitive learning system that includes many of the known anatomical and physiological properties of piriform cortex.[17] Their model includes a learning rule that incorporates what is known about plasticity in piriform cortex and model neurons that incorporate known detail about piriform neuronal activity. However, many of the important properties of the system can be understood by using the simple example shown in figure 8.10.

The network model in figure 8.10 consists of two interacting systems: a layer of nodes representing the olfactory bulb and a layer representing pyramidal cells in superficial piriform cortex. These pyramidal nodes are organized into small clusters (typically 10–20 nodes per cluster), each of which functions as a small competitive network. When an olfactory input arrives, the nodes in a cluster are differentially activated. One node in each cluster is most strongly activated; this node wins the competition and outputs its response, while feedback inhibition silences the nonwinning nodes (figure 8.10A). One of the unique features of the piriform model is that the input classification does not stop here. The piriform activity feeds back to inhibit the olfactory bulb, specifically suppressing the parts of the input pattern that activated the winning nodes (figure 8.10B). This allows new parts of the input pattern to activate new piriform nodes, which win the second round of the competition. The entire process may be repeated a number of times until all the olfactory input is suppressed and the network becomes quiescent.

Now suppose another input is presented that shares some features with the first odor (figure 8.10C); the common features will tend to activate the same initial response. Once these are masked out, the secondary response may be different (figure 8.10D). Thus, this network is capable of performing **hierarchical clustering** of inputs. The initial response to a stimulus is a coarse

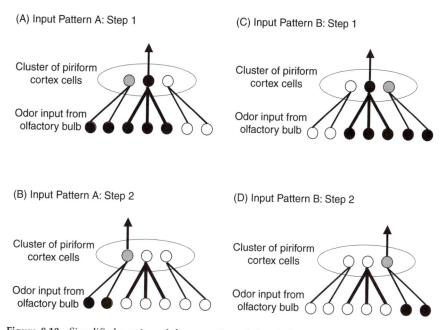

(A) Input Pattern A: Step 1

Cluster of piriform
cortex cells

Odor input from
olfactory bulb

(C) Input Pattern B: Step 1

Cluster of piriform
cortex cells

Odor input from
olfactory bulb

(B) Input Pattern A: Step 2

Cluster of piriform
cortex cells

Odor input from
olfactory bulb

(D) Input Pattern B: Step 2

Cluster of piriform
cortex cells

Odor input from
olfactory bulb

Figure 8.10 Simplified version of the operation of the piriform clustering model (Ambros-Ingerson, Granger, & Lynch, 1990). A series of inputs, representing odor information from olfactory bulb, connect to a large number of piriform cortex cells. Piriform cortex cells are organized into small clusters (one cluster is shown). (A) A familiar odor is presented to the olfactory bulb and elicits a pattern of activation in each piriform cortex cluster. Piriform nodes compete, the most strongly active node winning: It outputs maximally, and the other nodes are silenced. (B) Piriform activity feeds back to the bulb, masking out the portions of the input that activated the winning nodes. This allows the remaining input features to activate new piriform nodes on the next iteration. Many iterations may occur, each producing a different spatial activity pattern in the clusters. (C) A new odor input is presented that shares some features with the input in A. One piriform node wins the competition—the same as in A. This represents a coarse clustering, classifying the two odors into the same broad category of input. (D) After feedback masks the odor input, however, the remaining features activate a new piriform node. Thus, a finer classification is made that differentiates the current odor from the odor in A.

classification, which may not distinguish between several similar inputs. However, successive responses do become more and more fine-grained.

Conceptually, the network might first recognize a food odor, then recognize that this particular input is a cheese odor, and eventually identify a specific type of cheese. What is most interesting about this network is that this sophisticated analysis of an input in terms of successively finer-grained classification occurs without any external teaching signal; the network simply uses competitive learning to group similar inputs together.

There is a second important principle at work in the piriform cortex model: representational compression. If two stimuli co-occur, the network has no way of knowing this *a priori*. Instead, it will treat the two stimuli as a single, compound stimulus (figure 8.11A). For example, co-occurring floral and musk odors would be treated as a single odor with components of both floral and musky scents. The network will form a cluster in response to these features. If one of the component odors (e.g., floral scent) later appears alone, the network will recognize this as a degraded version of the compound odor,

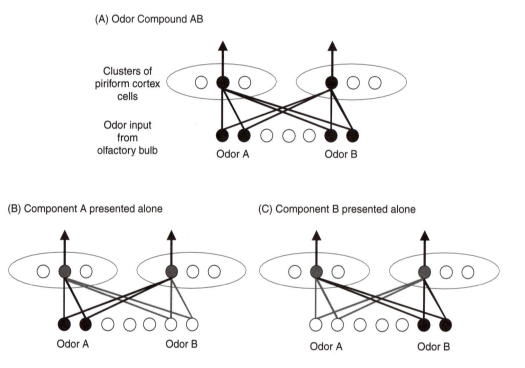

Figure 8.11 Co-occurring odors are compressed in the piriform model. (A) The network is trained on an input pattern that consists of two odor components A (e.g., a floral scent) and I (e.g., a musky scent). Within each node cluster (two are shown), one node wins the competition to respond to this compound odor, and the weights from active inputs to those nodes are strengthened. For simplicity, only strong connections are shown. (B) Later, one of the component odors is presented alone. This input will tend to activate the same nodes as the compound, along previously strengthened connections. The nodes will be less strongly activated by the individual odor, but as long as their activation is greater than that of any other node in the cluster, they will still win the competition. Thus, the network will tend to respond to the component odor in the same way as it did to the compound. (C) If component B is presented alone, the same response occurs. In effect, the representations of co-occurring odors A and B have been compressed, so the response to either component is similar.

and it will respond by activating the nodes coding that compound odor (figure 8.11B). *Thus, Granger and Lynch's model compresses the representations of co-occurring odors.*

From a computational perspective, this representational compression is essentially the same as that which occurs in our own cortico-hippocampal model.[18] The difference is that, while the hippocampal region processes a full range of polymodal information, the piriform cortex is limited (mainly) to processing odor stimuli. Furthermore, whereas the hippocampal region is hypothesized to both compress and differentiate representations as appropriate, the piriform model is capable only of representational compression.

This difference has several important implications, the most important of which is that once co-occurring odors are compressed, there is no way for the piriform model—working in isolation—to undo this compression. Thus, if odors A and B originally occur together (as in figure 8.11) and later need to be mapped to different responses, this mapping will be very difficult.

Of course, normal animals can learn to distinguish odors (and other stimuli) that have previously co-occurred. Apparently, some other mechanism is available to redifferentiate representations as needed. One possibility is the hippocampal region.

Piriform-Hippocampal Interactions

Our cortico-hippocampal model assumes that the hippocampal region can form new stimulus representations that compress redundant information while differentiating predictive information. Normally, the hippocampus receives highly processed, multimodal information from a whole range of stimulus modalities, and thus its representations can take into account the cross-modal features of individual stimuli or the co-occurrence of stimuli across different modalities. Sensory cortex, particularly primary sensory cortex, is largely limited to processing information in a single sensory modality. Thus, the piriform network described in the preceding section may compress the representations of co-occurring odors but not stimuli in other modalities. It is also unable to redifferentiate representations once they have been compressed.

One way to schematize the relationship between piriform cortex and hippocampal region is shown in figure 8.12A. Odor inputs are first processed by piriform cortex, which forms odor clusters and also compresses the representations of co-occurring odors. Because the piriform cortex has direct connections to the hippocampal region, these new odor representations are combined with highly processed information from other modalities. This, in

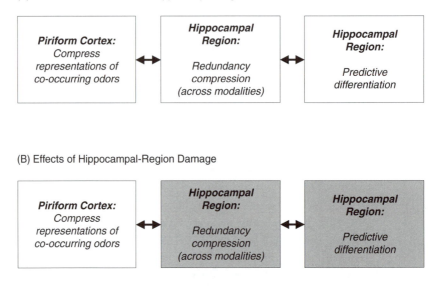

(A) Possible Normal Piriform–Hippocampal Region Interaction

Piriform Cortex:
Compress
representations of
co-occurring odors

Hippocampal
Region:

Redundancy
compression
(across modalities)

Hippocampal
Region:

Predictive
differentiation

(B) Effects of Hippocampal-Region Damage

Piriform Cortex:
Compress
representations of
co-occurring odors

Hippocampal
Region:

Redundancy
compression
(across modalities)

Hippocampal
Region:

Predictive
differentiation

Figure 8.12 Possible interactions between piriform cortex and hippocampal region. (A) Normally, the piriform cortex may tend to compress the representations of co-occurring odors. The hippocampal region also performs compression of stimuli that co-occur or are otherwise redundant; this may especially involve compression across stimulus modalities. The hippocampal region also performs predictive differentiation, pulling apart the representations of stimuli that are differentially predictive of future reinforcement. This serves as an opponent function for representational compression. Normally, the two processes are in balance. (B) Hippocampal-region damage removes the ability to perform cross-modal compression and the ability to perform predictive differentiation. The result is that undamaged compression processes in piriform cortex are allowed to proceed unchecked; overall, this will lead to a tendency to overcompress stimulus information, making it hard to distinguish stimuli which co-occur.

turn, generates new representations that compress redundant information while differentiating predictive information. In this case, hippocampal-region damage does not absolutely eliminate the ability to alter stimulus representations (figure 8.12B). The piriform cortex can still alter the representations of odor stimuli, as, presumably, other cortical areas do within their respective domains. But two abilities are lost. First, without the hippocampal region to integrate across modalities, there is relatively little ability to combine information across different sensory domains. Second, there is relatively little ability to differentiate representations, particularly representations that have previously been compressed. The net result is that cortical compression proceeds without the opponent process of differentiation, and, at least within a single sensory domain, there is a tendency to overcompress information, which in turn hinders subsequent differentiation. For the piriform cortex, this means that it will be very difficult to distinguish individual scents that have previously been presented together. Thus, we might expect that without hippocampal-dependent differentiation (due to brain damage), an animal might tend to overcompress or fuse stimuli that have appeared together in a compound.

In fact, exactly this kind of impairment *has* been observed in odor discrimination studies done in rats with hippocampal-region damage. Howard Eichenbaum and colleagues have extensively studied rat odor discrimination. In their laboratory, a rat is placed in a small chamber with a recessed port from which an odor is delivered as shown in figure 8.13A. Typically, one odor (e.g., A) is defined as positive. The rat's task is to learn to respond to A by pushing its nose into the port delivering A and holding this position for a few seconds. This behavior is rewarded by a small food or water reward. Then an elaborate vacuum system removes evidence of both odors from the chamber, and new odors are delivered for a new trial.

When a negative odor (e.g., B) is delivered, the rat must sample the odor, then withdraw its nose from the odor port to initiate the next trial. This kind of task is called **successive odor discrimination,** and normal rats can learn fairly easily, even if a large number of odors are used. Rats with a fornix

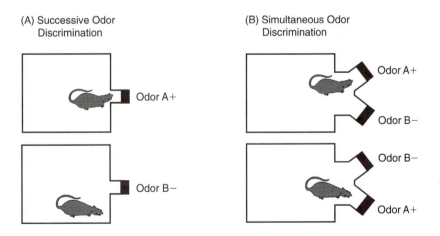

Figure 8.13 (A) Successive odor discrimination paradigm. The rat is presented with one of two odors from an odor port and must learn to poke its nose into the odor port in response to the rewarded odor A but not the nonrewarded odor B. (B) Simultaneous odor discrimination paradigm. Two odors arrive simultaneously; the rat must learn to nosepoke to the rewarded odor, regardless of spatial position. Hippocampal-region damage spares successive odor discrimination but impairs simultaneous odor discrimination (Eichenbaum et al., 1988). (Adapted from Myers & Gluck, 1996, figure 2.)

lesion (which severs an important pathway into and out of hippocampus) are also generally unimpaired at learning successive odor discriminations.[19]

Howard Eichenbaum and colleagues have considered a variation of this paradigm in which there are two odor ports that can simultaneously deliver separate odors (figure 8.13B); the rat must then nosepoke to the left-hand or right-hand odor port, depending on which port is delivering the positive odor. For example, given odor A+ at the left port and odor B− at the right port, the rat should nosepoke left to obtain water; given odor A+ at the right port and odor B− at the left port, the rat should nosepoke right to obtain water. This kind of task, called **simultaneous odor discrimination,** is severely impaired by fornix lesion.[20] Entorhinal lesion also disrupts retention of a similar task.[21] The lesioned animals' impairment cannot be ascribed to failure to nosepoke left or right, since under other circumstances, they can learn to do this;[22] therefore, the critical difference between the simultaneous and successive discrimination paradigms seems to be whether odors are presented singly or in pairs. The lesioned rats can cope with singly presented odors but not with odor pairs.

The schematized model shown in figure 8.12 suggests why this might be so. When odors are presented singly, as in successive discrimination, the piriform cortex will develop a representation for each; when odors are presented in compound, the piriform network will tend to compress representations of those component odors, making it harder to distinguish them—and therefore harder to learn to respond to one but not the other. Eichenbaum and colleagues have similarly suggested that hippocampal-region damage leads to a tendency to fuse representations of co-occurring odors.[23]

There is some evidence of this kind of overcompression or fusion deficit following hippocampal-region damage in other species. For example, retention and relearning of simultaneously presented odors is disrupted in monkeys with hippocampal-region damage.[24] It is less clear whether stimuli from other modalities are disrupted the same way. Thus, after hippocampal-region damage, choosing between two simultaneously presented visual cues is sometimes disrupted in monkeys and sometimes spared.[25] The data are similarly mixed for tactile and auditory discrimination in various species.

One possible explanation for these mixed results is that odor stimuli are, by their very nature, particularly prone to mix and blend, and therefore, co-occurring odors are especially subject to compression.[26] Visual stimuli, in contrast, may be prone to compression only if they are presented close together or if they are different features of the same object, such as color and form. Under these conditions, visual stimuli might be more likely to show compression—and more likely to show overcompression after hippocampal-region damage. This idea remains to be explored experimentally.

Integrating Piriform Cortex with the Cortico-Hippocampal Model

The idea that the piriform cortex compresses co-occurring odor stimuli while the hippocampal region compresses and differentiates all kinds of stimuli is relatively straightforward to instantiate within the general framework of our cortico-hippocampal model.[27] Two basic changes are required. The first, obviously, is the inclusion of a piriform network to perform preprocessing of odor stimuli. Nonodor inputs do not pass through this network; they are presumably preprocessed in other, nonolfactory cortical areas that are not included in the model (figure 8.14A). The outputs of the piriform network pass directly to the hippocampal-region network, consistent with the anatomical evidence.

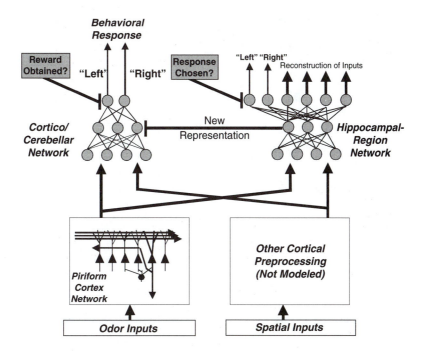

Figure 8.14 (A) The cortico-hippocampal model extended to allow odor preprocessing with a piriform network. Inputs encode odor quality and spatial arrangement. Odor inputs are preprocessed by the piriform cortex network, which clusters odors and compresses co-occurring odors. Other cortical areas may similarly preprocess spatial information, but this is not simulated here. The preprocessed inputs are provided to the cortico-hippocampal model. The cortico/cerebellar network learns to map from these inputs to a behavioral response (choose left or right). The hippocampal-region network learns to reconstruct its inputs and predict the behavioral response. As usual, new stimulus representations constructed in the hippocampal-region network are adopted by the cortico/cerebellar network. Full details of this model are given in the appendix to this chapter.

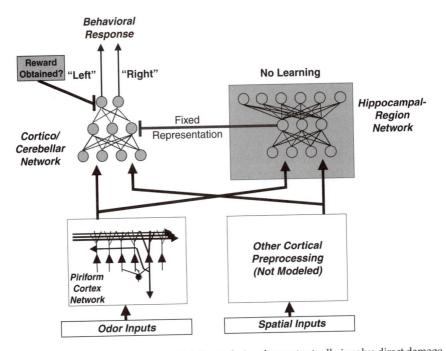

Figure 8.14   (B) The fornix-lesion model. Fornix lesion does not actually involve direct damage to the hippocampus but severs an important modulatory pathway connecting the hippocampus with structures such as thalamus and medial septum. Evidence suggests that this pathway may enable learning in the hippocampus. Thus, fornix lesion is modeled by eliminating learning in the hippocampal-region network. Information still passes through the network and is transformed into a representation in the internal node layer, according to random, fixed weighted connections; this representation is not subject to the usual hippocampal-mediated constraints of redundancy compression and predictive differentiation and instead is a random recoding of the input information. The cortico/cerebellar network must learn to map from these fixed representations to appropriate behavioral output. Full details of this model are given in the appendix to this chapter.

Second, unlike the prior application of our model to classical conditioning, in which the response was a single behavioral action (e.g., blink), in simultaneous odor discrimination the response is a choice between two or more responses (e.g., nosepoke left versus nosepoke right).

The cortico/cerebellar network (see figure 6.4 or figure 7.9) is easily generalized by giving it multiple output nodes, one representing each possible response. The hippocampal-region network is adapted to produce output that reconstructs its inputs and also predicts the behavioral response selected. This system can now be applied to simultaneous discrimination tasks such as those studied by Eichenbaum and colleagues.

A hippocampal-region (HR)-lesioned model could be generated by simply disabling the hippocampal-region network. In this case, odor inputs would be preprocessed by the piriform network and then project directly to the cortico/cerebellar network, as schematized in figure 8.14B.

However, in the relevant behavioral studies, Eichenbaum and colleagues generally did not consider HR lesions but rather fornix lesions. As we described earlier, a fornix lesion does not directly damage the hippocampus. Rather, it interrupts an important pathway connecting the hippocampus with subcortical structures such as the thalamus and septum.[28] Under some circumstances, fornix lesions may impair learning as much as outright hippocampal lesion,[29] although different lesions can and do have different effects;[30] we will return to this issue later, in chapters 9 and 10. For now, we merely note that fornix lesion destroys critical input to the hippocampus that is known to be important for hippocampal learning.[31]

Therefore, to implement a fornix-lesion model, we simply assume that the hippocampal-region network is not physically damaged, but rather is incapable of learning new information. Thus, information passes through the hippocampal-region network as usual, but the weights in the hippocampal-region network never change in response to input (figure 8.14B). The result is that the only representational changes that occur in the fornix-lesion model are those mediated by the piriform network, which tend to overcompress co-occurring odor stimuli. Full implementation details of the intact and fornix-lesion models are given in the appendix to this chapter.

Now the intact and fornix-lesion models can be applied to the simultaneous odor discrimination task shown in figure 8.13B. On each trial, two odors (e.g., A and B) are presented, together with information encoding their spatial location (i.e., left or right port). The piriform network clusters the odor information, and then the hippocampal-region network forms new stimulus representations that include both odor and spatial information. These new representations are adopted by the cortico/cerebellar network, which learns to map from them to the correct behavioral response (i.e., choose left or right). Figure 8.15B shows that the intact model can learn such a simultaneous discrimination quickly. In the intact model, the piriform network clusters the representations of odors A and B, which always co-occur. This information, together with the spatial information, is passed on to the hippocampal-region network. The hippocampal-region network forms new internal representations that differentiate the information needed to solve the task. In this case, the relevant information is which odors occur in which locations—in other words, whether odor A is on the left or the right. All other information, including the odor cluster

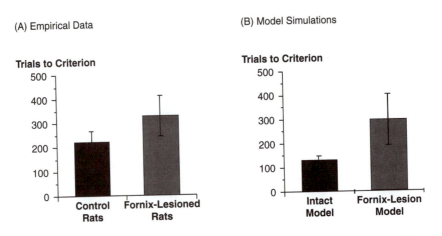

Figure 8.15 Simultaneous odor discrimination: Choose odor A over odor B, regardless of spatial ordering. (A) Control rats learn this task relatively quickly, while fornix-lesioned rats are slower. (Plotted from data presented in Eichenbaum et al., 1988.) (B) The intact and fornix-lesion models show a similar pattern. (Plotted from data presented in Myers & Gluck, 1996.)

information provided by the piriform network, is irrelevant for this end. The hippocampal-region representations therefore come to emphasize spatial information at the expense of the piriform clustering information. Figure 8.16 shows an example of such a representation. Initially, there are small weights to the internal-layer nodes from all inputs, both those from the piriform network and those detailing spatial information (figure 8.16A). By the end of learning, however, the weights containing information about the spatial locations of A and B (that is, whether each is arriving from the left or right port) have become heavily weighted (figure 8.16B); the weights from the piriform network—as well as those devoted to other odors such as C and D—remain low.

Figure 8.16 Magnitude of weights from each input to the internal-layer nodes in the cortico/cerebellar network, averaged across all internal-layer nodes. (A) In the intact model, all weights are initially random and small. (B) After training on A+, B−, the hippocampal-region network develops new internal representations that differentiate predictive information—namely, odor position—that are acquired by the cortico/cerebellar network. The new representations tend to strongly weight information detailing whether A and B appear on the left or right. To a lesser degree, some odor clustering information from the piriform network may be weighted as well. (C) The fornix-lesion model starts out with initial weights in the cortico/cerebellar model that are much like the initial state of the intact model. (D) However, the representations in the hippocampal-region network are fixed and do not come to emphasize relevant information. These are nonetheless adopted by the cortico/cerebellar network. Since no particular weight is given to predictive inputs, it is very difficult for the cortico/cerebellar network to learn the correct behavioral response on the basis of these representations. (Reprinted from Myers & Gluck, 1996, figure 9A,B,D,E.)

The situation is very different in the fornix-lesion model. The initial weights start out much the same as in the intact model (figure 8.16C), but since there is no hippocampal-region learning, representations are not adapted to emphasize predictive information. The random, fixed representations of the

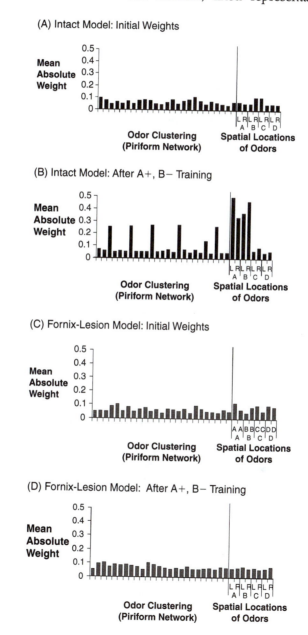

(A) Intact Model: Initial Weights

(B) Intact Model: After A+, B− Training

(C) Fornix-Lesion Model: Initial Weights

(D) Fornix-Lesion Model: After A+, B− Training

hippocampal-region network are adopted by the cortico/cerebellar network, but these tend not to contain much useful information (figure 8.16D). This makes it very difficult for the cortico/cerebellar network to map different odor locations to different behavioral responses, resulting in poor overall performance of the fornix-lesion model (figure 8.15B). This is consistent with the generally poor performance of fornix-lesioned rats on simultaneous odor discrimination.[32]

The average performance data shown in figure 8.15 hide some important individual differences. Figure 8.17A shows that most intact rats solve a simultaneous discrimination quickly, within a few hundred trials. Figure 8.17B shows similar performance in the intact model. On average, both the fornix-lesioned rats and fornix-lesion model do much worse. However,

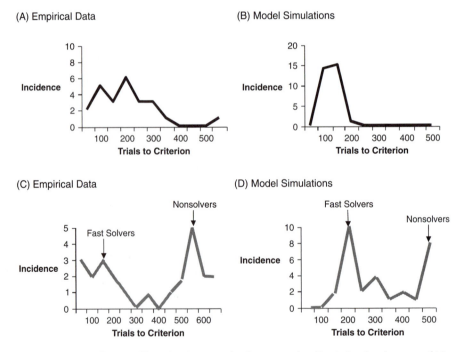

Figure 8.17 Distribution of learning times on simultaneous odor discrimination, in terms of trials to reach criterion, pooled over all tasks. (A) Control rats show a unimodal distribution, solving most tasks within fewer than 300 trials. (B) The intact piriform-hippocampal model shows a similar distribution of solution times. (C) Fornix-lesioned rats show a bimodal distribution, either failing to learn the discrimination within 500 trials or else learning just as quickly as control rats. (D) The lesioned model shows a similar bimodal distribution, most simulations solving tasks in about 200 or more than 500 trials. (Reprinted from Myers & Gluck, 1996; A and C are plotted from data presented in Eichenbaum et al., 1988.)

occasionally and seemingly at random, the fornix-lesioned rats do solve a simultaneous discrimination—and when they do, they do so just as quickly as control rats (figure 8.17C).

The fornix-lesion model shows similar performance, and our model provides an interpretation of the curious bimodality seen in the data from lesioned animals.[33] In our intact model, the hippocampal-region network constructs new stimulus representations that emphasize predictive information. In this case, the result is that internal-layer nodes come to respond strongly to information about the spatial layout of odors and largely ignore the overcompressed information from the piriform network.

Figure 8.18A shows an example of the kind of internal-layer node that tends to develop in the hippocampal-region network and then be adopted by the cortico/cerebellar network. The node is strongly active whenever a positive odor (A or C) is present at the left-hand port and a negative odor

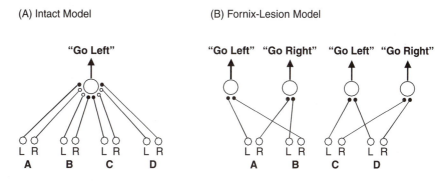

Figure 8.18 Even when an intact simulation and a fornix-lesioned simulation learn the same two problems (A+,B− and C+,D−), they do not learn them in the same way. (A) In the internal layer of the intact model, new representations are formed by the hippocampal-region network. The result is that internal-layer nodes develop such as the one shown here that learn general response rules: Go left whenever a positive stimulus is on the left (A or C) and a negative stimulus is on the right (B or D), and go right otherwise. Many of these nodes will develop in the intact model's internal layer, allowing the problem to be solved quickly. Further, when familiar odors are presented in novel recombinations (e.g., A versus D), this type of node continues to give the correct response. (B) Internal-layer nodes are fixed in the hippocampal-region network of the fornix-lesion model, meaning that nodes like the one in A cannot be constructed. In fact, the only way the fornix-lesion model can solve the discriminations is if initial, random weights fortuitously preserve some information about the spatial location of odors. If this happens at all, it is likely to be only about individual odors. Thus, a fornix-lesioned network that solves the two discriminations might have four internal-layer nodes, each of which responds to one spatial arrangement of one odor pair: go left for AB, go right for BA, go left for CD, go right for DC. This solution works well enough for the initial discriminations but will be of little help when the odors are recombined (e.g., A versus D).

(B or D) is present at the right-hand port; it is strongly inhibited by the reverse placements. Thus, this node should strongly activate the output node associated with a "go-left" response and strongly inhibit the output node associated with a "go-right" response.

The fornix-lesion network cannot construct new stimulus representations in the hippocampal-region network, and it is forced to learn on the basis of preexisting representations that will tend to include a large amount of compressed information from the piriform network. Generally, these preexisting representations will not preserve enough spatial information to allow an arbitrary odor discrimination to be solved. On occasion, however, the random initial weights in the fornix-lesion model's hippocampal-region network are such that they happen to preserve enough spatial information to solve a particular task. All it may take is a single internal-layer node that responds strongly when A is present on the left and B is on the right and responds weakly for the reverse ordering. Figure 8.18B shows an example of some internal-layer nodes that might exist in a fornix-lesion simulation. One node happens to respond when A is on the left and B is on the right (AB); another happens to respond to the reverse ordering (BA). By strongly weighting connections between these nodes and the output nodes in the cortico/cerebellar network, the model can learn to generate the correct response. If more nodes exist that similarly code CD and DC, the simulation will be able to learn that discrimination as well. In such a fortuitous case, the fornix-lesion model will be able to solve both discriminations—and solve them fairly quickly, as is shown in figure 8.15B.

This interpretation within our computational model is similar to the qualitative explanation suggested by Eichenbaum and colleagues. They argued that the fornix-lesioned rats could solve a discrimination only "as a fortuitous consequence of idiosyncratic perceptual variations."[34]

Although the fornix-lesioned rats and fornix-lesion model can occasionally solve a discrimination as quickly as their nonlesioned counterparts, this does not necessarily mean that they are using the same strategies. Eichenbaum and colleagues demonstrated such a difference in rats: Each fornix-lesioned rat was trained on various successive discriminations until the experimenters found two odor pairs (e.g., A+ versus B− and C+ versus D−) the rat could learn. A control rat was then trained on the same two odor pairs. Then the animals were presented with the familiar odors in novel recombinations (e.g., A versus D). Control rats continued to respond to the previously positive odor A instead of the previously negative odor D. Fornix-lesioned rats performed at chance, showing no preference for the previously positive odor, even though they continued to respond correctly when presented with the A versus B discrimination (figure 8.19A).[35]

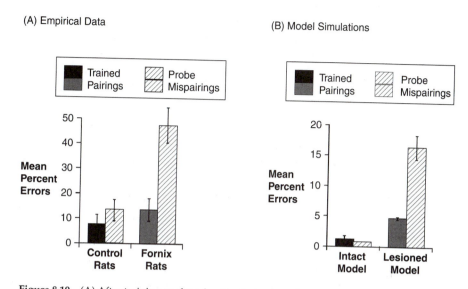

Figure 8.19   (A) After training on the odor discriminations A+ versus B− and C+ versus D−, rats were given test trials consisting of mispairings of the familiar odors: A+ versus D− and C+ versus B−. Control rats continued to perform very well on these probe mispairings. Fornix-lesioned rats, by contrast, performed near chance on these probe mispairings. (Plotted from data presented in Eichenbaum, Mathews, & Cohen, 1989.) (B) The piriform-hippocampal model shows a similar trend: The intact model performs well on both trained pairings and probe mispairings; the lesioned model shows a strong impairment on the probe mispairings. (Adapted from Myers & Gluck, 1996, figure 14.)

The intact and fornix-lesion models show the same effect (figure 8.19B): After training on two pairs that the lesioned model happens to master, the intact model performs nearly perfectly on the transfer test, while the lesioned model does not.[36] The internal-layer representations in figure 8.18 show why. When the intact network is presented with a novel recombination of trained stimuli (e.g., A versus D), internal-layer nodes such as the one in figure 8.18A can cope with the recombination: The node will still fire strongly to A on the right and D on the left and weakly to the other spatial arrangement, and therefore it is still useful as a "go-right" node. By contrast, the internal-layer node in figure 8.18B is activated by combinations of A and B and is only very weakly activated by either stimulus alone. Its output will not be very useful in gauging a response to the new combination. Further, because there is no new representational change in the fornix-lesion model's hippocampal-region network, the situation does not improve even after extensive training on the new combinations.

Thus, our model accounts for the subtle pattern of data seen in Eichenbaum's studies of olfactory discrimination in both the intact and lesioned rats.[37]

At the beginning of this section, we noted that the piriform clustering model of Granger and Lynch suggests that sensory cortices can adapt their representations to reflect superficial similarity between inputs. However, what these brain regions may not be able to do is to operate across sensory domains: for example, encoding both the visual and olfactory features of a stimulus into a unified compound percept. The sensory cortices may also not be able to differentiate stimulus representations based on meaning: For example, if both A and B (which are superficially similar cues) differentially predict the US, then their representations should be differentiated to facilitate mapping them to different responses. These kinds of multimodal and meaning-driven representational changes may lie uniquely within the domain of the hippocampal region. The next chapter reviews a model suggesting that a specific hippocampal-region structure, the entorhinal cortex, may be the locus of multimodal redundancy compression.

8.3   RELATIONSHIP OF COMPUTATIONAL MODELS TO QUALITATIVE THEORIES

So far, this chapter has discussed how primary sensory cortex may operate as a series of unsupervised networks, each of which forms topographic maps. These maps may provide preprocessed input to other cortical modules and to the hippocampal region. We focused on piriform cortex because of its simple paleocortical structure and its direct connection to the hippocampal region. However, there is evidence that similar general principles apply in other sensory cortices (refer to figure 8.3). In fact, topographic mapping may be a general principle of cortical organization. In primary sensory cortex, it is easy to see the topographic representation, because we know which sensory inputs drive individual cortical neurons. In later processing stages, where it is more difficult to know what inputs "mean," it may be more difficult to observe topographicity. And in cortical areas that are involved with abstract function such as planning or working memory, it is harder even to imagine what a topographic representation might look like. However, researchers are currently investigating these issues as well as other functions of cortex. There are also many computational models that address more complex aspects of cortical operation, including cell synchronization, inhibitory interneurons, and columnar architecture.[38]

In this chapter, the focus has been on representational plasticity in sensory cortex. The data and models that we have discussed so far deal with unsupervised plasticity, in which cortical representations are changed on the basis of stimulus frequency and the similarities between stimuli (stimulus clusters). However, there is another important factor governing cortical plasticity: stimulus meaning, such as whether a stimulus predicts future reinforcement (e.g., a US).

Norman Weinberger and colleagues have made extensive study of primary auditory cortex, recording from individual neurons in guinea pigs before and after the animals learn that a tone CS predicts some salient US.[39] Initially, each neuron in auditory cortex responds most to a particular tone: This is the cell's **best frequency;** the neuron responds in a decreasing fashion to tones that are increasingly different from this best frequency. For example, figure 8.20A shows the response of a single neuron when various tones are presented. This neuron's best frequency is around 0.75 kHz; the response drops off gradually as the frequency increases, and by 10 kHz, there is little or no response. Similarly, tones below the best frequency also generate weak responding. The best frequency of a neuron is not random, but relates to the neuron's position in the cortical map (refer to figure 8.3B). Thus, nearby neurons presumably have similar best frequencies.

Next, Weinberger and colleagues paired a 2.5-kHz tone CS with a US and observed what happened to the cortical neurons. Some neurons changed their best frequency in the direction of the CS, as is shown in figure 8.20B. That is, cells that previously responded only weakly to the CS now responded more strongly to it. If enough cells showed this type of change, the overall result might be a change in the cortical map: More areas of cortex would respond to the CS (compare figure 8.5). The changes were fast, occurring within as few as five training trials.[40] As long as eight weeks after training, many neurons maintained their new firing patterns.[41] However, if the CS is presented alone—not with the US—the changes may be absent or greatly reduced.[42] This implies that *stimulation alone doesn't drive cortical plasticity; instead, the stimulus has to be meaningfully related to reinforcement.*

Apparently, cortical plasticity occurs when a stimulus such as a CS is meaningfully related to (predictive of) a salient reinforcement such as a US. The next obvious question is: How does US information reach primary sensory cortex? USs often take the form of shock or food and are therefore perceived as somatosensory or gustatory stimuli; it is unlikely that this kind of information is accessible to primary auditory cortex, which is devoted to processing acoustic stimuli.[43] However, Weinberger's findings clearly indicate that the shock US influences plasticity in auditory cortex.

Weinberger and Merzenich have both suggested the same basic interpretation: They have argued that the auditory cortex does *not* receive information about reinforcing somatosensory or gustatory stimuli. Rather, they believe that it receives information only that a US of some kind has occurred. This

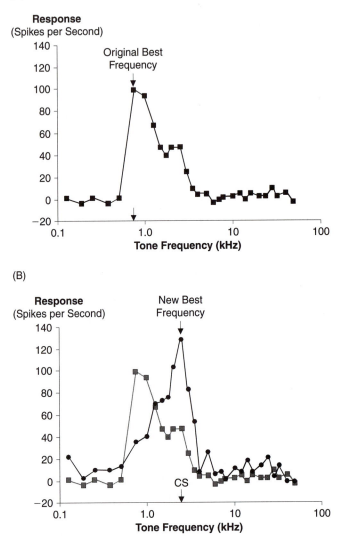

Figure 8.20 Responses of a single neuron in primary auditory cortex of guinea pig to various tone stimuli. (A) Originally, this neuron responds maximally to a tone at frequency 0.75 kHz; this is the cell's best frequency. The response drops off gradually for higher tones and precipitously for lower tones. Other neurons in auditory cortex respond preferentially to other tones. (B) After training that a 2.5-kHz tone CS predicted a shock US, the neuron's responses altered so that the new best frequency was the CS, and there was proportionately less responding to the previous best frequency. (Adapted from Weinberger, 1997, figure 2.)

information is enough to drive cortical remapping to expand the representation of the CS. Other brain areas (such as the amygdala, hippocampus, and polymodal cortex) may be responsible for encoding the memory linking this CS with a particular US—but not primary sensory cortex. Primary sensory cortex knows only which stimuli are worth expanded representation and which are not.

To implement this system, what is needed is a brain region that can signal importance to sensory cortex, giving warning that the current stimulus is worth remapping, without necessarily specifying exactly why. It turns out that several brain regions exist that could serve this kind of a function; both Weinberger and Merzenich have focused on the **nucleus basalis,** a small group of neurons located in an area known as the **basal forebrain** (figure 8.21). The nucleus basalis projects to all areas of the cortex and to the amygdala (though, interestingly, it does not project strongly to hippocampus). When nucleus basalis neurons are activated, they release a neurotransmitter called **acetylcholine** (abbreviated **ACh**). Acetylcholine has many functions in the brain, one of which is to enhance neuronal plasticity. Thus, a simplified view of the function of the nucleus basalis is that it could function as an enabler of cortical plasticity: *When a CS is paired with a US, the nucleus basalis becomes active and delivers acetylcholine to cortex, enabling cortical remapping to enlarge the representation of that CS.*[44]

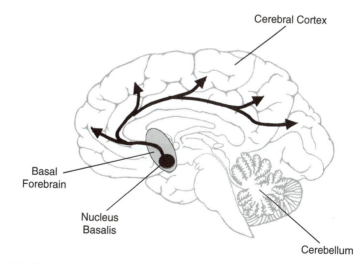

Figure 8.21   Cutaway view of the human brain showing approximate placement of the nucleus basalis within the general area denoted as the basal forebrain. Cholinergic neurons in the nucleus basalis project throughout the cerebral cortex.

Of course, this argument begs the question of how the nucleus basalis knows when to become active, and this is still a topic of intense current interest and research. However, the nucleus basalis does receive connections from areas such as amygdala that are known to receive information about USs such as shock and food.

Several studies have confirmed that the nucleus basalis can play a role in mediating cortical plasticity. Most important, when a tone CS is paired with nucleus basalis stimulation instead of a real US, cortical remapping occurs to that CS.[45] This lends strength to the argument that sensory cortex does not receive direct US information but only signals from the nucleus basalis that can initiate plasticity. Additionally, when the nucleus basalis is lesioned or the cholinergic projections are otherwise disrupted, cortical plasticity is greatly reduced.[46]

These findings are very exciting, not least because of their implications for rehabilitation after cortical damage. Perhaps it may eventually even be possible to use judicious stimulation of the nucleus basalis to encourage cortical remapping in individuals who have lost the use of one cortical area. Additionally, the idea of cholinergic mediation of cortical plasticity would be relatively simple to instantiate within a computational model. The competitive networks that we discussed in section 8.2 self-organize on the basis of stimulus frequency and stimulus similarity, without regard for stimulus meaning. It would be straightforward to add an additional assumption that plasticity is facilitated or increased in the presence of a cholinergic input that signals that a stimulus is associated with reinforcement.

8. 4   IMPLICATIONS FOR HUMAN MEMORY AND MEMORY DISORDERS

Most of the empirical work described in this chapter is based on animal research, but many of the same processes appear to operate in human cortex as well. This section describes one recent project using the principles of cortical remapping observed in monkeys to improve language skills in children.

Most children who are exposed to language throughout their infancy master the incredible complexities of speech generation and comprehension with seemingly little effort. A few children lag behind their peers in the development of language skills, and some of these children develop a cluster of impairments in language and reading that may be diagnosed as dyslexia. Some studies have estimated that 3–10% of all preschoolers have at least some language learning problems that are not attributable to known factors such as hearing impairment, mental retardation, or known brain lesion, and these children develop normally in other ways.[47]

Work by Paula Tallal and colleagues over the past twenty years has identified one subgroup of **language-learning impaired** (LLI) children who have normal intelligence but score well below normal on oral language tests. Tallal tested these children on tasks that required discriminating syllables such as /ba/ and /da/, which begin with consonant sounds that differ only in the initial few milliseconds (see MathBox 8.2). The LLI children were specifically impaired at making these fine temporal discriminations. Thus, Tallal hypothesized that what appeared to be a language-specific deficit in the LLI children might actually reflect a difficulty in processing information that was presented for only a few tens of milliseconds. Consistent with this idea, Tallal found that the LLI children had deficits in a wide range of nonspeech areas that involved such information. For example, if the LLI children were touched in rapid succession on two different fingers, they had trouble identifying which finger was touched first. Thus, LLI may be not a primarily linguistic impairment, but rather a problem in rapid sensory processing that has its most obvious expression in language difficulty.

The next step was to consider how LLI children could be helped. Michael Merzenich and other workers, studying animals, had shown that the cortex was plastic throughout life and that its ability to make distinctions between stimuli could be modified by experience—specifically by intense practice with those stimuli (refer to section 8.1). If that practice required making fine distinctions about temporal differences, then the cortex should remap to emphasize temporal information and facilitate the distinctions. Prior studies had already shown that normal adults who were given intense practice in recognizing extremely brief stimuli could demonstrate great improvements in their performance. Perhaps the same would be true with LLI children.

Tallal and Merzenich devised several computer games that were intended to drill LLI children in acoustic recognition of rapidly presented sounds. One game involved the presentation of two tones, each of which could be either high or low; the children were required to execute keyboard responses depending on the order of tone presentation. Initially, the tones were relatively long (60 msec) and had a brief interval between them (500 msec). The LLI children could master this task easily. As the drill progressed, the stimulus duration and intervals were gradually reduced.

In other games, the children were required to distinguish syllables that had been acoustically modified so that the difficult rapidly changing aspects (such as those differentiating /ba/ from /da/) were artificially extended—for example, from 40 msec to 80 msec. The syllables sound distorted but are easy to discriminate, even for LLI children. Again, the distorted aspects were gradually speeded up until they were as rapid as in normal speech.

Children were drilled on these games several times a day for several weeks, and by the end of this training period, many of the LLI children were able to play the games with the same speed and accuracy as non-LLI children. Following this training, the LLI children were given a test of their ability to process rapidly presented stimuli; performance improved dramatically relative to pretraining levels, and this improvement was still evident at a posttest six weeks after training.[48] More important, after a summer of practice, many teachers and parents reported improved performance when the LLI children returned to school in the fall.*

This study represents one example of how insights about cortical function discovered in animal research—specifically, that intensive training with particular stimuli could result in cortical remapping that made those stimuli more discriminable—could have clinical implications for humans with learning impairments. Potentially, the same idea could be applied to other domains of human learning impairment.

SUMMARY

• In mammals, cerebral cortex is mainly six-layered neocortex; a few areas such as primary olfactory (piriform) cortex are two-layered allocortex similar to the cortex found in reptiles and birds.

• For each sensory modality, the first cortical processing occurs in a specific region: primary visual cortex, primary auditory cortex, and so on. Primary sensory cortex is usually laid out in a topographic map, in which each subregion of cortex responds preferentially to a particular type of stimulus and neighboring cortical regions respond to similar stimuli.

• Cortical maps are plastic in adults, in response to dramatic changes in stimulation (such as deafferentation) and in response to learning (repeated pairing of a stimulus with reinforcement). Stimulus representations compete for cortical space, so as the area devoted to encoding one stimulus expands, the regions devoted to other nearby stimuli are shifted or compressed.

• Unsupervised or self-organizing networks are a class of neural network that discover underlying regularities in the input without generating any

*Tallal and Merzenich's learning games are commercially available under the product name Fast ForWord. They report that during two years of field testing by 35 speech pathologists and other clinicians, the program had a 90% success rate and helped to improve language processing in over 500 children with specific language impairments. Fast ForWord is marketed by the Scientific Learning Corporation. More information is available at the company's Internet Web site (http://www.scientificlearning.com) or by mail from Scientific Learning Corporation, 1995 University Avenue, Suite 400, Berkeley, CA 94704.

predefined output (such as a CR that anticipates the US). Competitive networks are a class of unsupervised network in which nodes compete to respond to inputs. Self-organizing feature maps are a kind of competitive network that can develop topographic representations similar to those developed in sensory cortex.

• Olfactory or piriform cortex may function as a competitive network that performs hierarchical clustering of odor inputs. In the process, it compresses co-occurring odors, meaning that it is harder later to distinguish the individual odor components.

• The cortico-hippocampal model assumes that one function of the hippocampal region is to differentiate the representations of predictive stimuli. This differentiation may ordinarily serve as an opponent process to combat piriform-mediated odor compression when needed. Hippocampal-region damage should then result in a tendency to overcompress co-occurring odors. This is consistent with data showing that rats with hippocampal-region damage have difficulties in simultaneous odor discrimination and in responding appropriately when familiar odors are presented in novel recombinations.

• Cortical plasticity reflects not only stimulus frequency and stimulus similarity but also stimulus meaning. Rather than receiving direct US inputs, sensory cortex receives cholinergic projections from the nucleus basalis that may signal that the current input is important—and representations should be enlarged—without specifying the exact nature of the associated reinforcement.

• Theoretical and empirical findings about cortical plasticity have lead to real-world advances, particularly in the treatment of language-learning impairments by intensive training with difficult speech elements.

APPENDIX 8.1   SIMULATION DETAILS

The model presented in the section beginning on page 241 was originally described in Myers & Gluck (1996). Full details of this model and its application to odor discrimination are given there.

The *external input* to the system is a 48-element vector. The first 12 elements represent 12 possible odors; each element is set to 1 if the corresponding odor is present on the current trial or to 0 otherwise. The remaining 36 elements make up a three-element subfield for each of the 12 odors, indicating whether the odor (if present) occurs at the left, center, or right odor port. In the experiments reported in the section beginning on page 241, two odors are presented on each trial, one each at the left and right odor ports.

The *piriform network* is a simplification of the piriform cortex model described in the section beginning on page 232.[49] It consists of a single layer of 25 nodes, each receiving weighted connections from all the inputs. There are 156 inputs: the 12 odor inputs each magnified to occupy a ten-element subfield and the 36 spatial inputs. The connection weights and node biases are initialized from the uniform distribution $U[0..1]$ and normalized so that the total weight to each node sums to 1.0. The nodes are divided into five groups of five nodes each. On each trial, each patch individually determines its winning node j with greatest activation V_j determined as $V_j = f(\Sigma_i w_{i-j} V_i + \theta_j)$, where $f(x) = 1/(1 + e^{-x})$, w_{ij} is the weight from input i to node j, V_i is the activation of input i, and θ_j is the bias of node j. The output o_j of each winning node j is set to 1.0, while the outputs of all other nodes in the cluster are set to 0.0. Each node j then updates its weights as $\Delta w_{ij} = \beta(o_j - V_j)V_i$ with learning rate $\beta = 0.005$. All weights are bounded between 0 and 1.

The *hippocampal-region network* is a predictive autoencoder with 61 inputs (the 36 external spatial inputs plus the 25 outputs of the piriform network), 25 internal-layer nodes, and 63 output nodes, which reconstruct the inputs and predict whether the behavioral response was "go left" or "go right." Weights and biases are initialized from a uniform distribution $U[-0.1..+0.1]$. (Randomly, two lower-layer weights into each internal-layer node are initialized from the uniform distribution $U[-1, +1]$.) Node activations are computed as in the piriform network; weights are trained by error back-propagation as described in MathBox 4.1 with learning rate $\beta = 0.25$ and momentum $\alpha = 0.9$.

The *cortico/cerebellar network* receives the same 61 inputs as the hippocampal-region network and contains 25 internal-layer nodes and 2 output nodes L and R, corresponding to the "go left" and "go right" responses. Weight initialization and node activation are identical to the hippocampal-region network. The behavioral response is computed from the two output nodes according to

$$\Pr(response = go - left) = \frac{1}{1 + e^{10(y_R - y_L)}}$$

The output nodes are trained according to the Widrow-Hoff rule (Math-Box 3.1) with $\beta = 0.5$. On each trial, only the weights from the output node associated with the behavioral response (L or R) are trained; if reward was trained, the desired output for that node was 1.0; otherwise, the desired output was 0.0. The internal-layer nodes are also trained by the Widrow-Hoff rule; the desired output of node j is the output of internal-layer node j in the hippocampal-region network.

The *fornix-lesion model* is identical to the intact model except that there is no learning in the hippocampal-region network; that is, $\beta = \alpha = 0$. As a result, the cortico/cerebellar network adopts hippocampal-region representations which are fixed and arbitrary.

9   Entorhinal Cortex

Chapter 8 argued that the anatomy and physiology of cerebral cortex was consistent with self-organization, including the development of topographic maps and clustered stimulus representations. Because so much of cortex shares a uniform stylized structure, it seems likely that other areas of cortex could perform similar functions. Various cortical regions differ chiefly in the kind of information they process, depending on their inputs and outputs.[1] Thus, primary auditory cortex processes sound because it receives sound inputs, while primary motor cortex guides movements because its outputs connect to motor neurons in the body. Although this scenario is doubtless oversimplified, it still provides a useful way for thinking about—and modeling—cortical function.

The hippocampal region as defined in this book includes the entorhinal cortex. Some definitions of the hippocampal region also include the nearby perirhinal and parahippocampal cortices. Each of these cortical areas may well perform information-processing functions similar to those described in chapter 8. The difference between, say, entorhinal and piriform cortex would be that, whereas piriform cortex receives and operates on odor inputs, the entorhinal cortex receives highly processed inputs covering the full range of sensory modalities. On the assumption that cortex is capable of self-organizing and clustering inputs, this would suggest that entorhinal cortex should be able to compress information across sensory modalities—for instance, combining the visual, auditory, olfactory, and other features of a stimulus.

This chapter considers three computational models that propose possible functions for entorhinal cortex and its interaction with other hippocampal-region and cortical structures. The first two concentrate on the entorhinal cortex as an input preprocessor for the hippocampus; the third is concerned with the storage of hippocampal-derived representations (or "memories") into cortical long-term storage sites. Finally, the chapter discusses a qualitative theory that focuses on the entorhinal cortex and that is consonant with some of the computational modeling.

9.1   ANATOMY AND PHYSIOLOGY OF THE HIPPOCAMPAL REGION

It sometimes seems as if every scientist studying the hippocampus has a different definition for specifying which structures constitute the hippocampal region (or hippocampal formation, hippocampal system, etc.). In this book, we have defined the **hippocampal region** to include the hippocampus (including subfields CA1 and CA3), dentate gyrus, subiculum, and entorhinal cortex (and possibly fimbria/fornix).* Other definitions would be equally valid for different anatomical, physiological, and behavioral purposes. Our definition of the hippocampal region as a functional unit is useful for two reasons. First, all the included structures appear to contribute to memory functions that are independent of sensory modality; thus, they appear to constitute a multimodal memory system. Second, until very recently, many techniques for "hippocampal lesion" actually involved damage to the broader hippocampal region. Hence, many early data on the effects of "hippocampal lesion" more accurately describe the effects of broader and more inclusive "hippocampal-region damage."

The basic routes of sensory information flow within the hippocampal region are schematized in figure 9.1. Sensory input, such as smell or auditory information, is processed first by primary sensory cortex and other cortical areas devoted to that modality (called **unimodal sensory cortices**) before progressing to **polymodal association cortices,** which integrate information across multiple sensory modalities. From there, information enters the entorhinal cortex. The one major exception to this rule, as we noted earlier, is that odor information from the piriform cortex travels directly to the entorhinal cortex. The entorhinal cortex also receives input from subcortical areas such as the septum, thalamus, hypothalamus, and amygdala.

Entorhinal cortex is intermediate in structure between six-layered neocortex and two-layered allocortex. For this reason, it is sometimes classified with the rather unwieldy name of **periallocortex.** For current purposes, it is sufficient to note that the cell layers in the entorhinal cortex are rather indistinct and clustered into **superficial layers** (layers II and III) and **deep layers** (layers IV–VI). Pyramidal neurons are located in both the superficial and deep layers. Sensory input projects largely to the superficial layers.

From superficial entorhinal cortex, axons project to the dentate gyrus and hippocampus (figure 9.2). The tract from entorhinal cortex to dentate gyrus is

---

*Our definition is roughly consistent with that of two premier hippocampal anatomists, David Amaral and Menlo Witter (1989), although they group the same structures under the term *hippocampal formation.*

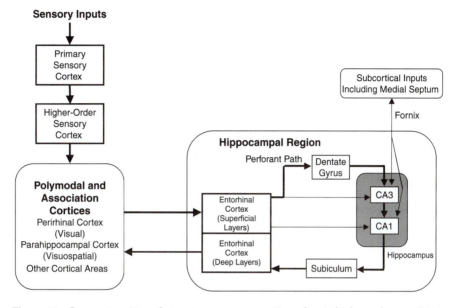

Figure 9.1 Sensory input travels to primary sensory cortices, then to higher-order association cortices, eventually reaching entorhinal cortex. There is also a direct path from primary olfactory (piriform) cortex to entorhinal cortex. Superficial layers of entorhinal cortex project to the dentate gyrus via the perforant path and also directly to hippocampal subfields CA3 and CA1. Information flows in a largely unidirectional fashion from dentate gyrus to CA3 to CA1, through subiculum, and back to the deep layers of entorhinal cortex. From there, information projects back to the cortical areas where it originated. There is also an input/output pathway through the fornix that connects hippocampus with subcortical areas including the septum, thalamus, hypothalamus, and amygdala.

known as the **perforant path,** because these fibers must travel through (perforate) the subiculum to reach their destination. From dentate gyrus, axons travel to hippocampal subfield CA3, which also receives a direct projection from entorhinal cortex. Recall from chapter 5 that the combination of strong dentate and weaker entorhinal projections to CA3, together with high recurrency among CA3 neurons, suggests that CA3 might function as an autoassociator.

Information next projects from CA3 to hippocampal field CA1, through the subiculum, back through the deep layers of entorhinal cortex, and finally back to the same cortical areas that gave rise to the information in the first place. There are additional pathways other than those described here or shown in figure 9.1, but this unidirectional flow from entorhinal cortex through dentate gyrus, hippocampus, and subiculum back to entorhinal cortex is a primary feature of the circuitry.[2]

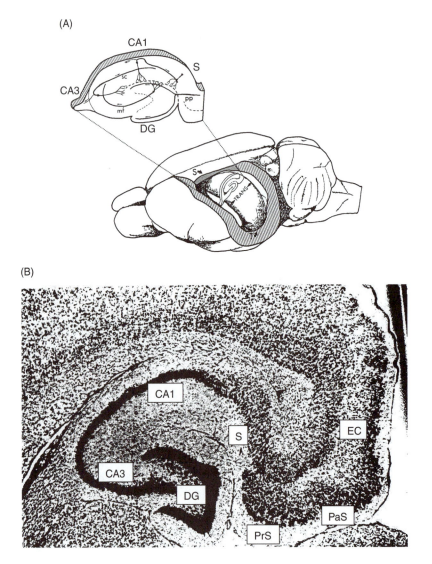

Figure 9.2   (A) Drawing of the rat brain, with cortical surface removed to show position of the hippocampus. A transverse slice through the hippocampus reveals the "C"-shaped organization (cutaway). Hippocampal fields CA1 and CA3, dentate gyrus (DG), and subiculum (S) are as shown. A few information pathways are drawn to illustrate the roughly unidirectional flow (pp = perforant path, mf = mossy fiber, sc = Schaeffer collaterals). (Reprinted from Amaral & Witter, 1989, figure 2.) (B) Photomicrograph of a section through the rat hippocampal region. The hippocampus (including fields CA1 and CA3) is visible as a "C"-shaped line of principal cells; the dentate gyrus (DG) is a backward "C"-shaped line of principal cells. Adjacent to hippocampal field CA1 is the subicular complex, including subiculum (S), presubiculum (PrS), and parasubiculum (PaS). The entorhinal cortex (EC) is the primary pathway for sensory information traveling into and out of the hippocampal region. (Adapted from Amaral & Witter, 1989, figure 1.)

For many years, it was believed that the hippocampal region functioned as a processing chain and that damage to any one link in the chain would disrupt processing in the entire chain. Further, there appeared to be a law of mass action, meaning that impairment increased in an orderly fashion as lesion size increased. Figure 9.3 shows one example of this apparent rule: On a battery of four measures of memory, there was progressively worse performance in monkeys with increasing hippocampal-region damage.[3] However, the story is not quite so simple; later studies have shown that there may be qualitative, not just quantitative, effects of different lesion extents.

An important methodological advance in recent years has been the development of **neurotoxic** lesions, such as the injection of **ibotenic acid,** which destroys neuron cell bodies near the injection site but spares nearby cell bodies as well as any axons that may be passing through the area.[4] This is in contrast to older lesion techniques, particularly surgical removal of tissue by **ablation** or **aspiration,** which not only removed all cells and fibers in the

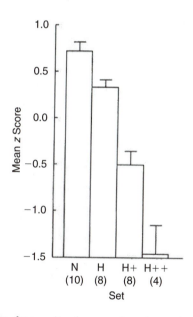

Figure 9.3 On many tasks, the severity of memory impairment is proportional to the extent of hippocampal-region lesion. On a battery of four measures, including delayed nonmatch to sample (DNMS) and delayed retention, monkeys show worse performance with increasing lesions. (Higher mean z-score indicates better performance over all four measures.) N = normal (ten monkeys); H = lesion of hippocampus, dentate gyrus, and subiculum (eight monkeys); H+ = H lesion plus adjacent entorhinal and parahippocampal cortices (eight monkeys); H++ = H+ lesion plus anterior entorhinal cortex and perirhinal cortex (four monkeys). (Reprinted from Zola-Morgan, Squire, & Ramus, 1994, figure 4.)

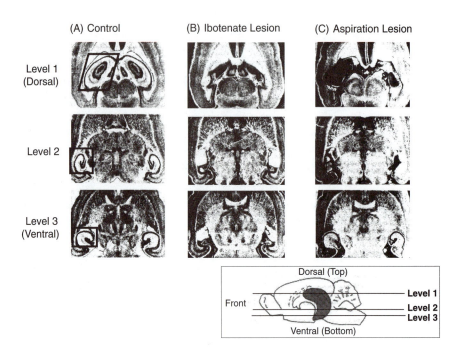

Figure 9.4 Photomicrographs of the rat brain, taken in a horizontal plane, at three levels ranging from dorsal (level 1) to ventral (level 3); the top of each picture is the front of the brain. Inset shows a schematic of a rat brain, with hippocampus in dark gray, illustrating the position of levels shown in A–C. (A) A control rat. Cell bodies in the hippocampus are visible at all three levels (left hippocampus is outlined in black at each level). (B) Hippocampal lesion by injection of ibotenic acid to destroy cell bodies. The lesion is visible in the picture as white spaces where the hippocampal cell bodies should be. Destruction of the hippocampus is relatively complete at all levels, and there is little damage to adjoining regions. (C) Aspiration lesion of the hippocampus. Areas where tissue has been removed are shown as black. Compared with the ibotenate lesion in (B), the aspiration lesion results in variable degrees of damage to the hippocampus; thus, while the dorsal hippocampus (top row) is largely destroyed, the ventral hippocampus (bottom row) is largely spared. Conversely, the aspiration lesion is apt to destroy nearby tissue; thus, in the top row, the black area extends beyond the hippocampus and into nearby tissue. (A–C adapted from Jarrard & Davidson, 1991, figure 4; inset adapted from West, 1990, p. 6, figure 1.)

target area, but also often involved cutting out significant portions of tissue overlying the target area.

Figure 9.4 compares ibotenic acid and aspiration lesions of hippocampus. The ibotenic acid lesion, shown in figure 9.4B, results in relatively complete destruction of cell bodies in the hippocampus and dentate gyrus (seen as white patches devoid of darkly stained cell bodies). In contrast, the aspiration lesion—visible as "empty" dark patches in figure 9.4C—results in a less accurate removal of tissue. In the example shown, the aspiration lesion generates nearly complete damage to the left dorsal (upper) hippocampus but incomplete damage to the left ventral (lower) hippocampus and much less damage to the right hippocampus. Additionally, the aspiration lesion extends somewhat beyond the hippocampus into nearby brain areas.

Thus, the behavior of an animal with aspiration lesions of hippocampus may be misleading for at least two opposing reasons: The residual hippocampal tissue may allow the animal to maintain some hippocampal-dependent processing, while ancillary damage to other nearby structures may result in deficits that are not hippocampal-related. Neurotoxic lesions, particularly ibotenic acid lesions, minimize these problems, allowing a more accurate analysis of how an animal behaves with specific and localized hippocampal damage. More recently, ibotenic acid has also been used to create specific and precisely localized entorhinal lesions.

By comparing memory deficits in animals with specific hippocampal (or entorhinal) lesions against animals with larger hippocampal-region lesions, researchers are beginning to understand how these separate structures interact in normal functioning. At the same time, these ideas are being explored via computational models. In the next section, we turn to review some models of entorhinal and hippocampal interaction in learning and memory.

9.2   COMPUTATIONAL MODELS

Only recently have computational models begun to address the individual functional roles of different hippocampal-region structures and how these structures might contribute to a coherent learning and memory system. As we discussed in chapter 5, hippocampal field CA3 has received extensive study owing, in part, to its physical resemblance to an autoassociative network. However, there has been much less consideration of how CA3 might interact with other hippocampal-region structures and with the rest of the brain. With a few notable exceptions, there has been even less study of the other hippocampal-region structures.

More recently, the entorhinal cortex has begun to receive attention from computational modelers for two reasons: first, because of its similarity to neocortex, which has already been extensively modeled, and second, because of exciting new empirical data, which suggest that many behaviors that were previously thought to depend on the hippocampus may actually be mediated by the entorhinal cortex.

In this section, we review three computational models of entorhinal cortex. The first is an elaboration of our own cortico-hippocampal model, which presumes that the entorhinal cortex plays a specific role in compression of redundant stimulus representations. The second is an extension of the Schmajuk-DiCarlo (S-D) model, which assumes that the entorhinal cortex is critical for stimulus configuration. Finally, a model proposed by Edmund Rolls suggests how information processed in the hippocampal region might be transferred from entorhinal cortex back to the neocortex.

Entorhinal Cortex and Redundancy Compression

In the rat, the piriform and entorhinal cortices lie adjacent to each other and are so similar anatomically that it is difficult to determine precisely where one structure ends and the other begins. The superficial layers of the piriform and entorhinal cortices are especially similar in anatomy and physiology, leading many researchers to suggest that the two structures may share a related function.[5] The most obvious difference between these two cortical areas is in their inputs: As was noted above, piriform cortex receives primarily olfactory input, whereas entorhinal cortex receives highly processed information from the full range of sensory modalities as well as from multimodal association areas (figure 9.1). In a sense, the entorhinal cortex represents the highest stage of cortical processing, in which all sensory information converges. Entorhinal cortex would thus be a logical place to perform clustering among stimuli in different modalities (e.g., smell and vision) or among the multimodal features of a single stimulus.

We have proposed that the entorhinal cortex can be modeled as follows:[6] The superficial layers of entorhinal cortex receive highly processed, multimodal stimulus inputs. Entorhinal cells are grouped together into clusters; within each cluster, cells compete to respond to the input (figure 9.5A). Cells that win this competition undergo plasticity, making them more likely to respond to similar inputs in the future (figure 9.5B). Meanwhile, losing cells also undergo plasticity, making them less likely to respond to similar inputs. These cells then become more likely to win the competition in response to very different inputs (figure 9.5C).

Our entorhinal network model performs unsupervised clustering of its inputs, just as the original piriform model did. Similar inputs evoke similar responses. Additionally, the network performs pattern compression or clustering. For example, suppose the pattern trained in figure 9.5C is really a compound stimulus consisting of three component stimuli that always co-occur. The network learns a response to the compound without distinguishing the components. Later, if one of the components is presented alone (figure 9.5D), it will tend to activate the same nodes as did the compound. Moreover, it may activate these nodes less strongly than did the compound.

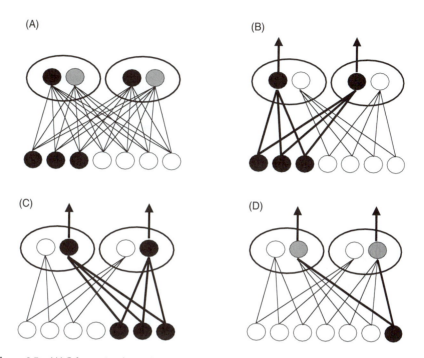

Figure 9.5 (A) Schematic of entorhinal cortex model. A layer of nodes is organized into clusters (two clusters containing two nodes each are shown; the full model consists of 100 nodes organized into five 20-node clusters). Within a cluster, nodes compete to respond to input patterns. If an input pattern is presented (the three black input nodes represent stimulus features that are present on the current trial), one node within each cluster responds most strongly: It wins the competition. (B) Winning nodes are allowed to output, while inhibition silences other nodes in the clusters. The winning nodes undergo plasticity, making them more likely to respond to similar inputs in the future, while losing nodes undergo plasticity to make them less likely to respond to similar inputs in future—and hence more likely to respond to different kinds of inputs. (C) When a very different input pattern is presented, other nodes are likely to win the competition. (D) The network has no way of knowing whether the trained pattern represents one complex stimulus with many different features or a compound of several individual stimuli. Suppose the pattern trained in (C) is really a collection of three different component stimuli. Now, if one component stimulus is presented, this will tend to maximally activate the same nodes in each cluster as the compound stimulus did. The activation may be weaker than that to the pattern trained in (C), but as long as it is stronger than the activation of other nodes in the cluster, it will be sufficient to win the competition. Hence, the network tends to generalize from compound stimuli to the components. This means that the network compresses together the representations of co-occurring stimuli (and stimulus features) into complex compound stimuli.

However, as long as these nodes are more strongly activated than other nodes in the cluster, they will continue to win the competition. Thus, the network tends to represent the components in the same way as it represented the compound. In effect, the network performs pattern completion; when presented with a component in isolation, it tends to evoke the representation of the full compound stimulus on which it was trained.

A Model of Selective Hippocampal Lesion That Spares Entorhinal Cortex. The implication of this network model is that the entorhinal cortex alone should be sufficient to implement one aspect of the hippocampal-region function proposed in our cortico-hippocampal model from chapter 6: representational compression of co-occurring (redundant) stimuli.[7] Other proposed hippocampal-region functions (particularly representational differentiation) would be mediated elsewhere in the hippocampal region; we will return to this issue later in this chapter.

For now, we consider how an entorhinal network might interact with cortical and cerebellar learning systems in the absence of other hippocampal-region processing. Figure 9.6 shows a schematic of information flow in the hippocampal region, simplified from figure 9.1. So far, we have focused mainly on the behavioral effects of a broad lesion of the entire hippocampal region extending from the entorhinal cortex through to the hippocampus (the **HR lesion;** figure 9.6B). But the entorhinal cortex has input and output connections with cortical areas that are independent of its connections with hippocampus. This implies that a selective lesion of the hippocampus and possibly dentate gyrus and subiculum (the **H lesion;** figure 9.6C) may spare some or all entorhinal processing. Note that the converse is not true: If the entorhinal cortex is lesioned (the **EC lesion;** figure 9.6D), the hippocampus may be functionally isolated from sensory input, and so the effects may be just as dramatic as a full HR lesion.

Recall that our intact cortico-hippocampal model of figure 9.7A assumes that all hippocampal-region representational processing takes place within a hippocampal-region network. This hippocampal-region network performs redundancy compression and predictive differentiation, creating new stimulus representations that are adopted by the cortico/cerebellar network. The HR-lesion model of figure 9.7B—which assumes that all of the hippocampal-region mediated processing is disabled—is really an "H + EC lesion" model. We can now consider an intermediate system: an H-lesion model, in which the hippocampus is lesioned but the entorhinal cortex is spared (figure 9.7C). Note that since the dentate gyrus, hippocampus, and subiculum form a largely unidirectional processing chain (refer to figure 9.1), damage to the hippocampus is liable to disrupt the dentate gyrus (by disabling its primary output pathway) and the subiculum (by disabling a primary input pathway). Hence, in the H-lesion model, the entorhinal cortex may be the only hippocampal-region structure that is still functional.

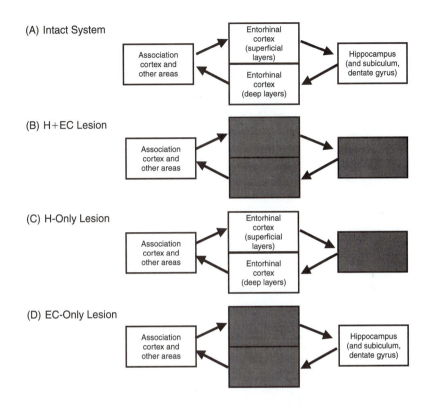

Figure 9.6 (A) In the normal, intact brain, information flows from cortical association areas and other cortical areas to entorhinal cortex to the hippocampus and back out through the entorhinal cortex. (B) Broad hippocampal-region damage (the H+EC lesion) is assumed to destroy processing in entorhinal cortex, hippocampus, and other hippocampal-region structures. (C) A more selective lesion of the hippocampus (H-only lesion) that leaves the entorhinal cortex intact may not totally disrupt processing in the entorhinal cortex; (D) however, a selective lesion of entorhinal cortex (EC-only lesion) functionally disconnects the hippocampus from its sensory input/output pathway. The behavioral effects of EC-only lesion may thus be comparable to those of a full H+EC lesion.

Therefore, in our H-lesion model of figure 9.7C, we assume that the entorhinal network performs stimulus compression and provides these compressed representations to the cortico/cerebellar network. Other representational changes, such as predictive differentiation, may depend on other hippocampal-region structures, such as the dentate gyrus and hippocampus. These functions would therefore be eliminated by a selective H-lesion in the model.

We will return later to the issue of which hippocampal-region structures may be involved in these other functions. For now, we expect the new

(A) Intact Model

(B) HR-Lesion Model

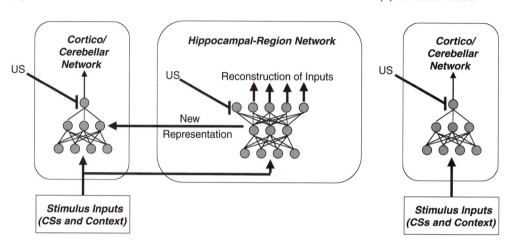

(C) Selective H-Lesion Model

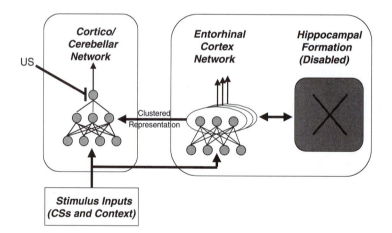

Figure 9.7 (A) The intact cortico-hippocampal model assumes that the operation of all hippocampal-region structures can be approximated by a single hippocampal-region network that produces new stimulus representations that are biased by redundancy compression and predictive differentiation. These new representations are then provided to the cortico/cerebellar network, which learns to map from them to a behavioral response. (B) Broad HR lesion is simulated by disabling all hippocampal-region processing; only the cortico/cerebellar network is assumed to operate. (C) A selective lesion of the hippocampus (the H lesion) may spare entorhinal processing, since the entorhinal cortex has reciprocal connections with other cortical areas that provide its major sensory input and receive its output (refer to figure 9.1). The H-lesion model assumes that only the entorhinal network is available to modify stimulus representations and provide these to the cortico/cerebellar network.

H-lesion model to be sufficient to show just those hippocampal-region-dependent behaviors that depend on redundancy compression but not those that depend on predictive differentiation. This model predicts that there should be a similar pattern of effects following selective H-lesion in animals.

Behavioral Predictions of the H-Lesion Model.   In chapter 7 we discussed how hippocampal-region damage disrupts **latent inhibition,** a behavioral paradigm in which learning a CS-US association is slower in animals that were given prior exposure to the CS (CS Exposure condition) relative to animals that were given equivalent exposure to the context alone (Sit Exposure condition). Hippocampal-region damage disrupts latent inhibition, so animals in the CS Exposure condition learn as fast as animals in the Sit Exposure condition.

In chapter 7, we simplified the story slightly: Although broad damage to the hippocampal region does indeed abolish latent inhibition, a more precise lesion that is limited to the hippocampus but spares the entorhinal cortex may spare or even enhance latent inhibition.*[8]

Furthermore, lesions that are limited to the entorhinal cortex (and possibly subiculum) but that spare hippocampus and dentate gyrus do suffice to disrupt latent inhibition (figure 9.8A).[9] Thus, it seems that while the hippocampus (and possibly dentate gyrus) are not necessary for latent inhibition, the entorhinal cortex is.

This finding is exactly as predicted by our cortico–hippocampal model. Recall from chapter 7 that the cortico-hippocampal model explains latent inhibition in terms of redundancy compression: During exposure, the representation of the CS is compressed together with the representation of the context in which it occurs, since neither predicts any US. Later, when the task is to respond to the CS but not the context alone, this compression must be explicitly undone, and learning is slowed while this redifferentiation takes

---

*One important exception to this rule is a study in which an ibotenic acid lesion that was limited to hippocampus and dentate gyrus impaired latent inhibition in rat appetitive conditioning; that is, lesioned rats learned equally quickly, whether or not they had previously been exposed to the CS (Han, Gallagher, & Holland, 1995). The reasons for this anomalous result are still unclear; one factor may be that Han, Gallagher, and Holland used a procedure in which animals were first exposed to the CS, then trained to approach the food cup for a reward, then trained that the CS predicted this reward. This paradigm contrasts with the more standard sequence in which animals are first trained to obtain food, then exposed, then given CS-US pairings (e.g., Honey & Good, 1993). Having a training session interposed between CS exposure and CS-US pairing may disrupt the effect, particularly in animals with hippocampal lesion, which may quickly forget the earlier exposure.

Latent Inhibition

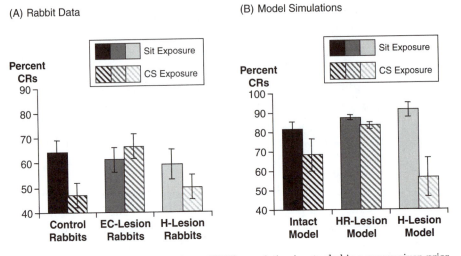

(A) Rabbit Data

(B) Model Simulations

Figure 9.8   Latent inhibition: Learning a CS-US association is retarded in a group given prior CS exposure compared with a group given equivalent exposure to the context alone (Sit Exposure). (A) Latent inhibition is eliminated by lesion that includes entorhinal cortex (ECL) but not by a selective hippocampal lesion (HL) that spares entorhinal cortex. (Data from Shohamy, Allen, & Gluck, 1999.) (B) The cortico-hippocampal model shows the same behavior: The H-lesion model but not the HR-lesion model shows latent inhibition. Note that in these and subsequent figures, the intact and HR-lesion models were simulated under slightly different conditions than the H-lesion model; for this reason, it is not appropriate to compare learning times, etc., between models (e.g., HR-lesion versus H-lesion), but only to compare a model's performance under one training condition with its own performance on a different training condition (e.g., exposed versus nonexposed).

place. Since this explanation of latent inhibition depends wholly on redundancy compression, it can be mediated by the entorhinal network alone; thus, the H-lesion model does show latent inhibition (figure 9.8B), though the HR-lesion model does not.[10]

A related effect is **learned irrelevance,** in which prior exposure to a CS *and* a US, uncorrelated with each other, slows subsequent learning of a CS-US association.[11] Again, our cortico-hippocampal model provides an account of this phenomenon in normal animals: During exposure, neither the context nor the CS is a good predictor of the US, so they become compressed together. As in latent inhibition, this compression hinders subsequent learning to associate the CS, but not the context alone, with the US.[12] Again, the model predicts that the learned irrelevance effect depends primarily on

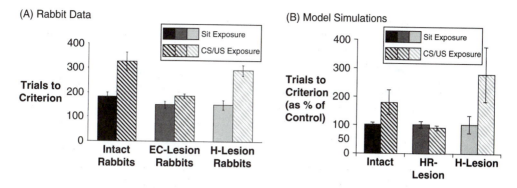

Figure 9.9 Learned irrelevance (retarded CS-US learning after exposure to CS and US, uncorrelated with each other). (A) Learned irrelevance is eliminated by lesion that includes entorhinal cortex (EC lesion) but not by a selective hippocampal lesion (H lesion) that spares entorhinal cortex. (Data from Allen, Chelius, & Gluck, 1998.) (B) The cortico-hippocampal model shows the same behavior: The H-lesion model but not the HR-lesion model shows learned irrelevance.

redundancy compression, and therefore the entorhinal cortex should be able to mediate learned irrelevance. In other words, HR lesion should disrupt learned irrelevance but H lesion might not, as is shown in figure 9.9B. In recent studies of rabbit eyeblink conditioning in our laboratory, we have now confirmed this prediction, as is shown in figure 9.9A.[13]

Several other novel predictions arise from our cortico-hippocampal model. For example, in **sensory preconditioning,** prior exposure to a compound AB increases the degree to which subsequent learning about A generalizes to B.[14] The intact model, but not the HR-lesioned cortico-hippocampal model, shows sensory preconditioning (figure 9.10A). The cortico-hippocampal model explains this effect in terms of redundancy compression: The representations of A and B are compressed during exposure to the compound, which increases later generalization between the components. Since this explanation involves redundancy compression, our model predicts that sensory preconditioning should survive selective H-lesion that spares the entorhinal cortex.[15] This is a prediction that remains to be tested in animals.

Easy-hard transfer of learning occurs when prior training on an easy discrimination facilitates learning a harder discrimination along the same stimulus continuum. For example, phase 1 might involve learning to discriminate a very low tone (S1+) from a very high tone (S4−). Phase 2 would involve transfer to a new discrimination along the same stimulus continuum—tone frequency in this case—such as discriminating a medium low tone (S2+) from a medium high tone (S3−). Prior training on the "easy" discrimination in

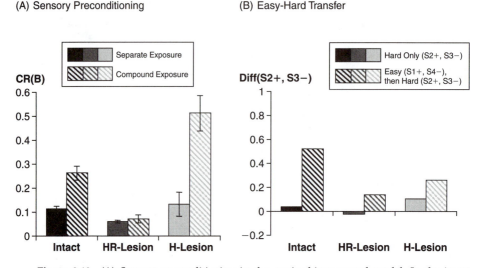

Figure 9.10 (A) Sensory preconditioning in the cortico-hippocampal model. In the intact model, exposure to the compound AB followed by A-US training leads to increased responding to B, compared with a control condition involving separate exposure to A and B. This sensory preconditioning effect is maintained in the H-lesion model but not in the HR-lesion model. (B) Easy-hard transfer (learning a hard discrimination, S2+, S3−, is facilitated by prior training on an easy discrimination, S1+, S4−, along the same stimulus continuum—more than equivalent amounts of prior training on the hard discrimination alone). The intact cortico-hippocampal model shows a strong transfer effect; after a fixed number of trials on the hard discrimination, the difference in responding to S2+ and S3− (Diff(S2+, S3−)) is stronger after prior training on the easy discrimination than after prior training on the hard discrimination itself. The HR-lesion model shows only a small (nonsignificant) easy-hard effect, which may be attributed simply to stimulus generalization. (The difference between the intact model and the HR-lesion model performance reflects the effect of representational changes in the intact model.) Similarly, the H-lesion model shows only a weak (nonsignificant) effect of prior easy training, again attributable to stimulus generalization.

phase 1 can often speed subsequent learning of the "hard" discrimination in phase 2—more than an equivalent amount of pretraining on the hard discrimination itself.[16]

We have hypothesized that this kind of easy-hard transfer would depend on predictive differentiation.[17] Learning about the easy discrimination in phase 1 results in differentiation of the representations of those stimuli, as more and more resources are devoted to encoding the relevant features. This differentiation will make all stimuli along the same continuum easier to distinguish, facilitating the hard task. As a result, the intact cortico-hippocampal model shows faster learning of the hard discrimination following prior training on the easy discrimination compared with a control condition given training on the hard discrimination all along, as is shown in figure 9.10B.[18]

The HR-lesion model shows only a minimal effect, and this is due to stimulus generalization whereby a response learned to S1+ generalizes partially to the nearby S2+. In contrast, the difference between the performance of intact and HR-lesion models in the easy-hard condition reflects the effect of representational changes in the intact model. Because the easy-hard effect is explained in terms of representational differentiation, rather than compression, the entorhinal network is not sufficient to mediate the effect. Thus, the H-lesion model does not show easy-hard transfer.[19] This prediction of the model remains to be tested in animals.

In sum, our model predicts that behaviors that depend on hippocampal-region mediation can be distinguished according to whether they primarily reflect representational compression, predictive differentiation, or both. Since the model expects that the entorhinal cortex is sufficient to mediate representational compression, behaviors that primarily reflect this process should survive selective hippocampal lesion. In contrast, behaviors that involve predictive differentiation may depend on other structures, such as the hippocampus and dentate gyrus, and may be eliminated following a selective hippocampal-region lesion.

Contextual Processing After H Lesion.   Chapter 7 focused on another class of behaviors that depend on the hippocampal region: contextual processing. Recall that after normal animals are trained to respond to a conditioned stimulus cue (e.g., tone) in a particular context X, there may be decreased responding when the tone is presented in a new context Y.[20] The intact cortico-hippocampal model shows a similar response decrement after context shift, as is seen in figure 9.11. In the intact model, the hippocampal-region network creates a new representation of the tone that includes information about the context X in which the tone occurs. This representation is acquired by the cortico/cerebellar network and then mapped to a behavioral response. When the tone is presented in a new context Y, the representation of tone-in-X is only partially activated, and so the response is only partially activated. This explanation assumes that the context-shift effect depends on hippocampal-region representational processes, and so our HR-lesion model does not show the effect.

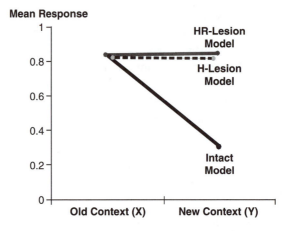

Figure 9.11   After training to respond to a cue A in a context X, the intact model but not the HR-lesion model shows a decrement in responding when A is presented in a new context Y. This is consistent with animal behavior (refer to figure 7.11A). The H-lesion model does not show a response decrement after context shift. Similarly, selective H lesion abolishes the context shift effect in rats (Honey & Good, 1993). (Adapted from Myers & Gluck, 1994, figure 3A, and Myers, Gluck, & Granger, 1995, figure 9.)

What about the H-lesioned model? The H-lesioned model does include representational compression in the entorhinal network, and as the tone is repeatedly presented in context X, the representations of tone and X should be compressed. Thus, at first glance, it might seem that the context shift effect should be mediated by entorhinal compression and should survive selective hippocampal lesion. However, the H-lesioned model does not include representational differentiation, a process that allows the representation of tone-in-X to be differentiated from that of X alone in the intact model. This makes all the difference.

For example, consider the simplified picture of the entorhinal network shown in figure 9.12. This network has four inputs: one representing the presence or absence of tone and three representing various features of the context. There are three patches of three nodes, each of which responds to this input. When context X is presented alone (figure 9.12A), one node in each patch wins the competition and becomes active. When the tone is presented in X (figure 9.12B), the input has considerable overlap with that encoding the context X alone; many of the clusters respond the same way to both. In this example, only one patch (the leftmost one) responds differently to X and tone-in-X.

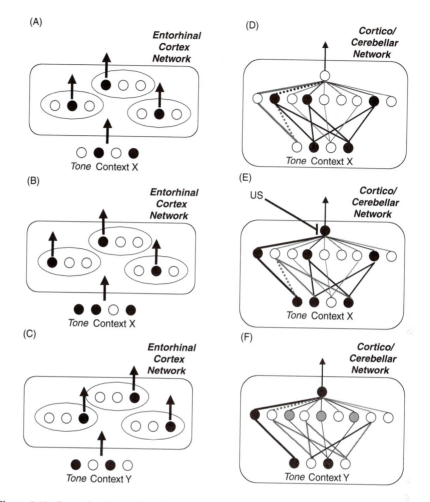

Figure 9.12 Loss of contextual sensitivity in the H-lesion model. For example, assume that the entorhinal network consists of nine nodes organized into three clusters. During tone+ training in context X, tone-in-X+ and X− trials are intermixed. Because of representational compression in the entorhinal network, the responses to tone-in-X+ and X− are liable to become similar. Thus, X− evokes one set of responses from the cluster (A), while tone-in-X+ evokes a very similar response (B): Only one cluster outputs differently to tone-in-X+ (the leftmost cluster). The cortico/cerebellar model adopts these entorhinal representations and learns to map from them to the correct response. This can be done only by learning strong weights from the elements that are present in the entorhinal response to tone-in-X+ but not to X−: Namely, the leftmost internal-layer node (activated by the tone) has a strong positive connection to the output (E), while the neighboring internal-layer node (active when the tone is absent) has a strong inhibitory connection to the output (D). Now the response of the network depends wholly on whether the tone is present; the internal-layer nodes encoding context information are ignored at the output level. When the tone is presented in a very different context Y, the entorhinal network will generate a very different pattern of responses (C), but these are adapted by the cortico/cerebellar network only over a series of many trials. On the initial presentation, the presence of the tone in the input is enough to drive a strong response (F). Hence, the H-lesion model continues to generate a strong response when the tone is presented in a new context: The context-shift effect is eliminated.

In the H-lesioned model, there is no hippocampal-mediated differentiation mechanism to pull these representations of X and tone-in-X apart. They are passed as is to the cortico/cerebellar model. In this simple example, there are nine internal-layer nodes in the cortico/cerebellar model—the same as the number of nodes in the entorhinal network—and so the internal-layer nodes eventually come to exactly mimic the entorhinal activations. Thus, the internal-layer activations for X alone (figure 9.12C) are the same as the entorhinal activation for X alone (figure 9.12A), and the internal-layer activations for tone-in-X (figure 9.12D) are the same as the entorhinal outputs for tone-in-X (figure 9.12B)

Now the cortico/cerebellar network must learn to map from these representations to the correct responses. Since there is such a high overlap between the representations of tone-in-X and context X alone, the cortico/cerebellar network must assign high weights to exactly those internal-layer nodes that are different between the two representations. In this case, that is only the leftmost internal-layer node (which responds to tone-in-X but not X alone) and its neighbor (which responds to X alone but not to tone-in-X). By assigning a strong positive weight to the leftmost node (and a strong negative weight to its neighbor), the network can learn to generate a behavioral response to tone-in-X but not to X alone. In effect, the cortico/cerebellar network of the H-lesion model learns to ignore the context and produce a response that depends only on whether the tone is present or absent.

Now suppose that the same tone is presented in a novel context Y that is very different from X. The entorhinal network will generate a new set of responses, as is illustrated in figure 9.12E, but these will be adopted by the cortico/cerebellar network only over the course of many repeated trials. On the very first presentation of tone-in-Y, Y will activate some subset of internal-layer nodes in the cortico/cerebellar network, and by virtue of prior training, the tone will continue to activate the leftmost internal-layer node, as is seen in figure 9.12F. But this leftmost node has a strong positive connection to the output, and so there will be a strong behavioral response—even in the new context Y, as is shown in figure 9.11.

The H-lesion model therefore predicts that selective hippocampal lesion that spares the entorhinal cortex should disrupt this context-shift effect.[21] Indeed, rats with selective hippocampal lesions do show no decrement in responding with context shift,[22] just as is expected by our model.

This finding of no context-shift effect in the H-lesioned model is particularly interesting because it is a model prediction that was not immediately obvious from the qualitative statement of theory. Only by implementing and observing the model in action does the full range of predictions become apparent. This is one reason why computational modeling is often valuable: It can help to make explicit the subtle implications of a theory.

The H-lesion model is similarly insensitive to contextual effects in latent inhibition. Recall that, in intact animals (and the intact cortico-hippocampal model), latent inhibition is disrupted if there is a context shift between exposure and training phases (figure 7.11). The H-lesion model shows latent inhibition (figure 9.8B) but does not show disrupted latent inhibition after context shift. Once again, exposure results in a compression of a stimulus cue with the context in which it occurs; this retards subsequent learning to respond to the cue but not to the context alone. Exposure also results in an overall reduction of the representational space allocated to the cue. Shifting to a new context for training can alleviate the former but not the latter. Thus, the H-lesion model continues to show latent inhibition even in a new context.[23] This is consistent with the finding that selective hippocampal lesions reduce the context sensitivity of latent inhibition.[24]

In general, the H-lesion model predicts that selective H lesion will greatly disrupt the contextual sensitivity of learned associations—just as HR lesion does. This prediction is consistent with two existing studies, as was mentioned above, but further empirical studies are needed to test this prediction fully.

Other Hippocampal-Region Subfunctions.   At this point, the entorhinal network and the H-lesion model that incorporates it are still largely speculative. The entorhinal network appears to be compatible with known features of the anatomy and physiology of entorhinal cortex, and the H-lesion model appears to account for what data exist regarding the effects of selective hippocampal lesion on classical conditioning. However, these data are relatively scant. There is clearly much more empirical work to be done—for example, testing the predictions described early for lesion studies of sensory preconditioning and easy-hard transfer. Our model also predicts that there should be a distinction between multimodal compression, which ought to depend on entorhinal cortex, and unimodal compression, which might be done in sensory cortices and thus survive entorhinal lesion. To date, there is little information comparing multimodal and unimodal stimulus processing in H-lesioned animals.

Our H-lesion model also begs an important question: If the entorhinal cortex is performing redundancy compression among co-occurring stimuli, where are the remaining postulated hippocampal-region functions localized? The original specification of our cortico-hippocampal model proposed that the hippocampal region was involved in compressing representations of stimuli that co-occur or have similar meaning while

Table 9.1 Summary of Representational Biases Assumed by the Cortico-Hippocampal Model to Reflect Hippocampal-Region Mediation

	Bias to Compress	Bias to Differentiate
Stimulus-Stimulus Relationships	Compress representations of co-occurring stimuli	Differentiate representations of stimuli that don't co-occur
Stimulus-Outcome Relationships	Compress representations of stimuli that predict similar outcomes	Differentiate representations of stimuli that predict different outcomes

differentiating the representations of stimuli that do not co-occur or that have different meanings.[25] These four representational constraints are summarized in table 9.1.

The entorhinal cortex can perform representational compression of co-occurring stimuli, termed stimulus-stimulus compression in table 9.1. Another kind of representational compression involves stimuli that have the same meaning. For example, if two stimuli, such as a tone and a light, both reliably predict a food US, then our theory argues that the representations of the tone and the light should be compressed, so that subsequent learning about the tone will generalize to the light. In fact, such an effect is seen in normal animals: If a tone is subsequently paired with a shock US, animals will tend to generalize this new learning to the light as well. This effect is termed **acquired equivalence.**[26] It is still an open question whether HR-lesion impairs acquired equivalence, but the cortico-hippocampal model predicts that it should.

Differentiation and the Dentate Gyrus.   The other type of representational recoding that occurs in our intact cortico-hippocampal model is representational differentiation. Differentiation requires decreasing the overlap in representation between two stimuli so that they never co-occur or so that they predict different future reinforcement. The easiest way to differentiate representations is to ensure that any nodes (or neurons) that respond to one stimulus do not respond to the other and vice versa. Several researchers have proposed that the dentate gyrus, which lies between entorhinal cortex and hippocampus in the processing chain of figure 9.1, could perform such a function.[27] The first reason to suspect that the dentate gyrus may perform differentiation of representations is anatomical. In the rat, there are about 100,000 pyramidal cells in entorhinal cortex, and these project to about one million neurons in dentate gyrus (called **granule cells**). This means that

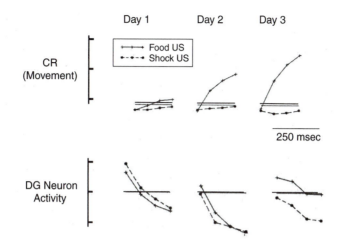

Figure 9.13   Neurons in the dentate gyrus come to differentiate stimuli that are mapped to different responses. Each graph shows the average response pattern to each CS on a given day of training. Top row: Rats are trained that one CS predicts a food US while another tone CS predicts a shock US. On day 1 of training, rats respond similarly to both; by days 2 and 3, rats show head movement responses to the CS that predicts food but not to the CS that predicts shock. Bottom row: activity recorded from cells in the dentate gyrus. On day 1, there is a brief increase in responding when either CS is presented, which lasts for about 250–500 msec and is followed by below-baseline activity. By day 3 (after the behavioral response has been acquired), there is a differential response to the CSs: excitation in response to the CS associated with food and inhibition in response to the CS associated with shock. (Adapted from Segal & Olds, 1973, figure 3.)

information fans out in a ratio of about 1:10 as it travels from entorhinal cortex to dentate gyrus, and this alone could help to increase the difference between stimulus items because more neurons yield more possible patterns.*[28]

Thus, the anatomy of the dentate gyrus would be consistent with automatically differentiating the representations of any random inputs. But there is also evidence that the dentate gyrus actively differentiates inputs that predict different outcomes.

In one study by Segal and Olds, rats were trained that one tone predicted a food US while a different tone predicted a shock US.[29] Figure 9.13 (top row)

---

*Another clue that the dentate gyrus might participate in representational differentiation comes from physiology: In the dentate gyrus, granule cells fire very infrequently; for any single stimulus, only a small percentage of granule cells respond (Treves & Rolls, 1992, 1994; Jones, 1993). This would be consistent with the idea that the dentate gyrus is orthogonalizing inputs, meaning that it reduces the representational overlap.

shows that on day 1 of training, rats responded to neither tone. However, by days 2 and 3, rats were showing reliable head-movement responses to the tone that predicted food but not to the tone that predicted shock. During learning, the experimenters recorded granule cell activity in the dentate gyrus. Figure 9.13 (bottom row) shows that on day 1 of training, the granule cells exhibit a short (250–500 msec) excitatory response to either CS, followed by a short (250–500 msec) inhibitory response. This pattern of responding was sensory-evoked, meaning that it depended on presentation of a tone CS rather than on that tone's meaning. By day 3, however, the response changed, and granule cells gave differential responses to the two tones: The positive CS (associated with food) evoked a short excitatory response, while the negative CS (associated with shock) evoked a short inhibitory response. This differentiated response occurred only after the behavioral response was well learned, and it did not occur unless the CSs were associated with different outcomes.[30]

In a related experiment by Deadwyler and colleagues, rats were again trained that one cue (e.g., tone) predicted a US while a second (e.g., light) did not.[31] Again, the dentate granule cells developed differential responses to the two cues, responding to the tone but not the light. Next, the experimenters reversed the contingencies so that the light but not the tone predicted the US. Gradually, the granule cells reversed their activity to reflect the new situation, developing responses to the light but not the tone.

Perhaps most significant of all, these differential responses to the two CSs were *not* visible in the entorhinal cortex, from which dentate gyrus receives most of its input regarding sensory stimuli.[32] This implies that the patterns of activity in the dentate gyrus were not just copies of distinctions made elsewhere in the brain, but that the dentate gyrus itself is integrally involved in differentiating the representations of stimuli that make different predictions about upcoming reinforcement.

Thus, in the same way that entorhinal cortex may perform representational compression, there is emerging evidence that dentate gyrus may perform representational differentiation. These two structures together could perform most or all of the representational processing that we have assumed takes place in the hippocampal region. Other hippocampal-region areas, such as CA3 and CA1, may be more integrally involved in short-term storage of this information and overseeing its eventual consolidation to cerebral cortex. A major focus of current and future modeling work will be expanding the cortico-hippocampal model to include both entorhinal and dentate (and CA3 and CA1) components and studying the manner in which they could interact to provide a more complete account of hippocampal-region function.

Stimulus Competition in Entorhinal Cortex

A very different conception of entorhinal cortex has been proposed by Nestor Schmajuk and colleagues. Figure 9.14A contains the simplified drawing of the Schmajuk-DiCarlo (S-D) model discussed in chapter 6.[33] As a brief re-view, the basic idea in this model is that the hippocampal region has two

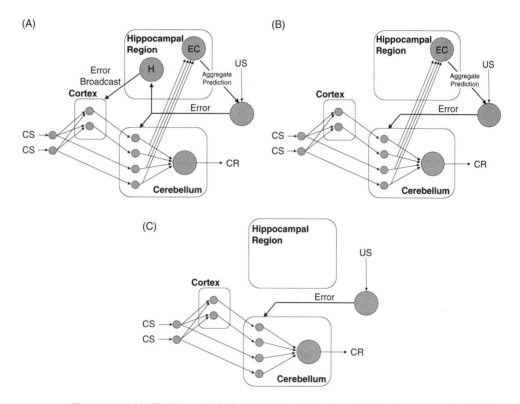

Figure 9.14   (A) The Schmajuk-DiCarlo (1992) model assumes that the hippocampal region has two basic functions. First, it is responsible for calculating the aggregate prediction of the US. This information is used to calculate overall prediction error (the difference between aggregate pre-diction and actual US). Second, the hippocampal region is assumed to be responsible for broad-casting this prediction error to the cortex. It is in the cortex that nodes learn to respond to configurations of stimuli. Later, Buhusi and Schmajuk (1996) proposed that the aggregate predic-tion could be mapped onto the entorhinal cortex and the error broadcast onto the hippocampus. (B) Selective H lesion would therefore disrupt learning in the cortex but not in the cerebellum. The resulting network could still learn direct CS-US associations but not configural CS-CS asso-ciations. (C) Broad HR lesion would disrupt both functions, disrupting configural learning in the cortex and also stimulus competition in the cerebellum. Direct CS-US associations could still be learned, but stimulus competition effects such as blocking would be disrupted.

functions. First, it is responsible for calculating the aggregate prediction of the US: On the basis of all available information (i.e., what CSs are present), how strongly is a US expected? The difference between this aggregate prediction and the actual US is the prediction error. Their second putative function for the hippocampal region is to broadcast this prediction error back to the cortex.

Hippocampal-region damage is assumed to damage both the aggregate prediction and error-broadcast functions (figure 9.14C). Without the aggregate prediction, the system no longer performs functions such as blocking that depend on how well the US is predicted by all available cues; without the error broadcast, the configural nodes in the cortex cannot be trained, and so learning is limited to direct CS-cerebellar projections.

In later work, Schmajuk and colleagues have considered how various components of their models can be mapped onto individual brain structures.[34] Specifically, Schmajuk and colleagues have suggested that the hippocampus might be principally involved in the error broadcast function, while the entorhinal cortex might compute the aggregate prediction. Thus, a selective lesion of hippocampus that spared entorhinal cortex might eliminate the ability to learn about cue configurations (figure 9.14B), while a broader HR lesion that included entorhinal cortex might also eliminate the ability to do cue competition (figure 9.14C).

Schmajuk and colleagues' proposal that the entorhinal cortex mediates cue competition is very different from the implications of our own proposal that the entorhinal cortex performs redundancy compression. As a result, the two models make some opposing predictions about the effects of selective H lesion. One example is sensory preconditioning. Figure 9.10A illustrated the prediction of the cortico-hippocampal model that selective H lesion should spare sensory preconditioning. The Schmajuk et al. model makes the opposite prediction. In this model, phase 1 exposure to a stimulus compound AB normally results in the formation of a configural node in the cortex that responds to this configuration (figure 9.15A). Next, in phase 2, A is paired with the US. Most associative weight accrues to a direct connection between A and the US (figure 9.15B), but A also partially activates the AB configural node, and so the weight from AB to US is also partially strengthened. Finally, when B is presented in phase 3 (figure 9.15C), it partially activates the AB node, which in turn activates a prediction of the US. Thus, in the Schmajuk model, sensory preconditioning depends on configural learning. According to the model, configural learning in turn depends on error broadcasts by the hippocampus. If this is removed, then there is no way to form configural nodes in the cortex (figure 9.15D). The model can still learn that A predicts

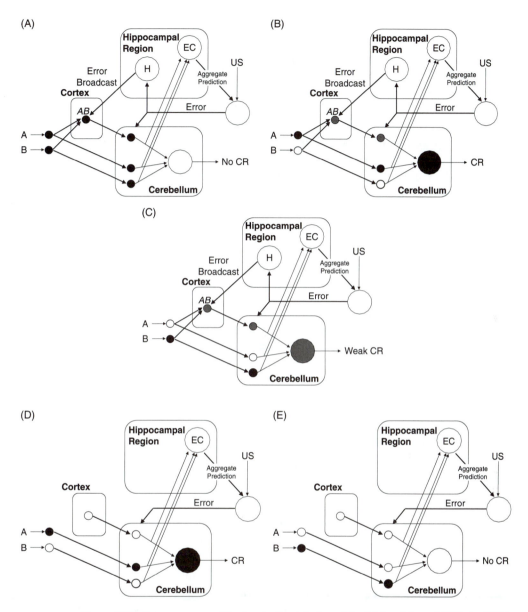

Figure 9.15 Sensory preconditioning in the intact model of Schmajuk and DiCarlo (1992). (A) In phase 1, CSs A and B are presented together. A configural node forms in cortex to encode the AB pairing; this and the components both project to the cerebellum, where they are not associated with any response. (B) In phase 2, A is paired with the US. The AB configural node is partially activated and acquires some association with the US. (C) In phase 3, B is presented alone, partially activates the configural AB node, and evokes a weak CR. (D) Selective H lesion eliminates the hippocampal error signal, meaning that the cortex cannot form new configural nodes. Phase 1 exposure to the compound AB does not result in formation of an AB node in cortex. In phase 2, only the direct A-US association is learned. (E) When B is presented alone, little or no response is evoked.

the US in phase 2, but when B is presented (figure 9.15E), little response is evoked.

Thus, the S-D model predicts that selective H lesion should disrupt sensory preconditioning.[35] This is the opposite prediction from our cortico-hippocampal model. Empirical studies are needed to determine which model's predictions are accurate on this issue. Currently, the only available data show that both fimbrial lesions and kainic acid injections into hippocampal field CA1 abolish sensory preconditioning. However, neither of these lesions provides the sort of precise hippocampal lesions that are created by ibotenic acid, as illustrated in figure 9.4B.[36]

Another interesting feature of the Schmajuk et al. model is that it contains several separate substrates that all contribute to a latent inhibition effect. Thus, different kinds of hippocampal-region lesions may have inhibitory effects, no effect, or even facilitatory effects on latent inhibition.[37] These arguments depend on extrahippocampal structures that are beyond the scope of the simple illustration in figure 9.15. Nonetheless, the model provides a large set of predictions that should keep empirical researchers busy for some time.

Backprojections from Entorhinal Cortex

The previous two sections described computational models that consider how the entorhinal cortex could operate on stimulus inputs. Both our cortico-hippocampal model and the models of Schmajuk and colleagues assume that the hippocampal-region operates on sensory information and then transmits its output back to cortex. In our cortico-hippocampal model, this takes the form of stimulus representations to be acquired by cortex. In the models of Schmajuk and colleagues, this takes the form of an error broadcast from the hippocampal region to cortex. In either case, an important question is to consider projections from the hippocampal region—specifically, from entorhinal cortex—back to other cortical areas.

Figure 9.16 shows a schematized drawing of cortico-cortical information flow, including both feedforward (solid) and feedback (dotted) pathways.* Sensory information reaches pyramidal neurons in the neocortex: first primary sensory cortex, then higher-order sensory cortex, and eventually polymodal association areas. This information contacts dendrites of pyramidal neurons in both the superficial and deep layers of cortex; neurons in the

---

*This simplified drawing, which follows Rolls, 1996, illustrates only the major projections under discussion. Additional neuron types and intrinsic projections are not shown.

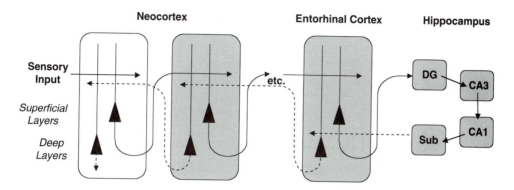

Figure 9.16 Schematic of sensory information flow through cortical areas as envisioned by Rolls (1996). Sensory inputs from previous cortical processing stages contact dendrites of pyramidal cells in superficial and deep layers of neocortical association areas. Axons from neurons in the superficial layers provide output that travels to subsequent cortical processing areas. This *feedforward* process is repeated through various neocortical sensory and association areas until information reaches the entorhinal cortex and then the dentate gyrus, hippocampus, and subiculum (additional intrinsic connections not shown). Information returns through a *feedback* pathway to deep layers of entorhinal cortex (dotted line) and then back to areas of cortex representing progressively earlier processing stages. DG = dentate gyrus; Sub = subiculum.

pyramidal layers continue the feedforward pathway, sending output on to other cortical areas that represent subsequent processing stages. Eventually, the information reaches entorhinal cortex and, from there, dentate gyrus, hippocampus, and subiculum. From there, information is projected back to cells in the cortical areas associated with earlier processing stages. This appears to be an anatomical pathway by which hippocampal-region processing can influence cortical areas.

Edmund Rolls has developed a theory of how these feedback projections could allow representations developed in hippocampus to drive cortical storage.[38]

Events might occur along the lines shown in figure 9.17. Pyramidal neurons in an area of cortex receive feedforward projections carrying sensory information from other (earlier) cortical areas and also feedback projections from other (later) cortical areas (figure 9.17A). In turn, they themselves send output on to later cortical areas and back to earlier cortical areas. In the case of entorhinal cortex, for example, feedforward inputs detail the highly processed, multimodal features of current input (vision and taste are shown in figure 9.17A), while feedback inputs carry information about the hippocampal region's rerepresentation of this information. Initially, these inputs

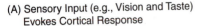 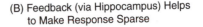

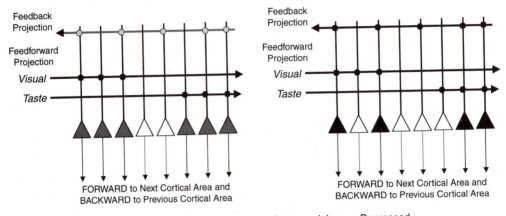

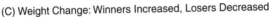

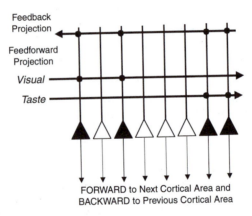

Figure 9.17 How cortical backprojections might transfer hippocampal representations to cortex, along the lines proposed by Rolls (1989, 1996). (A) Pyramidal neurons in an area of cortex receive both feedforward projections from earlier cortical processing areas and feedback projections from later cortical processing areas. Neurons that receive feedforward inputs become partially active and project to subsequent processing areas. In the case of the entorhinal cortex, for example, feedforward inputs specify highly processed multimodal features of stimuli, such as sight and taste; feedback inputs specify hippocampal-region representations of these inputs. (B) The hippocampal region provides the last processing step in the chain, and information begins to flow backward. Where feedforward and feedback projections converge, neurons are strongly activated. In general, the hippocampal-mediated feedback tends to make cortical activity sparse,[3] reducing the number of active neurons. (C) Following the rules of a competitive network, cortex undergoes plasticity: Neurons that are most active win, and their weights from active inputs are strengthened. Weights to nonwinning nodes are weakened.

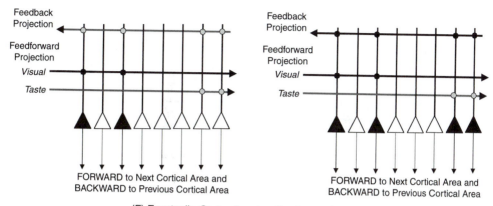

(D) Partial Sensory Input Is Provided
(e.g., Visual Only)

(E) Feedback Completes the Pattern

FORWARD to Next Cortical Area and
BACKWARD to Previous Cortical Area

FORWARD to Next Cortical Area and
BACKWARD to Previous Cortical Area

(F) Eventually, Cortex Acquires the Connections

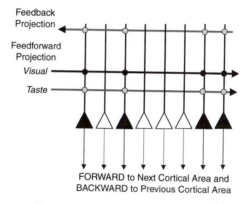

FORWARD to Next Cortical Area and
BACKWARD to Previous Cortical Area

Figure 9.17 (*continued*)   (D) Later, a partial version of the familiar pattern is presented; a subset of previously trained neurons become active. (E) This partial pattern is eventually transmitted to hippocampus, which completes the pattern. Feedback projections carry the complete representation back to cortex, completing the pattern in cortex. The pattern is recalled. (F) Eventually, local connections between coactive neurons in cortex are strengthened, and cortex can recall entire patterns without the help of hippocampal feedback: The memory is consolidated.

make random weighted synapses on the pyramidal neurons (shown as circles). In general, feedback from the hippocampal region is assumed to sparsify the pattern, as outlined previously in this chapter. Where feedforward and feedback inputs converge (figure 9.17B), neurons are strongly activated. Under the assumption that the cortex performs competitive learning, strongly activated "winning" neurons undergo plasticity—strengthening the weights from active inputs—while the remaining neurons undergo weight decreases (figure 9.17C). At this point, the pattern and its hippocampal representation are stored.

Consider now what happens when a partial version of a stored pattern is presented to the network: for example, the sight of a stimulus without its taste, as schematized in figure 9.17D. A subset of neurons that were previously trained become active. This partial pattern is projected forward to the hippocampal region and eventually returns as feedback projections (figure 9.17E); the additional feedback input is enough to reconstruct the original stored pattern in cortex. The complete pattern is recalled. Eventually, local recurrent connections between neurons (not shown in the figure) become strengthened, so cortex can recall entire patterns on its own without the help of hippocampal feedback (figure 9.17F); at this point, the memory is consolidated in cortex, and hippocampal-region damage will not disrupt recall.

This basic plan of cortical backprojection has several important implications. First and most important, it provides a plausible interpretation of how sensory representations from the hippocampal region could eventually be adopted in cortex. One problem in theorizing about hippocampal-region function has always been in understanding how very specific activation patterns (e.g., episodic memories) encoded in hippocampus could be transferred to cortical storage. In a computational model, it is easy to hardwire appropriate connections between a hippocampal-region module and a cortical module. However, in the brain, it is less likely that there exists a predetermined blueprint ensuring that, for any neuron X in the cortex that projects to neuron Y in another region, there is a reciprocal connection from Y to X. Worse, even if every neuron in hippocampus did have such reciprocal connections with the rest of the brain, there is huge convergence from the entire brain onto a relatively small number of hippocampal-region cells. How would the hippocampus "know" which of these backprojections were appropriate for the current information? The mechanism of figure 9.17 neatly sidesteps this issue. In Rolls's model, the hippocampus doesn't "know" where to project information; it simply projects everywhere, and storage occurs automatically wherever conjoint feedforward and feedback projections converge.

A second implication of Rolls's theory concerns the mechanism of storage. Assuming that the hippocampus projects to the right place in cortex, how is information stored there? It does not seem likely that, as many computational models propose, the hippocampal output acts as a teaching signal, forcing cortical cells to respond to particular inputs. As we described in previous chapters, such teaching inputs require very specific anatomical properties that appear to exist in only a few places in the brain (e.g., the mossy fiber connections from dentate gyrus to CA3 and the climbing fiber inputs to cerebellum). The Rolls scenario requires no more than the ubiquitous Hebbianlike learning, in which plasticity occurs to strengthen the connections between any two coactive inputs. Neurobiological mechanisms for Hebbian learning have indeed been observed in superficial layers of cerebral cortex, right where Rolls's model requires that they should be.[39]

One limitation of the system illustrated in figure 9.17 is that it may learn too much: Every time a new input is presented, the hippocampal region will develop a new representation of that input and backproject that representation to cortex for storage. But such constant learning will quickly overload the network, leading to catastrophic interference in which new information overwrites old. Rolls notes that there is a fairly simple way to avoid this problem, and that is to assume that the system does not learn arbitrary information, but only information that is "significant."[40] Other brain areas, such as the amygdala (which is involved in learning the emotional significance of stimuli) and basal forebrain (which is involved in signaling stimulus novelty), could provide this information through projections to cortex. Only in the presence of one or more of these signals would cortical storage be enabled. The next chapter will return to this issue of how subcortical inputs might modulate memory storage for especially significant events.

9.3   RELATIONSHIP TO QUALITATIVE THEORIES: STIMULUS BUFFERING AND CONFIGURATION

Howard Eichenbaum and colleagues Tim Otto, Neal Cohen, and Mike Bunsey have addressed the problem of distinguishing entorhinal hippocampal function on the basis of behavioral and neurophysiological data. They divide the hippocampal region into two basic components: the **parahippocampal region,** which includes entorhinal cortex and nearby perirhinal and parahippocampal cortices (called postrhinal cortex in rats), and the **hippocampal formation,** which includes the hippocampus and the dentate gyrus.

The subiculum appears to be transitional between the two areas. In rats and monkeys, damage to the parahippocampal region devastates the ability to perform tasks such as delayed nonmatch to sample (DNMS) that require maintaining stimulus information over a short interval (e.g., 30–120 seconds). Recordings of neuronal activity in the parahippocampal region during such a task suggest that cells hold firing patterns during the interval.[41] On the basis of these and related data, Eichenbaum and colleagues have suggested that the parahippocampal region operates as an intermediate store of stimulus information.[42]

One aspect of this storage is the ability to fuse co-occurring stimuli and to allow configuration of stimuli that co-occur with slight temporal displacement (e.g., a lightning flash and a thunderclap). The hippocampal region, by contrast, is hypothesized to play a largely antagonistic role: learning about relationships between individual items. Selective removal of the hippocampus thereby results in a system that tends to overcompress stimulus information at the expense of recognizing individual components. A broader lesion that included the parahippocampal region would eliminate this compression, leaving only the ability to form simpler stimulus-response relationships.

Eichenbaum and Bunsey tested these predictions in a rat odor discrimination paradigm.[43] In these studies, a rat was presented with odor stimuli (e.g., A, B, C, and D) and had to choose whether to respond. The odors were presented in sequential pairs: one odor followed by a second odor. Some odor pairings (e.g., AB+ and CD+) were rewarded; recombinations or **mispairs** of these odors (e.g., AC−, BD−) were not rewarded. Thus, this task required rats to learn about configurations of odors, because any individual odor could be rewarded or nonrewarded, depending on its companion odor.

Figure 9.18A shows the empirical results. Control rats learned to respond to pairs but not mispairs within about 21 training sessions. In contrasts, rats with parahippocampal-region lesion (PRER) did not learn even within 35 sessions.[44] This is consistent with the hypothesis that the parahippocampal region is involved in compressing or configuring stimuli. Most interestingly, rats with selective hippocampal lesions were *facilitated* relative to controls.[45] Once the putatively antagonistic hippocampus was removed, the parahippocampal region was free to work its compression unfettered, and since compression of odor pairs facilitated learning this particular task, learning was speeded.

At the same time, the rats were trained to discriminate odor pairs from **nonpairs,** in which one odor was never associated with reward (e.g., AX−, BY−). To solve this task, the rats needed only to learn never to respond on any trial involving the nonrelational odors X and Y; it was not necessary to attend to stimulus configurations. All that was needed was strong inhibitory weights from X and Y. In this case, the control, PRER, and H-lesion rats all learned at the same speed (figure 9.18B).[46] Again, these results supported the theory: The parahippocampal region (and hippocampus) are needed only for learning involving relationships between cues, not for simple stimulus-response learning.

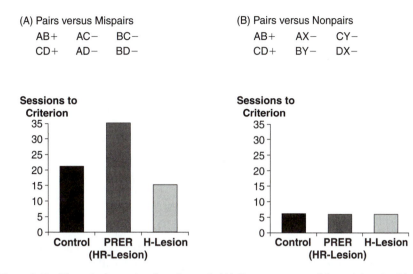

(A) Pairs versus Mispairs

AB+	AC−	BC−
CD+	AD−	BD−

(B) Pairs versus Nonpairs

AB+	AX−	CY−
CD+	BY−	DX−

Figure 9.18   The paired associate learning task. (A) One component of the task involved learning to respond to odors when presented in particular pairs (e.g., AB+, CD+) but not when recombined into mispairs (e.g., AC−, BD−). Note that this task cannot be solved by assigning weights to individual components but only by assigning weights to compounds: Thus, A is sometimes positive (when paired with B) and sometimes negative (when paired with C or D). Control rats learned the distinction within about 21 training sessions. Rats with lesions of the perirhinal and entorhinal cortex (PRER), which also disconnect the hippocampus from its primary sensory input and output, were greatly impaired; most did not learn within 35 sessions. This is consistent with the idea that the entorhinal cortex (or, more broadly, the parahippocampal region) compresses the representation of co-occurring stimuli into compound stimuli. By contrast, rats with selective hippocampal lesions (H lesion) were facilitated in learning this discrimination. This is consistent with the idea that the hippocampus normally performs a function antagonistic to the entorhinal cortex; its removal disinhibits entorhinal function. (B) A similar discrimination, with the same odor pairs but with contrasting nonpairs, which include one odor that is not part of a reinforced pair (e.g., X, Y). Note that this task can be solved by attaching strong negative weights to nonpair odors. Control, PRER, and H-lesion rats all learn at equivalent speeds. (Plotted from data presented in Bunsey & Eichenbaum, 1993; Eichenbaum & Bunsey, 1995.)

By now, the reader will have noticed a strong similarity between Eichenbaum and colleagues' account of parahippocampal and hippocampal interplay and that embodied in our own cortico-hippocampal model.[47] Whereas Eichenbaum and colleagues propose that the parahippocampal region configures stimuli, the cortico-hippocampal model assumes that the entorhinal cortex compresses stimulus representations. The chief differences are that Eichenbaum and colleagues include a temporal dimension and that they consider the entire parahippocampal region, not merely the entorhinal cortex. Otherwise, the two statements of function are quite compatible.

This correspondence is especially encouraging, since these parallel ideas emerged from two very different research traditions: one based on behavioral and neurophysiological observations of rat odor discrimination and the other from computational modeling constrained by anatomical data.

9.4   IMPLICATIONS FOR HUMAN MEMORY AND MEMORY DISORDERS

One of the most pressing reasons for trying to understand hippocampal-region function is that hippocampal-region dysfunction may be an important contributor to the cognitive impairments of Alzheimer's disease. **Alzheimer's disease (AD)** is a progressive, degenerative neurologic illness that may afflict up to four million adults in the United States alone. Currently, it is a leading cause of death among Americans over the age of 60, afflicting an estimated 25% of Americans over age 85. The causes of the disease are unknown, although there appears to be a genetic component, but abnormal elements called **plaques** and **tangles** accumulate in the brain. Neurons begin to degenerate, losing synapses and eventually dying (figure 9.19A). As this occurs, the brain itself begins to shrink or **atrophy** (figure 9.19B), causing behavioral impairments and eventually death.

One of the earliest deficits in AD is memory decline. This is evidenced by failure on such tasks as the **paragraph delayed recall** test, in which the experimenter reads a short story aloud and asks the subject to repeat the story back. The subject gets a point for every item in the story that is repeated correctly (typically, there are about 25 such items). Next, there is a delay of 5–15 minutes, and then the subject is asked to repeat the story once more from memory. A normal young or middle-aged subject may be able to recall most of the paragraph, while a normal elderly subject may recall ten or eleven of the story items. Subjects with AD may do substantially worse. Even a very mild impairment on this kind of test may indicate an increased risk for developing AD.[48] Interestingly, this kind of task—which involves the recall of factual information over a time span of a few minutes—is exactly the kind of memory task that is disrupted in amnesic subjects with medial temporal lobe damage. Therefore, one might suspect that hippocampal damage or dysfunction underlies some of the cognitive deficits in early AD.

As Alzheimer's disease progresses to later stages, the symptoms become devastating, including memory loss, personality changes, loss of initiative (apathy), poor judgment, disorientation of time and place, and depression. Individuals with AD experience a gradual decline in abilities until they

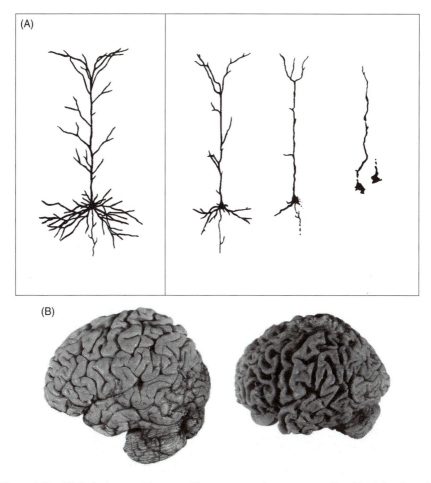

Figure 9.19   (A) Left: A neuron in normal human cortex has processes (dendrites) that branch multiply and widely. Other neurons make synapses on these dendrites, allowing information transfer. Right: Cells from the same area of patients with Alzheimer's disease show progressive degeneration, especially in terms of shrinking of dendritic branches. (Adapted from Kalat, 1995, p. 463, figure 138.) (B) The cerebral cortex of a normal person (left) shows a characteristic wrinkled appearance as the cortex folds in on itself. The cerebral cortex of a patient with Alzheimer's disease (right) is shrunken, with exaggerated spaces between folds of cortex. Atrophy occurs in other brain areas too, including the hippocampal region. (Adapted from Kalat, 1995, p. 462, figure 13.7, which reprinted the pictures courtesy of Dr. Robert Terry.)

eventually require round-the-clock care, including assistance with eating, dressing, bathing, and other daily activities.

Currently, there is no cure for AD. The few medications that are available treat the symptoms. At best, the medicines temporarily arrest the progress of the disease; they cannot reverse the damage or prevent further decline.

Because of this, it is vital to identify individuals who are at risk to develop AD before they begin to show cognitive decline and memory impairments. Memories, once lost, are gone forever.

Recent research has produced findings that may allow early detection of which individuals are most at risk to develop AD in the future. In some elderly individuals, the hippocampus and entorhinal cortex show atrophy while other nearby brain structures appear intact. This can be seen by using neuroradiography such as **magnetic resonance imaging (MRI).** These techniques provide a picture of a slice through the brain (or body) without harming the individual being imaged. Figure 9.20 shows two MRIs of human brains, taken in the horizontal plane, meaning that they would parallel the floor if the individual were standing. Figure 9.20A shows a normal brain; the two hippocampi are in the boxed areas. Figure 9.20B shows an individual with hippocampal atrophy; the hippocampi are considerably shrunken.[49] There is little visible shrinkage of other nearby areas; the atrophy appears to be largely confined to the hippocampus itself.

The kind of hippocampal atrophy that is shown in figure 9.20B has been observed both in patients diagnosed with mild AD and in elderly individuals who have cognitive impairments that are suggestive of possible AD.[50] Thus, hippocampal atrophy may be an indicator of which individuals are most at risk to subsequently develop AD.[51] Not every individual with

(A) Normal (No Hippocampal Atrophy)   (B) Moderate Hippocampal Atrophy

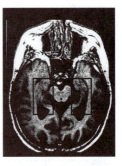

Figure 9.20 Two magnetic resonance images (MRIs) of the human brain, showing slices through the brain that would be parallel to the floor if the subject was standing upright. The nose is at the top of the images, and the back of the head is at the bottom. The hippocampi lie in the areas outlined in black. (A) Normal (nonatrophied) hippocampi. (B) Moderately atrophied hippocampi. The kind of atrophy shown in B could indicate that the individual is at risk for future development of the kind of cognitive impairments that are associated with AD (Golomb et al., 1993). (Images adapted from de Leon et al., 1993a.)

hippocampal atrophy will go on to develop AD, but hippocampal atrophy may be one warning sign; individuals with atrophy could then be monitored closely to see whether there are further signs of decline, and these individuals could be started on drug therapies as early as is appropriate.

If hippocampal atrophy is indeed a predictor of cognitive decline and AD, then it ought to be possible to estimate hippocampal atrophy by behavior alone: If an individual starts to perform poorly on hippocampal-dependent tests, then that might indicate that the individual is experiencing hippocampal atrophy. One example is the paragraph recall task described above; poor performance on this test is correlated with hippocampal atrophy.[52] However, this task is sensitive to many different kinds of brain dysfunction that result in memory impairments.

What is really needed is a task that is specifically designed to tap into hippocampal-region function. Then, poor performance on this task would be a much better indicator that hippocampal atrophy—rather than some other kind of damage or disease—was present.

Behavioral Measures of Hippocampal Atrophy

The cortico-hippocampal model suggests that selective hippocampal damage might lead to overcompression deficits: a tendency to perceive co-occurring stimuli (or stimulus features) as compound objects, leading to a difficulty in subsequent discrimination. Further, the previous chapter noted that broad HR lesion that includes the entorhinal cortex might have a similar effect, at least for tasks involving compression within a single modality that might be mediated by unimodal sensory cortices. The implication is that hippocampal damage (with or without conjoint entorhinal damage) might lead to an overcompression deficit. Given training with co-occurring stimuli, lesioned subjects will tend to overcompress and therefore perform poorly when familiar stimuli are presented in novel recombinations. The same logic will hold true for stimulus features. Remember that the cortical network has no *a priori* way of knowing whether two co-occurring inputs are different stimuli or different features of the same stimulus.

For example, consider the visual discrimination task shown in figure 9.21, which was developed in our laboratory as a test of hippocampal-region function.[53] There are eight pairs of objects (four are shown in figure 9.21A), and each object has the features of color and shape. (In figure 9.21, colors are approximated as gray levels.) Within each discrimination, only one feature varies across the object pair: The first two discriminations differ in color but not shape, and the last two differ in shape but not color. Subjects in our study

(A) Phase 1: Training   (B) Phase 2: Transfer

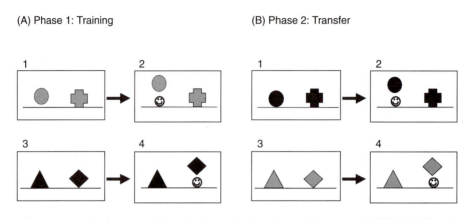

Figure 9.21   A color-shape discrimination task from Myers, Kluger, et al. (1998). (A) Phase 1 (training phase) consists of eight pairs of colored shapes (here, colors are approximated by gray levels). For example, one pair might consist of a same-colored circle and cross (1). The subject saw the two objects on the computer screen (1) and chooses one. The chosen object is raised (2), and if the subject's choice was correct, a smiley face is revealed underneath. Here, the circle is always the correct choice. Another pair might consist of a same-colored triangle and diamond (3), with the diamond always correct (4). For both these discrimination pairs, the shape but not the color is relevant with respect to predicting the smiley face's location. Other discrimination pairs differ in color but not shape (e.g., a red spiral versus a yellow spiral). Phase 1 continues until the subject reaches criterion performance, correctly responding on all eight of discrimination pairs. (B) Phase 2 is a transfer phase. Here, objects are recombinations of familiar colors and shapes, maintaining the relevant features from phase 1. Thus, given the circle-cross discrimination pair (1), the circle is still the correct choice (2). Given the triangle-diamond discrimination pair (2), the diamond is still the correct choice. Color is still irrelevant in these discriminations. Subjects who learn to pay attention only to the relevant features in phase 1 (e.g., choose circle over cross, regardless of color) should perform close to perfectly in phase 2. By contrast, subjects who learn responses based on all (relevant and irrelevant) features of the objects in phase 1 (e.g., choose gray circle over gray cross) should be at a loss when new combinations (e.g., black circle versus black cross) are presented in phase 2.

are shown discrimination pairs, one at a time over many trials, and must learn to choose the rewarded object of each pair, regardless of the objects' left-right position. Eventually, normal subjects come to give the correct response on each trial.

There are at least two strategies that a subject may adopt to solve this kind of task. The first strategy is to notice that, within each discrimination, one stimulus feature is relevant and one is irrelevant. Thus, in discrimination 1 of figure 9.21A, color is relevant and shape is irrelevant. A rule that would guide correct responding is: Choose the red object over the yellow object, regardless of shape. Similar rules can govern responding in the other discriminations.

Note that it is not necessary that subjects explicitly form a verbal rule; a simple associative learning system (such as the Rescorla–Wagner model) will also learn to weight relevant inputs heavily and to ignore irrelevant inputs.

An alternative strategy for solving this discrimination task would be to treat all stimulus features equally and compress them into compound percepts. In effect, subjects might learn to choose the red-square over the yellow-square. This kind of solution requires the ability to form compressed or configured representations of stimulus inputs.

Either strategy can yield perfectly accurate performance on the original discriminations. However, in our studies, we included a second, transfer phase as schematized in figure 9.21B. Here, the familiar stimulus features are recombined into novel objects. The recombination is done according to strict rules: Features that were relevant in phase 1 have the same meaning in phase 2, but now they are paired with different irrelevant features. Thus, whereas the red square but not the yellow square predicted reinforcement in phase 1, the red arrow but not the yellow arrow predicts reinforcement in phase 2.

Now the strategy used to solve phase 1 makes a critical difference. If a subject had learned to ignore the irrelevant features in phase 1, phase 2 performance should be close to perfect. The original rule to choose red over yellow (regardless of shape) in phase 1 still yields the correct answer in phase 2. However, if a subject had learned about stimulus configurations in phase 1, phase 2 performance should be close to chance. The original rule to choose a red-square over a yellow-square is of little use when one is confronted with a red-arrow and a yellow-arrow—two new objects. To master phase 2, the subject would have to learn an entirely new set of rules, and phase 2 learning might take fully as long as the original phase 1 learning.

On the basis of the predictions of our cortico-hippocampal model, we conjectured that normal subjects, with functioning hippocampal regions, would tend to favor the more general solution: Hippocampal-mediated representations would differentiate predictive cues (such as the color in discrimination 1) and de-emphasize or ignore redundant ones (such as the shape in discrimination 1).

Moreover, we expected that irrelevant features should be largely ignored in phase 1 learning, leading to very good phase 2 transfer performance. In contrast, our cortico-hippocampal model predicts that hippocampal-region damage should impair this differentiation process, while cortical compression would proceed unchecked. Thus, we expected that subjects with hippocampal damage might tend to respond to stimulus compounds in phase 1, leading to poor phase 2 performance.

To test our hypothesis, we tested a group of twenty elderly individuals on this task, recruited through an aging study at New York University. All had been given thorough psychological testing as well as neuroimaging like that in figure 9.20. All the individuals were judged cognitively normal on the basis of their performance on the psychological tests, but twelve individuals showed signs of very mild atrophy to one of their hippocampi, much like that seen in figure 9.20B.

Figure 9.22A shows that there was no significant difference between the atrophy and no-atrophy subjects in terms of performance on psychological tests such as the paragraph recall test. Therefore, the subjects with atrophy were not yet showing cognitive decline on standard measures of memory.

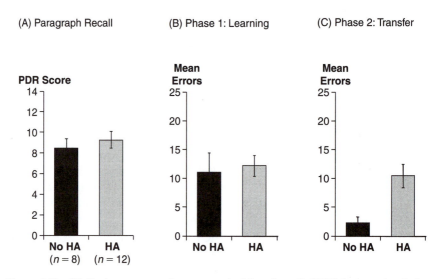

Figure 9.22 (A) Performance on the paragraph delayed recall (PDR) has previously been shown to correlate with (and therefore predict) hippocampal atrophy. In the current study, however, PDR did not discriminate between subjects without hippocampal atrophy (noHA) and those with mild hippocampal atrophy (HA). All subjects averaged recall of about eight to ten items from the paragraph after a 5- to 10-minute delay; this performance is about normal for elderly subjects. (B) Performance on phase 1 of the colored shape discrimination, in terms of total errors, is not significantly different between the subjects with no hippocampal atrophy (noHA) and with mild hippocampal atrophy (HA). (C) However, there is a dramatic difference on performance in phase 2: Subjects with no atrophy performed close to perfect, as expected, while subjects with mild atrophy performed significantly worse. Thus, this simple transfer task may discriminate between subjects with and without hippocampal atrophy. (From data presented in Myers, Kluger, et al., in prep.)

When tested on the visual discrimination task, all twenty subjects were able to master the first phase of learning with the original eight discriminations with the colored shapes. Figure 9.22B shows that there was no significant difference between atrophy and no-atrophy subjects in terms of total errors to reach criterion performance on this phase.

On the other hand, there was a dramatic difference on the transfer phase (figure 9.22C).[54] Subjects with no hippocampal atrophy performed close to perfect on this phase, averaging only about two errors. Subjects with hippocampal atrophy performed very differently. These subjects averaged about twelve errors—approximately as many as in phase 1. This suggests that these subjects had to learn phase 2 from scratch—The prior experience in phase 1 was no help at all. This in turn suggests that the subjects with hippocampal atrophy may have formed overcompressed rules in phase 1 that did not apply to the recombined features in phase 2.

Tasks such as our transfer test described above may represent a possible way to identify which elderly individuals may have hippocampal atrophy before they begin to exhibit serious cognitive decline. This classification is made on the basis of abnormal behavior on a task that may reflect hippocampal dysfunction. Our hope is that this and similar tasks may eventually be used in general practice to evaluate nondemented elderly individuals. Elderly individuals could receive this kind of simple test as a part of their annual checkup. When and if an individual's performance begins to show signs of hippocampal dysfunction, this would signal that the individual should undergo more elaborate testing, including MRI analysis and other means to determine risk for AD.

At present, though, the results described above represent only the first step in developing such a diagnostic test. Only a small sample of elderly subjects have been tested, and among these, even those described as having hippocampal atrophy have only very mild degrees of atrophy. We do not yet know how individuals with more pronounced atrophy may perform. More important, even if the task is reliable in detecting hippocampal atrophy, we do not yet know whether it is reliable in predicting risk for AD. The subjects here might indeed have hippocampal atrophy, but as a result of some other disease or prior trauma. For instance, some kinds of stroke can result in hippocampal atrophy; in that case, the presence of atrophy would not necessarily mean that the individual was at risk to develop AD. For now, one important project in our laboratory is to track the individuals who participated in our original study and find out which of them do go on to show cognitive decline and eventually develop AD. Only then can we fully evaluate the clinical potential of this approach.

Entorhinal Versus Hippocampal Atrophy in AD

A final important issue concerns the relative contributions of the hippocampus and entorhinal cortex. So far, we have described only atrophy of the hippocampus as an early indicator of AD. However, the entorhinal cortex also shows signs of pathology early in AD—perhaps even before hippocampal atrophy becomes apparent.[55] Entorhinal atrophy is harder to evaluate than hippocampal atrophy, for anatomical reasons.

As is evident in figure 9.20, the hippocampus is visibly different from its surrounding structures. It is possible to precisely delineate the hippocampus's boundaries for the purposes of calculating its volume and estimating shrinkage. The entorhinal cortex, by contrast, does not have a precise boundary. It is difficult to tell where it ends and the next cortical area begins. Many researchers are currently working to develop procedures for reliably measuring the precise volume of the entorhinal cortex.

SUMMARY

• The entorhinal cortex is a periallocortical structure within the hippocampal region, meaning that its form is intermediate between six-layered neocortex and two-layered allocortex. It receives highly processed, multimodal sensory input and projects to the hippocampus; in turn, hippocampal outputs project to entorhinal cortex and from there back to the cortical areas where they arose.

• On some tasks, memory impairment simply grows as a function of how much hippocampal-region tissue is lesioned. But more recent studies have suggested qualitative differences in impairment based on precise lesion extent, suggesting that a lesion that is precisely limited to hippocampus may spare some entorhinal function.

• A simple entorhinal model may be constructed similar to the piriform cortex model: Clusters of nodes complete to respond to inputs; representations of similar and co-occurring (redundant) inputs are compressed.

• The cortico-hippocampal model suggests that this entorhinal compression may survive selective hippocampal damage, which disables a normally competing hippocampal differentiation function. The result is that selective hippocampal lesion results in a tendency to overcompress information, and this is consistent with existing data.

• Other computational models have suggested that the entorhinal cortex is involved in stimulus configuration and the backprojections from hippocampus to entorhinal cortex and beyond provide a possible substrate for memory consolidation.

• Eichenbaum and colleagues have suggested that the entorhinal cortex is an intermediate-term buffer, one aspect of this buffer is the ability to configure representations of items that occur with slight temporal displacement. This proposal is quite consonant with the cortico-hippocampal model's account.

• A discrimination task, based on the model predictions and animal data, shows some promise for detecting the very mild hippocampal atrophy that may be an indicator of risk for subsequent development of Alzheimer's disease.

APPENDIX 9.1   SIMULATION DETAILS

The H-lesion model of figure 9.7C, including entorhinal network, was originally presented in Myers, Gluck, and Granger (1995).

Briefly, the entorhinal network consists of a single layer of 100 nodes, divided into five nonoverlapping patches of 20 nodes each. Nodes in one patch are all reciprocally connected with a single local inhibitory feedback cell. Each node receives weighted connections from all external inputs, and the weights are initialized from a uniform distribution and normalized so that the sum of all weights to one node equals 1.0. On each trial, each node n computes activation V_n as a weighted sum across all external inputs i:

$$V_n = \sum_i w_{in} y_i$$

In each patch, the node with maximal activation is the winner. The output of the winning node w is set to $y_w = 1.0$, while the local inhibitory cell silences all other nodes in the patch (output $y_j = 0.0$ for all $j \neq w$). The winning nodes (one per patch) update their weights as

$$\Delta w_{iw} = \alpha I_i (y_w - V_w)$$

where $\alpha = 0.001$ for winning nodes and $\alpha = 0.0001$ for all other nodes.

In the H-lesion model of figure 9.7C, the entorhinal network output provides the training signal for the internal-layer nodes of the cortico/cerebellar network. For each internal-layer node in the cortico/cerebellar network, the desired output is a weighted sum of the activations of the nodes in the entorhinal network. These weights are initialized from a normal distribution and fixed thereafter. Otherwise, the cortico/cerebellar network is similar to that found in previous chapters. (Full details of the entorhinal network and H-lesion model are given in the appendix to Myers et al., 1995.)

10 Cholinergic Modulation of Hippocampal-Region Function

Previous chapters have discussed various aspects of the interaction between the hippocampal region, cortex, and cerebellum. An emerging theme is that the hippocampal region does not operate in isolation. Areas such as cortex provide input to the hippocampal region and are the eventual targets of its output.

Other brain structures modulate hippocampal-region processing. These other structures provide chemical messengers—**neurotransmitters** and **neuromodulators**—that affect how hippocampal-region neurons behave. One of the principal neuromodulatory systems arises in the **medial septum,** a small group of cells that project to the hippocampus. Some of these cells are **cholinergic** neurons, meaning that they produce the neurotransmitter **acetylcholine** (abbreviated **ACh**).

This cholinergic input is critical for normal hippocampal function. When the septohippocampal cholinergic pathway is disrupted through damage to the medial septum or with drugs that affect ACh efficacy, hippocampal-region function is disrupted. In many cases, *hippocampal-region disruption has qualitatively different effects on learning and memory behavior than direct hippocampal-region damage.*

This chapter begins by first providing a brief review of neurotransmission and neuromodulation, with particular attention to acetylcholine and how it affects memory. Next, the chapter discusses computational models suggesting that acetylcholine provided from medial septum to hippocampus is integral in mediating hippocampal function and a model that addresses the effects of changes in acetylcholine levels on learning and memory. Finally, the chapter discusses how these models relate to other theories of septohippocampal modulation and how they may apply to research with various patient populations.

10.1   ACETYLCHOLINE AS A NEUROMODULATOR

Back in chapter 3, we discussed the basic anatomy of neurons that receive inputs through their dendrites and send output via axons to other neurons (figure 10.1A). To review, the small gap between neurons is called a **synapse;** when a sending (or **presynaptic**) neuron becomes sufficiently activated, it releases chemicals called **neurotransmitters** into the synapse. The receiving (or **postsynaptic**) neuron contains **receptors,** each keyed to respond to a particular kind of neurotransmitter. *Different neurotransmitters have different effects on the postsynaptic neuron, and the postsynaptic neuron's response depends on the sum of all these effects.* Any neurotransmitter that does not attach to a receptor is quickly cleaned out of the synapse; lingering

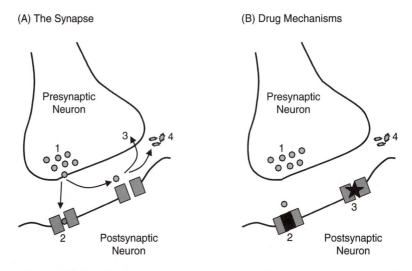

Figure 10.1   (A) Schematic of synaptic transmission. A sending (presynaptic) neuron releases chemicals called neurotransmitters (1) from its axon into a small gap (synapse). The receiving (postsynaptic) cell contains receptors (2), which are activated by specific neurotransmitters. Any remaining neurotransmitter is cleaned out of the synapse—either taken back into the presynaptic cell and recycled (3) or broken down into chemical components (4). (B) Drugs work by altering synaptic transmission. Presynaptically, drugs may alter the rates at which transmitters are produced or released (1). Postsynaptically, drugs may block receptors (2), preventing neurotransmitters from reaching their destination and interfering with transmission. Drugs may mimic neurotransmitters (3), even activating receptors more efficiently than the neurotransmitter itself. Other drugs act by affecting the rate at which neurotransmitter is removed from the synapse (4); neurotransmitter that remains in the synapse longer has more chance of eventually activating a receptor. Thus, a drug that decreases synaptic cleanup facilitates transmission.

neurotransmitter molecules are either reabsorbed by the presynaptic neuron and recycled for future use or broken down into smaller chemical components.

Drugs can affect neurotransmission by altering any step of this process (figure 10.1B); **agonists** facilitate transmission while **antagonists** impede transmission. Some drugs act presynaptically, altering the rate at which neurotransmitter molecules are produced or released. For example, botulinum toxin, the substance that causes botulism, is a cholinergic antagonist that prevents the release of ACh. The venom of the black widow spider is a cholinergic agonist, which causes an equally lethal overrelease of ACh—flooding the system. Alternatively, some drugs act postsynaptically. Nicotine is a cholinergic agonist that can activate one kind of cholinergic receptor, "tricking" the postsynaptic cell into thinking that it has received ACh. Drugs can also block receptors, preventing neurotransmitters from attaching to the postsynaptic cell. Scopolamine—once used as an analgesic during childbirth and currently marketed as a motion-sickness remedy—is a cholinergic antagonist that blocks cholinergic transmission in this way. *Finally, other drugs affect the cleanup process:* If the rate of molecular breakdown or recycling is reduced, neurotransmitters remain in the synapse longer and have more of a chance to attach to receptors. The drugs tacrine (brand name Cognex) and donepezil (trade name Aricept), which are currently marketed for treating Alzheimer's disease, work by slowing down the processes that cleans up unused ACh from the synapses, thereby allowing the existing ACh molecules to linger, increasing the chances that they will contact a postsynaptic receptor.

Neuromodulation

Neurotransmitters carry specific neural "messages" from one neuron to another. An excitatory neurotransmitter increases the probability that the postsynaptic neuron will become active (passing the message on), and an inhibitory neurotransmitter decreases this probability. A different means of neuronal communication is via **neuromodulators.** *Whereas neurotransmitters carry the messages between neurons, neuromodulators affect how those messages are processed.* For example, a neuromodulator might increase the overall responsiveness of a postsynaptic neuron to other, incoming neurotransmitter messages.

A simple metaphor for these processes is radio transmission. The neurotransmitters carry the signal being broadcast—the words or music. Neuromodulators act like the volume control on the radio receiver. The volume control adjusts how the message is transmitted without changing the content of that message.

Neuromodulators activate receptors according to the same basic principles of neurotransmission shown in figure 10.1. In fact, a single chemical substance can sometimes act as either a neurotransmitter or a neuromodulator. Acetylcholine has this dual role: Outside the brain, ACh acts as a neurotransmitter, carrying specific commands from the spinal cord to muscles throughout the body. Inside the brain, ACh acts like a neuromodulator, broadcasting general information across wide areas.

Acetylcholine (ACh) and Memory Function

In this chapter, we focus on the neuromodulatory effects of acetylcholine; some of the basic principles are similar for other neuromodulators.[1] Neurons that contain acetylcholine (cholinergic neurons) exist in several areas of the brain, including the **basal forebrain,** shown in figure 10.2. Within the basal

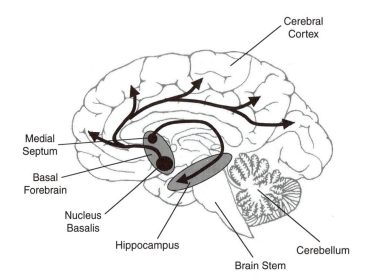

Figure 10.2 Schematic of some important cholinergic projections in the human brain. The basal forebrain is a small region that includes the medial septum, nucleus basalis, and other cell groups. The medial septum sends a cholinergic projection to hippocampus, while the nucleus basalis sends cholinergic projections throughout cortex. Other basal forebrain areas project to other brain structures. Some structures in the brain stem also send cholinergic projections to subcortical areas and out of the brain to neurons in the spinal cord that innervate muscles and control movements.

forebrain, one group of cells, called the **nucleus basalis,** projects ACh throughout the cortex, while another cell group, the **medial septum,** is a primary source of cholinergic projections to the hippocampus.* These latter pathways are often termed the **septohippocampal projection.**

Acetylcholine has a number of neuromodulatory effects.[2] These effects are varied, and not all their implications are yet clear. For example, application of acetylcholine itself (or cholinergic agonists that enhance the efficacy of ACh) can lead to a general increase in activity in pyramidal neurons. At the same time, ACh increases the spontaneous firing rates of inhibitory cells while decreasing the responsiveness of these cells to synaptic transmission. In addition, ACh appears to facilitate synaptic plasticity and hence to facilitate learning.

One of the reasons that acetylcholine has received so much attention is that disruption of the cholinergic system can have a devastating effect on memory. Disrupting the septohippocampal projection disrupts hippocampal function[3] and can cause memory impairments.[4] Drugs that are cholinergic antagonists, blocking the efficacy of ACh receptors in the brain, can also cause memory disruption.[5]

One well-known cholinergic antagonist is **scopolamine.**[6] Scopolamine can temporarily disable cholinergic pathways, including those from medial septum to hippocampus. The behavioral effect is a form of temporary amnesia. For example, normal human volunteers may be given a dose of scopolamine and then presented with information to study. Later, when the drug has cleared out of their systems, the volunteers have little or no memory of the information—or indeed of the study episode.[7] In effect, scopolamine induces temporary anterograde amnesia in subjects with no hippocampal-region damage.

However, the effects of cholinergic disruption are not identical to the effects of hippocampal lesion.[8] One example is classical conditioning of motor reflexes. Direct damage to the hippocampal region does not affect acquisition of a conditioned eyeblink response in animals or humans (figure 10.3A).[9] However, scopolamine does disrupt eyeblink conditioning (figure 10.3B).[10] Removal of the medial septum—which permanently disrupts the septohippocampal cholinergic projections—has an even more devastating effect on acquisition of eyeblink conditioning (figure 10.3C).[11] Thus, in classical

*In humans, the primary cholinergic input from basal forebrain to hippocampus comes from a nearby structure, called the diagonal band of Broca. The diagonal band and medial septum are so interrelated that they are often conceived as a single, compound structure (i.e., the medial septum/diagonal band complex).

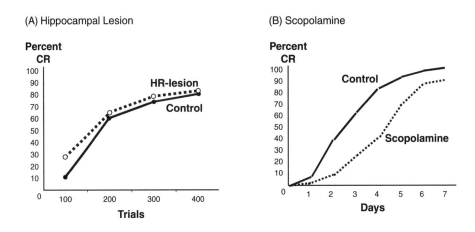

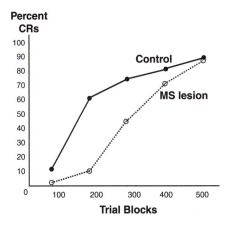

Figure 10.3 (A) Direct lesion to the hippocampus or hippocampal region does not impair acquisition of a conditioned eyeblink response in rabbits (Allen, Chelius, & Gluck, 1998). (B) Disruption of hippocampal function by administration of a cholinergic antagonist (scopolamine) to disrupt septohippocampal cholinergic projections does slow eyeblink conditioning, although subjects eventually reach normal performance levels (Solomon et al., 1983). (C) Lesion of the medial septum also disrupts conditioning (Ermita et al., 1999).

eyeblink conditioning, disrupting the hippocampus is actually worse than removing it altogether. In the next section, we will present computational models that address some of these behavioral data and provide an interpretation of these seemingly paradoxical findings.

10.2 COMPUTATIONAL MODELS

Acetylcholine in the Hippocampal Autoassociator

Many computational models, including some discussed in chapter 5, assume that hippocampal field CA3 functions as an autoassociator. That is, a pattern of input activations is stored in the CA3 network by strengthening connections between pairs of nodes that are simultaneously active, as shown in figures 10.4A and 10.4B. Later, when a partial or distorted version of a stored pattern is presented as input (figure 10.4C), this activates the corresponding subset of the nodes in the stored pattern, and from these nodes, activity will spread to the remaining nodes, retrieving the rest of the pattern (figure 10.4D).

However, there is a conceptual problem with this kind of autoassociator network, one that is often glossed over in the literature. Suppose that a pattern has previously been stored in the network that activates nodes A, B, C, and D and the connections between these nodes are strengthened as illustrated in figure 10.5A. Now a second pattern is presented for storage; this pattern activates

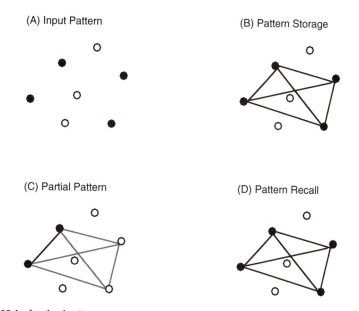

Figure 10.4 In the basic autoassociator, patterns are stored by strengthening associations between coactive nodes. (A) A pattern is presented that activates a subset of nodes (dark circles); (B) the pattern is stored by strengthening associations between these coactive nodes (shown as lines connecting active nodes). (C) Later, when a partial version of the pattern is presented (dark circles), activation spreads along these connections to recall the original stored pattern (D).

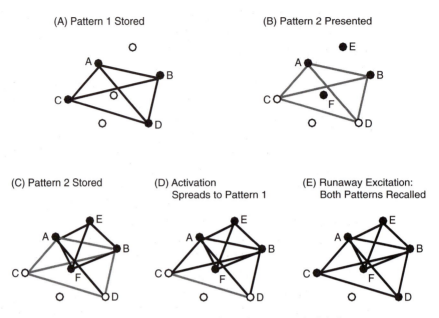

Figure 10.5 Runaway excitation in an autoassociative network. (A) Suppose one pattern (which activates nodes A, B, C, and D) has been stored by strengthening connections between coactive nodes (heavy lines). (B) Now a second pattern (which activates nodes A, B, E, and F) is to be stored. (C) First, associations between coactive nodes are strengthened. (D) However, the activation of nodes A and B will also spread along previously strengthened connections to activate nodes C and D. (E) Once C and D are activated, connections will be strengthened between them and other coactive nodes. The result is that a pattern is stored that is an amalgam of the two original patterns. In computational models, runaway excitation is often prevented by assuming that recall and storage are separate phases. Thus, the spreading activation shown in D does not occur during a storage phase. However, most models do not consider how such a restriction might be implemented physiologically.

nodes A, B, E, and F, partially overlapping with the first stored pattern (figure 10.5B). Connections between coactive nodes will be strengthened, storing the second pattern (figure 10.5C), *but* at the same time, activity will spread along connections that were previously strengthened, activating nodes C and D (figure 10.5D). When nodes C and D become active, connections between those nodes and other coactive nodes will be strengthened (figure 10.5E), creating a new pattern that is an amalgam of the two stored patterns. This process is known as **runaway excitation:** Presentation of one pattern for storage will activate all other patterns that share common elements. If storage occurs under such conditions, the result will be **runaway synaptic modification** as weights between all coactive nodes are strengthened.

To avoid this problem, computational modelers working with autoassociative networks have usually assumed that there are discrete storage and recall phases of the network's operation; during the storage phase, plasticity takes place between coactive cells, but this activity is not allowed to spread to other cells within the network. In other words, using the example of figure 10.5, the chain of events would proceed from figure 10.5A through 10.5C , but the spread of activation along previously strengthened connections (figure 10.5D) would be prevented.

This solution works well enough in a computational model because the human programmer can decide which state the network is in (recall or storage) and therefore which connections should be active or inactive at any given point. But in the brain there is no programmer who can decide when storage should take place and helpfully disable inopportune pathways. If a biological network indeed functions as an autoassociator, there must be a biological mechanism that can guide storage, allowing synaptic plasticity along new pathways (figure 10.5C) while preventing synaptic transmission along old pathways (figure 10.5D).

Michael Hasselmo and his colleagues have suggested a possible mechanism for these two processes to work together within the same circuit.[12] Hasselmo's idea is based on a curious feature of acetylcholine: It has different effects on different portions of a neuron. In general, ACh suppresses synaptic transmission; that is, given a fixed amount of excitatory neurotransmitter released from the presynaptic neuron, ACh makes the postsynaptic neuron less likely to become active in response to that input. But the specific amount of suppression varies for different kinds of inputs.

As is shown in figure 10.6, pyramidal cell bodies lie in one layer (called the *stratum pyramidale*, or pyramidal layer) of hippocampal field CA3, but their dendrites and axons extend into other layers. The inputs making synapses on the dendrites are largely segregated by layer. Inputs from the entorhinal cortex tend to synapse far from the cell bodies, in the *stratum lacunosum-moleculare*. Inputs from other CA3 neurons tend to synapse near the cell bodies, in the *stratum radiatum*. In other words, **extrinsic inputs,** arising outside the hippocampus, synapse in one layer, while **intrinsic inputs,** from inside the hippocampus, synapse in another layer.

When a cholinergic agonist is applied to CA3, its effects on suppressing synaptic transmission are much more pronounced in stratum radiatum than in stratum lacunosum-moleculare.[13] *That is, ACh appears to suppress intrinsic inputs more than extrinsic inputs* (figure 10.7).

A similar pattern of connectivity is seen in hippocampal field CA1:[14] ACh suppresses intrinsic inputs (from elsewhere in the hippocampus) more than

Hippocampal Field CA3

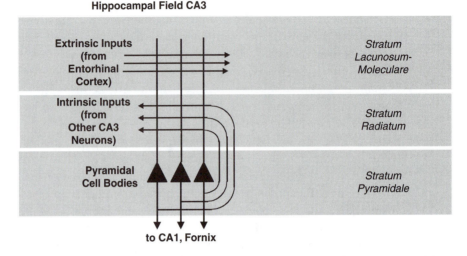

Figure 10.6 Schematic representation of hippocampal field CA3. CA3 is segregated into several layers, each defined by what types of cell bodies and inputs it contains. Pyramidal cells are located in the *stratum pyramidale,* and their dendritic processes reach up into *stratum radiatum* and *stratum lacunosum-moleculare.* The inputs that make synapses in *stratum lacunosum-moleculare* are largely extrinsic inputs from entorhinal cortex, whereas *stratum radiatum* contains intrinsic inputs, synapses from other CA3 cells. Acetylcholine acts selectively to suppress the intrinsic inputs more than the extrinsic inputs.

Hippocampal Field CA3

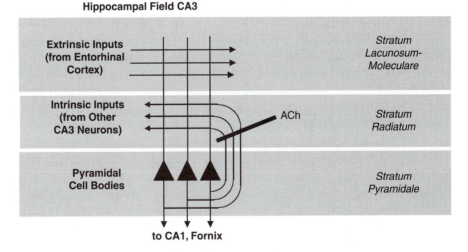

Figure 10.7 Hasselmo and colleagues have demonstrated that acetylcholine (ACh) has a suppressive effect on neuronal transmission that is more pronounced in *stratum radiatum* than in *stratum lacunosum-moleculare* in CA3. This means that ACh selectively suppresses intrinsic inputs (from other CA3 neurons) more than extrinsic inputs (from outside the hippocampus).

extrinsic inputs (from the entorhinal cortex). Other studies have demonstrated similar selectivity of cholinergic effects in dentate gyrus and cortex.[15] Thus, a basic principle of cholinergic function may be that ACh and cholinergic agonists exert a strong suppressive effect on *intrinsic* inputs but have little effect on *extrinsic* inputs.

Hasselmo has suggested how this property of ACh can be used to guide an associative network between storage and recall processing whereby *high levels of ACh suppresses intrinsic inputs, allowing storage, and low levels of ACh allow activity among intrinsic inputs, allowing recall.* This means that when cholinergic input is present, the hippocampus can store new patterns; when this ACh is absent, the hippocampus can retrieve patterns that were previously stored.

Figure 10.8 shows an example. A pattern is presented for storage to the CA3 network (figure 10.8A). The input activates a subset of the entorhinal afferents (e.g., a and b), which in turn activate a subset of CA3 pyramidal neurons (e.g., A and B). Acetylcholine suppresses activation along the recurrent collaterals (figure 10.8B) so that no additional CA3 pyramidal neurons are activated. However, enough activation passes to allow strengthening of connections between coactive CA3 neurons. At this point, the pattern AB is stored. Now suppose that a subset of the entorhinal inputs are presented—such as just afferent a (figure 10.8C). Node A is activated, and in the absence of acetylcholine, activation spreads along recurrent collaterals (figure 10.8D). The previously weighted connection between A and B allows node B to become active: The stored pattern is recalled. Finally, suppose another pattern is presented for storage. Entorhinal afferents b and c activate CA3 neurons B and C (figure 10.8E). In the presence of acetylcholine, activation is not allowed to spread along the previous connection from B to A, and so A does not become active. Thus, only the current pattern is stored; pieces of previous patterns do not intrude.

The basic assumption underlying the model in figure 10.8 is that acetylcholine should project from medial septum to hippocampus when novel input is to be stored but not while familiar input is being recalled. Important evidence of this effect has recently emerged. These data were obtained through microdialysis, an elegant technique for measuring local changes in neurotransmitter levels, and showed that the amount of acetylcholine in the ventral hippocampus increases during CS-US learning and decreases after the CR is well learned.[16] This is consistent with Hasselmo's assumption that acetylcholine levels should be high during learning and low thereafter.

Behavioral Predictions.   Hasselmo's model expects that new information is stored in the presence of acetylcholine. Therefore, drugs that reduce brain

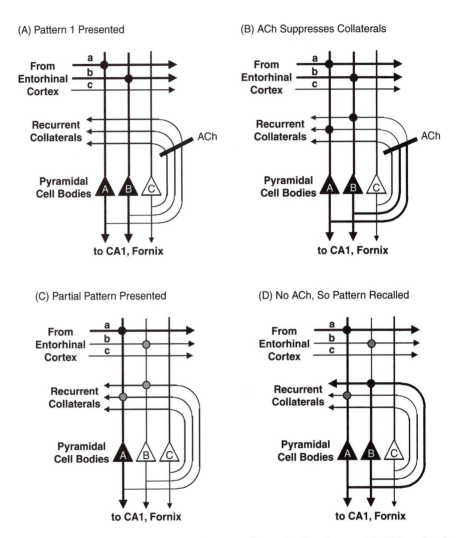

Figure 10.8 Storage of a new pattern in CA3, according to the Hasselmo model. (A) Entorhinal afferents provide information about a pattern to be stored (e.g., ab). These afferents activate a subgroup of the CA3 pyramidal cells (e.g., AB). Synapses from active entorhinal afferents to active CA3 neurons are strengthened (black circles). Acetylcholine (ACh) generally suppresses activity along recurrent collaterals. (B) Enough information passes to allow strengthening of connections between coactive CA3 neurons (gray circles) but not to activate any additional CA3 neurons. (C) When a partial version of the stored pattern is presented along the entorhinal afferents (e.g., a), this activates a subset of the CA3 neurons (e.g., A). (D) In the absence of acetylcholine, activation spreads along recurrent collaterals, activating the CA3 neurons to complete the pattern (e.g., B).

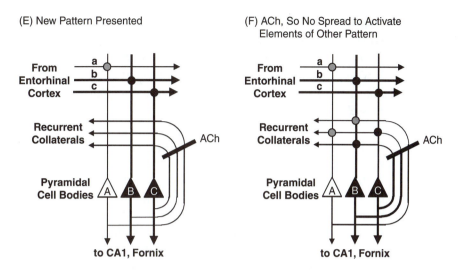

Figure 10.8 *(continued)*   (E) A new pattern is presented for storage (e.g., bc) that shares some elements with the previously stored pattern. It activates a subset of the CA3 neurons (e.g., BC). (F) In the presence of acetylcholine (ACh), recurrent activation is not allowed to spread and activate additional neurons. Thus, although node B has a weighted connection to node A as part of the previously stored pattern, node A is not activated in the current context, and so no erroneous connection is made between A and C.

acetylcholine levels should impair the ability of the hippocampus to store new information, leading to a kind of temporary, reversible amnesia while the drug is in effect. On the other hand, because acetylcholine is not needed for recalling information in the model, cholinergic antagonists should not impair the recall of previously stored information.

This prediction has been experimentally confirmed. Rabbits and humans given the anticholinergic drug scopolamine are indeed strongly impaired in learning (storage) of new information, as was shown in figure 10.3B. However, scopolamine does not abolish execution (recall) of a trained response, indicating that the subjects can still recall previously learned information while under the influence of scopolamine.[17]

In humans, scopolamine can likewise affect the ability to learn and remember various sorts of information.[18] For example, subjects who were given scopolamine before presentation of a list of words displayed very poor performance when they were later asked to recall the words. These subjects recalled only about 6 out of 128 words, in contrast to control subjects who were not given scopolamine, who were able to recall about 45 words. However, in another study, subjects were first presented with the words, then given scopolamine, and then asked to recall the words from the original list. For these subjects, there was no retrieval deficit; they could recall just as many words as control subjects. Together, these studies show that scopolamine selectively impairs encoding (storage) of new information but does not impair recall (retrieval) of previous information as suggested by Hasselmo's model.[19]

Cholinergic Modulation of Cortico-Hippocampal Interaction

As the preceding section described, Hasselmo has suggested that the cholinergic input from medial septum to hippocampus modulates storage in the hippocampus. Specifically, when ACh is high, the hippocampus tends to store new information; when ACh is low, the hippocampus tends to retrieve previously stored information. Another way of saying this is that the rate of hippocampal storage is proportional to the amount of ACh received.

Our cortico-hippocampal model can be extended to capture the effects of cholinergic modulation in a very straightforward way. Recall from chapter 6 that our model includes a hippocampal-region network that learns to reconstruct its inputs. In the process, new representations are formed in the internal layer that are biased to compress redundant information while preserving and differentiating predictive information. Weights in the hippocampal-region network are adjusted on the basis of the error between the input and output patterns. This adjustment can go quickly or slowly, depending on a variable in our model: a global **learning rate** (called β) specifying the magnitude of change to a weight.

Note that there are three separate and independent learning rates in our model, one corresponding to each brain region being modeled. Thus, there is one learning rate in the hippocampal-region network, one for the cortical (lower) layer of the cortico/cerebellar network, and one for the cerebellar (upper) layer of the cortico/cerebellar network; these three learning rates may be modified independently.

When the hippocampal-region network is presented with an input pattern (figure 10.9A), a representation is activated in the internal-layer nodes, which in turn activates an output pattern. This output pattern is the network's attempt to reconstruct the input. If the input pattern is familiar, the output will be an accurate reconstruction. If a novel input pattern is presented that shares some elements with a previous pattern (figure 10.9B), it may activate a similar internal representation and, in turn, generate output that is consistent with the previously learned pattern. This is the network's attempt at pattern retrieval. However, because the output is incorrect, learning occurs in

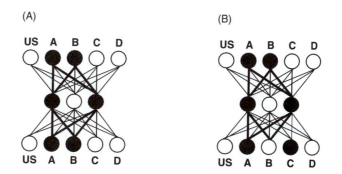

Figure 10.9 Storage versus recall in the hippocampal-region network of the cortico-hippocampal model. Activated nodes are shown as dark circles; previously strengthened connections are shown as thick lines. (A) Assume that the network has been well trained that two stimuli (A and B) are often presented together and do not predict the US. When these stimuli are presented, a particular pattern of activities is evoked in the internal layer: the representation of the compound stimulus AB. This in turn has been mapped onto outputs that reconstruct the inputs. In this case, the pattern of output activities perfectly reconstructs the inputs, and so reconstruction error is zero. (B) Now the network is presented with a new input pattern: stimuli A and C. Previously strengthened weights (thick lines) from stimulus A tend to activate the old representation, which in turn tends to activate the output pattern AB. This is incorrect: Two nodes in the output layer (B and C) have activations that do not match the input pattern, so reconstruction error equals two out of the five output nodes. At this point, learning may occur to adjust the weights to make the output look more like the input. The rate of weight change is set by the network's learning rate.

the network's weights so as to store the new pattern. This learning process causes weights to be changed to make this new pattern generate appropriate output. The magnitude of weight change on any one trial is proportional to the network's learning rate parameter. If the learning rate is high, then the network tends to always store new information. However, if the learning rate is low, the network will tend to continue to produce previous patterns in response to novel inputs.

Thus, in our model of learning in the hippocampal region, the learning rate parameter determines whether the network performs pattern storage or pattern retrieval. This is essentially the same as the storage-mediating function that Hasselmo proposes for acetylcholine. Thus, *Hasselmo's theory of ACh can be instantiated within Gluck and Myers's cortico-hippocampal model by assuming that acetylcholine from medial septum determines the hippocampal region's learning rate*, as is shown in figure 10.10.[20]

When this cholinergic input is high, hippocampal storage takes place; when the cholinergic input is absent, there is no storage at all. Between these two extremes, hippocampal storage proceeds at intermediate rates. In effect,

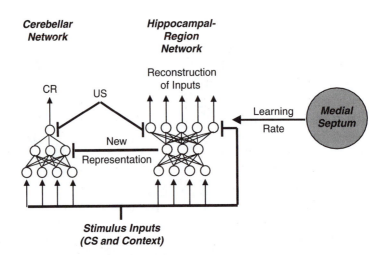

Figure 10.10 Myers et al.'s (1996) hypothesis that septohippocampal cholinergic projections modulate the amount of hippocampal storage can be implemented in the cortico-hippocampal model by assuming that the medial septum determines the hippocampal-region network's learning rate.

we have argued that the medial septum provides a "volume control" governing the degree of hippocampal learning of new stimulus representation.[21] Note that changing the hippocampal-region learning rate does not directly affect the learning rate in the cortico/cerebellar network or the rate at which hippocampal-region representations are adopted by the cortico/cerebellar network.

Cholinergic Antagonists (Scopolamine). The effect of explicitly lowering the hippocampal-region network learning rate in our model is shown in figure 10.11B. Suppose a "normal" learning rate is defined as $\beta = 0.05$. With this learning rate, the intact cortico-hippocampal model learns to respond to a CS within about 50 trials. If the learning rate is lowered by a factor of ten (to $\beta = 0.005$), learning is dramatically slower: About 125 trials are required to learn the response. The response is learned just as strongly in the end, but the system takes longer to get there. This is the same kind of slowing that is seen in rabbits that are given the cholinergic antagonist scopolamine during eyeblink conditioning: Animals that are given the drug take over twice as long to learn the conditioned response (figure 10.11A).[22] For this reason, we call the cortico-hippocampal model with the lowered learning rate a **scopolamine model;** its performance on a variety of tasks can be compared to that of animals given scopolamine.[23]

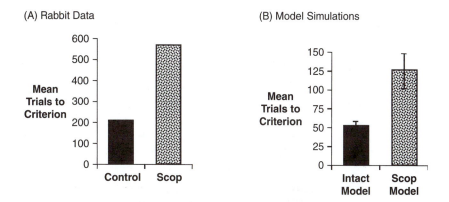

Figure 10.11   (A) The cholinergic antagonist scopolamine slows acquisition of a conditioned eyeblink response in rabbits, compared with control animals that are given an injection of saline. This is reflected in longer learning times for scopolamine (Scop) versus control animals. (Plotted from data given in Solomon et al., 1983.) A similar effect occurs in human eyeblink conditioning (Solomon et al., 1993). (B) The cortico-hippocampal model assumes that scopolamine lowers the learning rate in the hippocampal-region network. For example, whereas the hippocampal-region network in the intact model has a learning rate of $\beta = 0.05$, a scopolamine model may have a learning rate of $\beta = 0.005$. The result is that learning of a conditioned response is considerably slower in the scopolamine model than in the intact model (Myers, Ermita, et al., 1998).

In our scopolamine model, lowering the learning rate in the hippocampal-region network means that it takes longer for the model to develop new, stable stimulus representations. Because the cortico/cerebellar network—wherein long-term memories are stored and the learned response is produced—is continually working to adopt these representations, it cannot make much progress until the hippocampal region's representations have stabilized. Thus, even though learning in the cortico/cerebellar network is not slowed per se, the slow representational learning in the hippocampal-region network has the effect of retarding associative learning in the cortico/cerebellar network. However, once the hippocampal representations are stabilized, the cortico/cerebellar network can adopt these new representations—and learn behavioral responding at its normal rate. Thus, the eventual performance of the scopolamine model is just as good as the (normal) intact model; it just takes longer to get there.

Cholinergic Agonists (Physostigmine) and Dose-Response Relations. Whereas the cholinergic antagonist scopolamine slows learning, cholinergic agonists have the opposite effect. For example, **physostigmine** is a cholinergic agonist that retards the rate at which ACh is cleaned out of the synapse.

In one study, monkeys were given physostigmine and then trained on delayed nonmatch to sample (DNMS).[24] As we described in chapter 2, DNMS is a learning task in which animals see a sample object, followed by a short delay, and then must choose the novel object from a set including the original sample object. Monkeys that are given a moderate dose of physostigmine performed this task significantly better than animals that were given a low dose or no physostigmine at all, as shown in figure 10.12A. Interestingly, if the dose was high, the benefits of the drug disappeared: These monkeys learned no better than normal.

A similar phenomenon was recently shown in rabbit eyeblink conditioning.[25] Rabbits were given doses of **metrifonate,** another cholinergic agonist that works by interfering with removal of ACh from the synaptic gap. Moderate doses of metrifonate improved learning more than high doses of the drug, as is shown in figure 10.12B. In other studies, very high doses of cholinergic agonists were shown to impair learning.[26] *Thus, it appears that moderate doses of cholinergic agonists can facilitate learning, while higher doses do not facilitate learning and may even interfere with learning.*

This phenomenon may seem counterintuitive, but the cortico-hippocampal model provides an interpretation of why different doses of cholinergic agonists might have qualitatively different effects on learning. Figure 10.12C shows that lowering the hippocampal-region network's learning rate (e.g., from $\beta = 0.05$ to $\beta = 0.005$) can slow learning, whereas raising the learning rate (e.g., to $\beta = 1.0$) can facilitate learning. The faster the hippocampal-region network constructs representations, the faster these are acquired and used by the cortico-cerebellar network. However, if the hippocampal-region network's learning rate is raised still further (e.g., to $\beta = 2.0$), weights are changed so dramatically on every training trial that the hippocampal-region network begins to fluctuate wildly. It may never stabilize, or it may stabilize only after a long period. Such poor learning with an overly high learning rate is a general property of neural networks.[27] Since the hippocampal-region network never stabilizes, the cortico/cerebellar network can never stabilize either, and its ability to produce a reliable response is greatly impaired. Thus, in our cortico-hippocampal model, a very high learning rate can be just as detrimental as a very low learning rate.[28]

This principle has important implications for the development of "memory-enhancing drugs" in humans. Individuals who have chronically reduced levels of ACh—for example, after lesion to the basal forebrain structures (including medial septum)—often show improved memory function when they are given cholinergic agonists such as physostigmine.[29] Since normal aging also can reduce brain ACh levels, administering a cholinergic

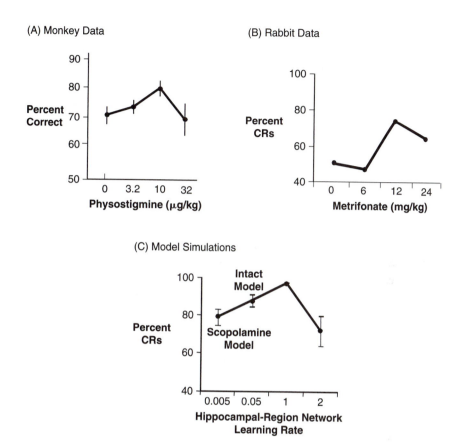

Figure 10.12 (A) Whereas a cholinergic antagonist (such as scopolamine) may slow learning, a cholinergic agonist (such as metrifonate or physostigmine) may speed learning—up to a point. Monkeys that are given a moderate dose of physostigmine (3.2 µg per 1 kg of body weight) showed improved learning compared to control monkeys that were given an injection of saline. A higher dose of physostigmine (32 µg/kg) did not improve learning (Ogura & Aigner, 1993). In other studies, high doses of physostigmine can actually impair learning (e.g., Dumery, Derer, & Blozovski, 1988; Miyamoto et al., 1989; Ennaceur & Meliani, 1992). (B) Rabbits that are given a moderate dose of metrifonate (e.g., 12 mg/kg of body weight) show faster learning than control rabbits that are given an injection of saline. Rabbits that are given a low dose (6 mg/kg) do not show the effect. A high dose of the drug (24 mg/kg) is less effective than the moderate dose. (Plotted from data presented in Kronforst-Collins et al., 1997.) (C) The cortico-hippocampal model shows a similar dose-dependent effect of increasing the hippocampal-region network's learning rate. Whereas lowering the learning rate from its normal value of $\beta = 0.05$ to $\beta = 0.005$ produces a scopolamine-like retardation in learning, increasing the learning rate to $\beta = 1.0$ produces a physostigmine-like improvement in learning. However, if the learning rate is increased too far ($\beta = 2.0$ or greater), learning begins to degrade as the hippocampal-region network becomes unstable. (A and C adapted from Myers, Ermita, et al., 1998, figure 5; B adapted from Myers et al., 1996, figure 8B.)

agonist can often improve memory in aged animals.[30] In all these cases, when brain ACh is low, a cholinergic agonist may increase the amount of available ACh and improve function. However, *in normal young subjects, whose ACh levels are presumably already optimal, further increases in ACh may not have a beneficial effect.* Thus, physostigmine given to normal young humans causes little or no improvement in memory, just as predicted by our model.[31]

Latent Inhibition and Learned Irrelevance. As we described above, our cortico-hippocampal model expects that cholinergic disruption via cholinergic antagonists will slow hippocampal-region learning. It is important to note that this is qualitatively different from the predicted effects of a hippocampal-region lesion that eliminates all hippocampal-region processing. Thus, on a behavior such as conditioned acquisition that is *not* dependent on the hippocampal region, hippocampal-region disruption (via scopolamine) may be *more* disruptive than outright hippocampal-region lesion as was seen in figure 10.3.

There is also a second, and complementary, implication of our model of cholinergic function in the hippocampal region: On behaviors that *do* require hippocampal-region processing, disruption with scopolamine may be *less* disruptive than hippocampal lesion. Scopolamine will slow hippocampal-region processing but will not eliminate it. Given enough time, the hippocampal region will still accomplish its task, and hippocampal-dependent learning will still be demonstrated, even though the entire process may be slowed.

For example, recall the phenomenon of **latent inhibition:** Prior unreinforced exposure to a cue retards subsequent learning about that cue. Our cortico-hippocampal model explains these latent inhibition behaviors in terms of redundancy compression: Cue and context are compressed together during exposure, and this impairs subsequent learning to respond to the cue but not to the context alone. Because this redundancy compression depends on the hippocampal region, damage to the hippocampal region disrupts latent inhibition (figure 10.13B).

However, we assume that scopolamine slows, but does not eliminate, hippocampal-region processing. What effect would this have on latent inhibition? During exposure, when the CS occurs in the experimental context and neither the CS nor the context predicts any US, the hippocampal region should compress their representations. Under scopolamine, this compression will proceed more slowly than normal, but it will still go on. If the exposure period is long enough, the representations of CS and

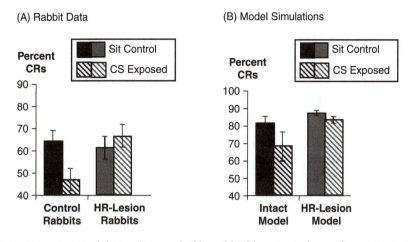

Figure 10.13 Latent inhibition: In normal rabbits, CS-US learning is slower after prior exposure to the CS (CS Exposed group) than after equivalent exposure to the context alone (Sit Control group). (A) Lesion of the hippocampal-region (including entorhinal cortex) attenuates or abolishes latent inhibition in rabbit eyeblink conditioning (Shohamy, Allen, & Gluck, 1999). (B) Similarly, there is latent inhibition in the intact model but not in the lesioned cortico-hippocampal model.

context may become just as compressed as in the normal model. Then, when the CS is paired with the US, learning will still be retarded. Under scopolamine, *any* CS-US learning is slow, of course, but prior exposure to the CS will slow learning even further. Thus, our cortico-hippocampal model expects that scopolamine should not eliminate latent inhibition (figure 10.14B).[32]

In fact, this prediction of the model appears to be borne out by data from at least one animal study: Although scopolamine slows eyeblink conditioning overall, prior exposure to the CS slows learning even further (figure 10.14A).[33]

Other studies have examined latent inhibition after injection of a toxin such as 192 IgG-**saporin,** a substance that selectively destroys cholinergic neurons. Unlike scopolamine, which merely *reduces* available ACh, saporin completely *destroys* cholinergic neurons. Thus, injecting saporin into the medial septum completely destroys the cholinergic projections to the hippocampus. In this case, the model predicts that hippocampal learning will be eliminated, and so latent inhibition will likewise be eliminated. As expected, the animals given saporin showed just this effect: Pre-exposure to the CS had no effect on subsequent CS-US learning.[34]

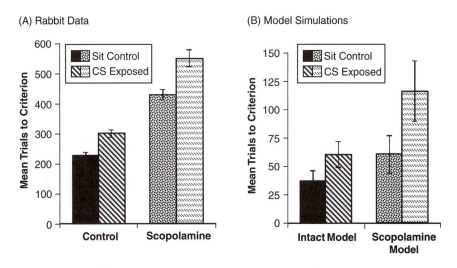

Figure 10.14 (A) The latent inhibition effect is maintained under scopolamine: Rabbits that are given scopolamine learn more slowly overall, but CS exposure slows learning still more. (Plotted from data presented in Moore et al., 1976.) (B) The cortico-hippocampal model shows a similar effect. The intact model shows latent inhibition: Exposure to the CS slows learning more than equivalent exposure to the context alone. This effect is maintained in the scopolamine model (Myers, Ermita, et al., 1998).

Learned irrelevance is a related behavioral paradigm, in which prior uncorrelated exposure to CS and US retards subsequent learning that the CS predicts the US. In previous chapters, we described data that show that learned irrelevance in rabbit eyeblink conditioning is eliminated by hippocampal-region damage (figure 10.15A). Our intact cortico-hippocampal model shows learned irrelevance because of representational changes in the hippocampal-region network; thus, learned irrelevance is also eliminated by hippocampal-region damage in our model (figure 10.15B).

Like latent inhibition, learned irrelevance is not abolished by scopolamine. In one study, experimenters administered scopolamine to a group of rabbits and then exposed them to the CS and US, uncorrelated. Later, when the effects of the drug had worn off, the rabbits received CS-US training. Learning the CS-US association was slower in these rabbits than in rabbits that had not received exposure (figure 10.16A). Thus, learned irrelevance was preserved under scopolamine.[35]

Again, our cortico-hippocampal model shows the same effect (figure 10.16B).[36] Although the hippocampal network is slowed by scopolamine during the exposure phase, representational changes do eventually occur. These are sufficient to slow later CS-US learning.

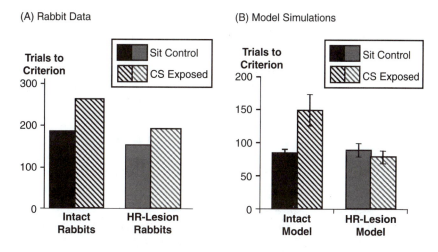

Figure 10.15 Learned irrelevance is the phenomenon whereby prior uncorrelated exposure to CS and US slows subsequent CS-US association. (A) Hippocampal-region damage (specifically entorhinal lesion) disrupts learned irrelevance in rabbit eyeblink conditioning. (B) The cortico-hippocampal model shows the same effect. (A is from Allen, Chelius, & Gluck, 1998.)

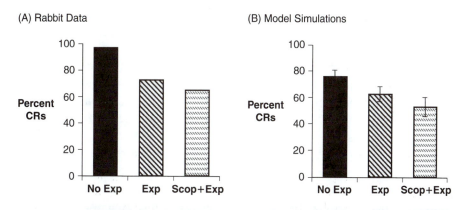

Figure 10.16 (A) Scopolamine does not disrupt learned irrelevance. Among rabbits that are given a control injection, exposure to uncorrelated CS and US (Exp group) slows subsequent CS-US learning relative to a group that received equivalent exposure to the context alone (No Exp group). To test the effects of scopolamine, rabbits were given uncorrelated exposure to CS and US while under the influence of the drug (Scop+Exp group); later, when the drug had washed out, these rabbits showed learning that was just as slow as or slower than that of the Exp group. (Plotted from data presented in Harvey et al., 1983.) (B) The cortico-hippocampal model shows the same effect. The intact model shows learned irrelevance: Uncorrelated exposure to CS and US slows subsequent learning, compared with simulations that were given equivalent exposure to the context alone. If the hippocampal-region network's learning rate is lowered during exposure (Scop+Exp condition), learning is still slowed. (Plotted from data presented in Myers, Ermita, et al., 1998.)

Scopolamine and the Hippocampus.   All the empirical data reported so far involve **systemic administration** of drugs, meaning that a drug is injected into the bloodstream or otherwise allowed to spread throughout the body. This means that the drug could be acting at any of a number of places, since cholinergic receptors are located throughout the brain and throughout the body. We have assumed that the important effects are taking place in the cholinergic projections from medial septum to hippocampus, but this is only an assumption in dealing with a drug that has been administered throughout the body and brain.

What is needed is a way to determine whether the important effects of scopolamine really take place in the medial septum and hippocampus. One way to investigate this is by combining drug studies with selective lesion studies. If scopolamine disrupts learning by disrupting cholinergic projections from medial septum to hippocampus, then scopolamine should have no effect in a hippocampal-lesioned subject.

This prediction of our model has also been verified in rabbit eyeblink conditioning:[37] Rabbits with hippocampal-region damage learn a conditioned response at the same speed with and without scopolamine (figure 10.17A). Again, our cortico-hippocampal model shows the same effect, as is seen in figure 10.17B.[38] These data on the effects of scopolamine in lesioned animals are in contrast to the effects of the same drug in intact animals and the intact model (figures 10.17C&D, reproduced from figure 10.11).

In our model, the effect of scopolamine is to retard hippocampal-region learning. If the hippocampal region is removed, then scopolamine has no effect on learning in the model. Thus, the empirical data and model behavior are consistent in implicating scopolamine as acting to disrupt hippocampal processing.

A second way to investigate where scopolamine has its effect is to administer the drug via localized injection to a particular brain region. Of course, any drug that is so injected may well spread somewhat to adjacent areas, particularly if the injection size is large and the brain area is small; still, this is a more precise method than systemic administration. Here, the questions of interest are: What happens when a cholinergic antagonist such as scopolamine is directly injected to the hippocampus? And what if it is injected directly to the medial septum? Our cortico-hippocampal model predicts that *any* interference with septal-hippocampal cholinergic processes might retard learning.

Up to a point, this has been shown to be the case. Scopolamine that is injected directly into the medial septum does slow eyeblink conditioning.[39] Scopolamine that is injected into the nearby lateral septum, which does not

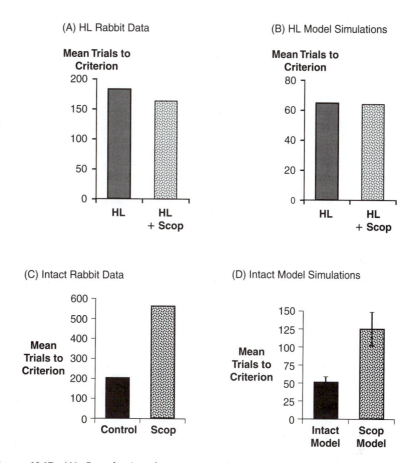

Figure 10.17 (A) Scopolamine does not retard eyeblink conditioning in rabbits with hippocampal lesion (HL). (Plotted from data presented in Solomon et al., 1983.) (B) Since the scopolamine model involves reduced hippocampal-region network learning rates, it is also trivially true that scopolamine does not affect learning in the HR-lesion model. Compare to Figure 10.11A, reprinted here as (C). The cholinergic antagonist scopolamine slows acquisition of a conditioned eyeblink response in rabbits, compared with control animals that are given an injection of saline. This is reflected in longer learning times for scopolamine (Scop) versus control animals. (Plotted from data given in Solomon et al., 1983.) A similar effect occurs in human eyeblink conditioning (Solomon et al., 1993). (D) The cortico-hippocampal model assumes that scopolamine lowers the learning rate in the hippocampal-region network. For example, whereas the hippocampal-region network in the intact model has a learning rate of $\beta = 0.05$, a scopolamine model may have a learning rate of $\beta = 0.005$. The result is that learning of a conditioned response is considerably slower in the scopolamine model than in the intact model (Myers, Ermita, et al., 1998). (A and B are adapted from Myers, Ermita, et al., 1998, figure 10.)

project to the hippocampus, does not affect eyeblink conditioning.[40] Thus, the medial septum does seem to be critically involved in the effects of scopolamine on learning.

However, when scopolamine was injected directly into the hippocampus, eyeblink conditioning was not slowed.[41] At first glance, this result appears to suggest that the hippocampus is *not* the site where scopolamine has its effect.

There are several possible explanations for this anomalous empirical finding. The first is that these studies did not inject scopolamine throughout the hippocampus, but only in the dorsal hippocampus; this is approximately the top half of the "C" formed by the hippocampus (figure 10.18; also refer to figure 8.2A). However, in rabbits, large portions of the septohippocampal cholinergic projection terminate in the ventral hippocampus.[42] It is possible that dorsal injections disrupted cholinergic function in one half of the hippocampus but left enough ACh in the lower (or ventral) hippocampus to allow learning. We conjecture that if the experiments were repeated, with scopolamine injected throughout the hippocampus, the hippocampus might be sufficiently disrupted to impair learning.

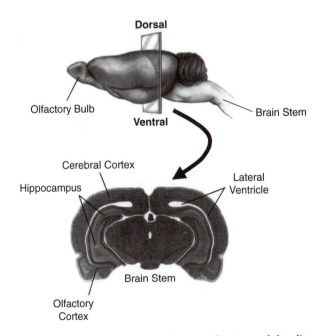

Figure 10.18 Top: Drawing of the rat brain, showing placement of the slice shown below. Bottom: Slice through the rat brain. At this point, the hippocampus has a long vertical extent and a rough "C" shape. A "dorsal" hippocampal lesion would remove only the top half of the "C," while a "ventral" lesion would destroy the lower half. The white areas are fluid-filled ventricles. Dark regions are cell bodies. (Adapted from Bear, Connors, & Paradiso, 1996, p. 179.)

A second possible interpretation of the anomalous result is that scopolamine may not be the correct kind of drug to use for a study of hippocampal cholinergic processes. ACh, like many neurotransmitters, can activate a number of different kind of receptors, and various kinds of receptors respond differentially to different experimental drugs. Thus, a drug which blocks (or activates) one receptor type may not affect another receptor type. Cholinergic receptors come in two basic classes, called **muscarinic** and **nicotinic** receptors. These receptor types are so named because the chemical muscarine activates the first type while nicotine activates the second type. (This is a purified version of the nicotine found in tobacco products.) In contrast, the brain's natural ACh activates both types of receptors.

Scopolamine primarily blocks muscarinic receptors but has little effect on nicotinic receptors. The hippocampus has both muscarinic and nicotinic receptors, and only the muscarinic receptors would be blocked by scopolamine, leaving the nicotinic receptors to function normally. Perhaps the mediation of these nicotinic receptors is enough to allow learning even after the muscarinic receptors are blocked by scopolamine.[43] Thus, it might be important to try to replicate the experiment using a drug (or a cocktail of drugs) that blocks both muscarinic and nicotinic receptors. In contrast, when scopolamine is injected to the medial septum, this may reduce the overall levels of ACh provided to the hippocampus, which would reduce the activation of both muscarinic and nicotinic receptors.

In sum, then, despite a considerable amount of prior work, there is still need for further studies to confirm the exact mechanisms by which scopolamine impairs learning and the locations at which scopolamine has its strongest effects. Nonetheless, the idea that cholinergic disruption retards hippocampal learning, thereby retarding conditioning, seems to account for a broad range of existing data as well as being consistent with many anatomical and physiological observations.

Who Modulates the Modulator?

The previous section described how acetylcholine may modulate network dynamics in hippocampal field CA3 (and elsewhere), determining whether storage or retrieval dominates. But this begs an important question: How is the level of acetylcholine determined? How does the system know whether the pattern of inputs present along the extrinsic afferents represents a new pattern to be stored or a degraded version of an old input that should be retrieved from memory?

One clue comes from the finding that there is also a path from hippocampus *back* to medial septum.[44] When this hippocampal-septal pathway is electrically stimulated, this causes a decrease in medial septal activity.[45] This implies that activity in the hippocampus can turn off the medial septum, thereby cutting off the septohippocampal projections of ACh.

Hasselmo and colleagues have suggested that this backprojection forms a self-regulating feedback loop in hippocampal field CA1.[46] We will not go through the details of the CA1 model here,[47] but the basic idea includes the assumption that CA1 performs a comparison function: noting whether the output from CA3 matches the original entorhinal input.[48] When they do match, this indicates that the pattern has been successfully stored in CA3. When they differ, either the pattern is novel or it is incompletely stored; in either case, storage should be enabled.

Figure 10.19A illustrates Hasselmo's idea in which a familiar pattern is presented along the entorhinal inputs. CA3 responds, and CA1 compares this response against the original entorhinal inputs. If the match is good, CA1 activity is high. CA1 then inhibits the medial septum, which reduces ACh. Low ACh corresponds to recall mode, in which the recurrent collaterals connections between neurons are allowed to reverberate and storage is disabled.

However, if a novel pattern is presented along the entorhinal inputs—as shown in figure 10.19B—CA3 responds as best it can, and CA1 notes that this response is a poor match to the entorhinal inputs. CA1 activity drops, ceasing its inhibition of medial septum. The medial septum springs to life, projecting ACh to hippocampus. High ACh corresponds to storage mode in which the recurrent collaterals are suppressed and the new pattern is stored.

Hasselmo's model of feedback regulation of septohippocampal ACh is still a hypothesis that needs to be fully tested. However, one behavioral result is consistent with the model: Medial septal neurons respond strongly when an animal is presented with novel but not familiar stimuli—just as is expected by Hasselmo's model.[49]

Moreover, Hasselmo's self-regulation theory lends itself naturally to being incorporated into our cortico-hippocampal model of conditioning. Earlier in this chapter, we described how ACh levels could be functionally interpreted as hippocampal learning rates within the cortico-hippocampal model.*[50] More recently, we have extended this modeling to incorporate Hasselmo's ACh self-regulation theory into the cortico-hippocampal model.[51] The mismatch between CA3 output and entorhinal input proposed by Hasselmo as a

---

*Technically, the neurons recorded by Wilson and Rolls were in the diagonal band of Broca; this is a group of cells lying next to the medial septum in the basal forebrain. The diagonal band of Broca and medial septum appear to function as a single processing unit, and the fact that they are distinguished with different names may be misleading.

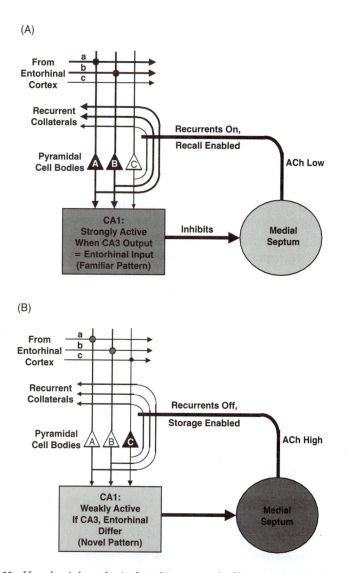

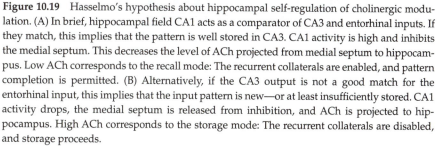

Figure 10.19 Hasselmo's hypothesis about hippocampal self-regulation of cholinergic modulation. (A) In brief, hippocampal field CA1 acts as a comparator of CA3 and entorhinal inputs. If they match, this implies that the pattern is well stored in CA3. CA1 activity is high and inhibits the medial septum. This decreases the level of ACh projected from medial septum to hippocampus. Low ACh corresponds to the recall mode: The recurrent collaterals are enabled, and pattern completion is permitted. (B) Alternatively, if the CA3 output is not a good match for the entorhinal input, this implies that the input pattern is new—or at least insufficiently stored. CA1 activity drops, the medial septum is released from inhibition, and ACh is projected to hippocampus. High ACh corresponds to the storage mode: The recurrent collaterals are disabled, and storage proceeds.

function for CA1 is very much like what happens in our autoencoder network when inputs and outputs are compared. As in Hasselmo's theory of CA1 as a novelty detector, the cortico-hippocampal model's autoencoder generates an input/output mismatch for novel stimuli.

We are currently analyzing a self-regulating version of the cortico-hippocampal model, based on Hasselmo's ACh self-regulation theory, in which the autoencoder mismatch error drives increases medial-septal activity, raising the hippocampal learning rate. Preliminary analyses of this generalized version of the cortico-hippocampal model indicate that it is consistent with both behavioral data on conditioning and electrophysiological data on medial septal activity during conditioning.[52] Interestingly, this biologically based model of learning rate regulation is very similar to algorithms that have previously been proposed within the neural network literature for optimizing network performance.[53]

10.3   OTHER THEORIES AND ISSUES

The models that we discussed in the previous section focus on the cholinergic projection from medial septum to hippocampus and how it can modulate hippocampal learning rates. This section reviews two related issues. First, acetylcholine is not the only chemical involved in the projection from medial septum to hippocampus; there are also neurons that project the neurotransmitter **GABA** (gamma-aminobutyric acid). This neurotransmitter may play an important role in how medial septum modulates hippocampal function. Second, acetylcholine functions as a neuromodulator in cortex, as well as in the hippocampus. Some of the same principles underlying cholinergic modulation of hippocampus may apply to cortex as well.

Finally, although this chapter focuses on neuromodulation involving ACh, it is important to note that ACh is not the only neuromodulator that affects hippocampal function. Other neuromodulators have received less study in terms of their effect on learning and memory, but one in particular—dopamine—has recently been the focus of interesting empirical and computational work. The interested reader is particularly referred to a model of dopamine modulation in predicting reward[54] and of norepinephrine in modulating sensitivity to behavioral context.[55]

Septohippocampal GABAergic Projections

As we mentioned above, the medial septum projects GABA as well as ACh to the hippocampus.[56] When the medial septum is lesioned or disrupted, this

GABAergic projection to hippocampus is also affected. Thus, some of the effects of septal damage or disruption may also reflect loss of GABAergic modulation in the hippocampus.

GABA is the major inhibitory transmitter in the brain, meaning that it tends to reduce activity in the postsynaptic neuron. In the hippocampus, GABA can be thought of as a neuromodulator that causes global changes in hippocampal processing. Specifically, the GABAergic septohippocampal projection is important in the generation of **theta rhythm,** a phenomenon in which large numbers of hippocampal neurons begin to fire in synchronous bursts, approximately four to eight times a second. Although the firing of any one neuron results in a minuscule electric charge, the synchronized activity of many thousands of neurons causes an electric charge large enough to be detected through the scalp. A procedure that records these group effects is the **electroencephalogram (EEG).** Figure 10.20 shows examples of an EEG recorded from a rat, during theta rhythm versus during a period of unsynchronized firing. During theta rhythm, periodic waves of GABA from medial septum arrive in the hippocampus. In turn, hippocampal pyramidal neurons go through rhythmic cycles of activity and inactivity.

In an animal such as a rat, theta rhythm typically occurs during exploratory behaviors, such as walking, rearing, and sniffing. Nonsynchronized firing occurs during consummatory behaviors, when the animal is sitting quietly and eating, drinking, or grooming. Perhaps not coincidentally, during exploratory behaviors, an animal has to organize and remember incoming

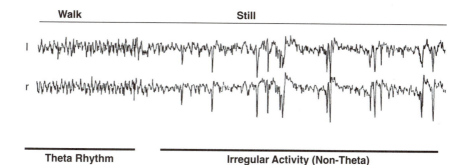

Figure 10.20   EEG recordings from hippocampal field CA1 in a rat during about 13 seconds; for the first 3 or 4 seconds, the rat was walking, and during the final 6 or 7 seconds, the rat was still. The top trace shows neuronal activity recorded from the left (l) hippocampus, and the lower trace is from the right (r) hippocampus. When the animal was walking, both traces showed regular, fast theta rhythm. When the animal became still, the trace showed large, irregular non-theta activity. (Adapted from Buzsáki, 1989, figure 1.)

sensory information—comparable to a learning or storage phase. By contrast, consummatory behaviors provide relatively less incoming sensory information and would be a good time for the brain to work on organizing and consolidating previous information.

György Buzsáki has interpolated from these data to propose that the two stages of neuronal activity might correspond to two different aspects of learning.[57] In brief, Buzsáki's theory proposes that theta rhythm occurs during exploration and other learning behaviors when new information is bombarding the brain and is being temporarily stored in the hippocampus. Theta rhythm serves the purpose of rhythmically silencing the hippocampus, breaking the steady stream of inputs into manageable 200-msec packets of information. Once exploration stops, there is time for the brain to "catch its breath" and analyze this information. The pattern of neural activity at this point is consistent with a recall and consolidation process: Recently active hippocampal neurons become active again and cause activation in the same entorhinal cells that excited them previously. This may allow the information that was temporarily stored in the hippocampus to be transferred out to cortical areas for long-term storage.

In short, Buzsáki's theory suggests that GABAergic septohippocampal inputs modulate hippocampal processing between storage (theta) and consolidation (non-theta). There is an obvious parallel between this theory and Hasselmo's proposal that cholinergic septohippocampal inputs modulate hippocampal processing between storage (high ACh) and recall (low ACh) states.

While GABA is a fast-acting neurotransmitter, the effects of ACh are slower. How do they interact? Perhaps slow-acting ACh might set the overall framework in which storage can occur: putting the hippocampus into a storage mode or a recall mode. Once the hippocampus is in storage mode, fast-acting GABA induces theta rhythm, modulating the storage of individual pieces of information. In this way, both cholinergic and GABAergic modulation might each contribute an important function to hippocampal dynamics (table 10.1).

Whether or not the relationship conjectured in table 10.1 is true, it is clear that an important avenue of future research will be to determine exactly how GABAergic and cholinergic inputs interact. Computational modeling may prove helpful here as a means of exploring prospective interactions.[58]

Cholinergic Modulation in Cortex

As we noted previously, acetylcholine projects throughout the brain and body. Near the medial septum in the basal forebrain is another group of cells, the

Table 10.1   Possible Synchrony Between ACh and GABA in Modulating Hippocampal Dynamics

	Exploring	Resting State
Observable Behavior	Incoming information to process and store	Little incoming information
Hippocampus	Rapidly *store* new information	*Recall* and consolidate to cortex
Acetylcholine	*High* → Enable hippocampal storage	*Low*→ Enable hippocampal recall
GABA	*Theta rhythm:* Break input into manageable packets	*Non-Theta activity:* Associated with recall and consolidation

nucleus basalis, which projects ACh throughout cortex (refer to figure 10.2). Just as acetylcholine promotes plasticity in the hippocampus, it also promotes plasticity in cortex. And just as acetylcholine suppresses extrinsic inputs more than intrinsic inputs in hippocampus, there is evidence that it behaves the same way in cortex.[59] This leads to the idea that if ACh modulates information storage in hippocampus, it might have a similar function in cortex. This would suggest that just as the medial septum drives hippocampal storage, cholinergic projections from nucleus basalis could drive cortical storage.

Recall from chapter 8 that stimulus representations in sensory cortex expand and shrink, depending on the meaning of stimuli. In particular, if a stimulus is paired with a US, its representation tends to expand, while the representations of other stimuli may compress to make room. Important (meaningful) stimuli win a larger portion of the cortical map. The available evidence suggests that the cortex does not know what kind of US a particular stimulus might be associated with, only that the stimulus is somehow significant. Apparently, some other parts of the brain are responsible for recognizing the CS-US association and signaling the cortex to adapt its stimulus representations accordingly.

Areas such as the amygdala are known to receive information about CS and US pairings and may be responsible for forming associations between them. These areas project to the nucleus basalis. Therefore, one plausible hypothesis is as follows: *When a CS is paired with a US, the amygdala (or other brain areas) activate the nucleus basalis, which in turn delivers acetylcholine to cortex, enabling cortical remapping to enlarge the representation of that CS.*[60]

If this hypothesis is true, then stimulating the nucleus basalis should cause cortical remapping. Several studies have shown just such an effect. When a tone CS is paired with nucleus basalis stimulation—instead of a real US—the representation of the CS in primary auditory cortex expands.[61] Additionally, when the nucleus basalis is lesioned or the cholinergic projections are otherwise disrupted, cortical plasticity is greatly reduced.[62]

These findings are very exciting, not least because of their implications for rehabilitation after cortical damage. Perhaps it may eventually even be possible to use judicious stimulation of the nucleus basalis to encourage cortical remapping in individuals who have lost the use of one cortical area. For now, though, we turn to some more immediate implications for human memory disorders.

10.4   IMPLICATIONS FOR HUMAN MEMORY AND MEMORY DISORDERS

Understanding cholinergic modulation of brain function is important with respect to understanding how normal learning and memory occur. Cholinergic modulation is disrupted in clinical syndromes that damage the basal forebrain, potentially damaging projections both from medial septum to hippocampus and from nucleus basalis to cortex. Understanding cholinergic modulation and its disruption in these syndromes may help in the development of pharmacological treatment and rehabilitation techniques.

Basal Forebrain Damage Following Cerebral Aneurysm

In rare instances, an individual may suffer selective damage to one or more basal forebrain structures, disrupting cholinergic projections with little collateral damage to nearby brain areas.[63] These individuals offer an opportunity for researchers to study how the human brain responds to loss of these cholinergic projections.

More often, the basal forebrain may be among the structures that are damaged in a stroke. A **stroke** occurs when blood flow is interrupted, through either occlusion (blockage) or rupture of a blood vessel. In either case, brain areas downstream, which depend on that blood vessel to supply oxygen and nutrients, are deprived; in the extreme, cells in the deprived areas will die. In an **aneurysm,** the walls of the blood vessel are weakened and may balloon out under pressure of the blood flow (figure 10.21A); in the extreme, the aneurysm may rupture. One of the most common sites of cerebral aneurysm is the **anterior communicating artery (ACoA),** a small blood vessel that interconnects the right and left anterior cerebral arteries. The ACoA provides oxygen and nutrients to the basal forebrain and frontal cortex (figure 10.21B), and ACoA aneurysm is a frequent cause of basal forebrain damage in humans.

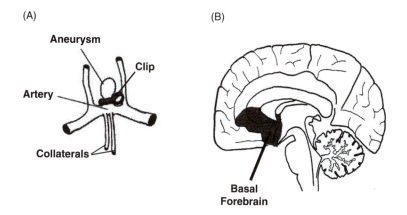

Figure 10.21   (A) An aneurysm is a weakening of the wall of an artery; under pressure of blood flow, the wall may balloon out. If the balloon ruptures, blood will leak out, decreasing blood flow in the artery. Structures downstream of the aneurysm, which depend on that artery for blood and nutrients, will be deprived. Surgery to repair an aneurysm may involve implanting a small clip at the neck of the aneurysm, preventing rupture and leakage. Blood resumes flowing through the artery and into the collateral branches that direct blood to its destinations. (B) The anterior communicating artery (ACoA) vascularizes a variably sized region that can include basal forebrain and parts of the frontal cortex. ACoA aneurysm and rupture can result in damage to these regions.

About 85% of individuals who survive ACoA aneurysm recover well enough to return to work or normal life, but about 5–15% have long-lasting impairments. The cluster of symptoms is called **ACoA syndrome,** and there are three basic components: (1) anterograde amnesia, (2) personality changes (such as loss of self-control, unpredictable aggression, or apathy), and (3) confabulation, or the spontaneous production of false memories.* Which components an individual displays and their severity may depend on the precise degree to which various brain structures have been damaged.

The anterograde amnesia that can follow ACoA aneurysm is superficially similar to the amnesia that follows medial temporal damage—except that the

---

*Confabulation should be distinguished from lying, in which an individual deliberately attempts to mislead others; confabulators are genuinely unaware that their memories are inaccurate. Confabulation should also be distinguished from false memory syndrome, in which an otherwise normal individual suddenly "remembers" a supposedly repressed memory of childhood abuse or other trauma. Confabulation is a clinical syndrome resulting from brain injury. A typical instance of confabulation would be if a patient, asked what he had for breakfast, gave a perfectly reasonable response (e.g., "cereal and toast") that just happened to be wrong.

ACoA aneurysm survivors have no direct hippocampal damage. This component of ACoA syndrome is believed to result from basal forebrain damage, which may disrupt hippocampal function in humans, much as it does in animals.[64] The animal studies—along with drug studies and computational modeling—suggest that the behaviorally superficial similarity between individuals with damage to the hippocampal-region lesion and damage to the basal forebrain lesion may be illusory. Underneath, the two amnesic syndromes may have subtle but important differences.

For example, recall that whereas direct hippocampal lesion spares eyeblink conditioning in rabbits, medial septal lesion impairs it. Similarly, humans and animals that are given the anticholinergic drug scopolamine show retarded eyeblink conditioning. Accordingly, we expected that ACoA amnesia, which involves basal forebrain damage, would also impair eyeblink conditioning. If so, this would be in contrast to the finding of spared eyeblink conditioning in medial temporal amnesia.

Recently, we have had the opportunity to test a small population of individuals who became amnesic following ACoA aneurysm. When we tested these individuals on the eyeblink conditioning paradigm, they showed a severe impairment relative to age-matched control subjects, as is shown in figure 10.22.[65] In contrast, individuals with medial temporal amnesia show relatively normal eyeblink conditioning.[66] Thus, eyeblink conditioning ap-

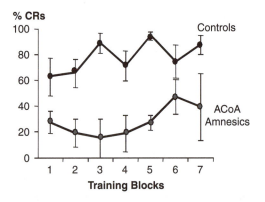

Figure 10.22 Eyeblink conditioning in individuals who became amnesic following aneurysm of the anterior communicating artery (ACoA) is strongly impaired relative to matched control subjects. The ACoA amnesics have presumed damage to basal forebrain, including medial septum and nucleus basalis. Their performance is in marked contrast to the performance of amnesic subjects with medial temporal (hippocampal-region) damage, who condition normally. (Drawn from data presented in Myers, DeLuca, et al., in preparation.)

pears to discriminate between amnesia caused by hippocampal-region damage and hippocampal disruption. These findings are exactly as predicted by the animal data and by our computational modeling.

This finding has important clinical implications. Although basal forebrain damage and hippocampal damage can both cause amnesia, the two amnesic syndromes are not identical. Eyeblink conditioning is differentially affected by the two lesion types, and other kinds of learning may be, too. Accordingly, patients with different etiologies may respond to different kinds of therapy, and a clinician might make use of this information to optimize rehabilitation programs.

Cholinergic Depletion in Alzheimer's Disease

As we described in chapter 9, **Alzheimer's disease (AD)** is a degenerative disease of the brain that leads to cognitive impairments, particularly memory decline. One anatomical hallmark of AD is the dysfunction and death of basal forebrain neurons, leading to cholinergic depletion throughout the brain.[67] Other neuromodulators, including dopamine, norepinephrine, and serotonin, are also reduced in the AD brain, but the cortical cholinergic systems seem to be affected earlier and to a greater extent than the other systems.

Cholinergic depletion may underlie some of the cognitive impairments associated with AD.[68] There is some similarity between the kinds of memory impairments seen in individuals who are given cholinergic antagonists (such as scopolamine) and individuals in the early stages of AD,[69] although scopolamine does not reproduce all of the symptoms of AD.[70]

If cholinergic depletion is responsible for some of the symptoms associated with AD, then administration of cholinergic agonists should provide some relief from these symptoms. In fact, some limited memory improvement has been observed in Alzheimer's patients who are given cholinergic agonists such as tacrine (brand name Cognex), physostigmine, or donepezil (trade name Aricept).[71]

The effectiveness of these drugs tends to be modest and short-lived; symptoms may be temporarily ameliorated but not reversed.[72] Additionally, there are often side effects: Liver and gastrointestinal problems are common in individuals taking tacrine. The limited success of cholinergic agonists in treating AD indicates that cholinergic depletion is only one piece of the AD puzzle.

On the other hand, the fact that cholinergic agonists have any success at all confirms that cholinergic systems do play an important role in AD.

Computational models of cholinergic modulation and AD may lead to a better understanding of the role of ACh in normal learning and in dementia.

SUMMARY

• Various neuromodulators, including acetylcholine (ACh), alter how neurons transmit messages—without altering the content of the message. The major cholinergic input to the hippocampus is from the medial septum in the basal forebrain.

• Disrupting the septohippocampal cholinergic projection (by damage to medial septum or through drugs that affect synaptic transmission of ACh) can lead to devastating memory impairment, presumably by disrupting hippocampal function. ACh depletion is also implicated in the memory impairments of Alzheimer's disease.

• Whereas direct hippocampal region spares classical conditioning, septohippocampal disruption impairs classical conditioning; thus, the effects of disrupting the hippocampus can be worse than outright removal.

• Hasselmo and colleagues, noticing that ACh has different effects on extrinsic than intrinsic inputs, suggested that ACh acts to modulate hippocampal dynamics between a storage mode and a recall mode.

• Building on this idea, we suggested that septohippocampal cholinergic input could specifically act to modulate hippocampal-region learning rates. This was implemented in the cortico-hippocampal model and accounted for the effects of various cholinergic drugs on classical conditioning.

• Other neuromodulators also have effects on learning; GABA from medial septum to hippocampus may also mediate hippocampal storage, while ACh from nucleus basalis to cortex may be important in cortical plasticity and the development of topographic maps.

APPENDIX 10.1   SIMULATION DETAILS

The computational model presented in section 10.2B was originally described in Myers, Ermita, et al. (1998). Full details of this model are given there (see also Myers et al., 1996).

In brief, the cortico-hippocampal model is generally the same as that described in other chapters (e.g., chapters 6 and 7). The hippocampal-region learning rate is set to a fixed parameter: $\beta = 0.05$ on trials in which the US is present and $\beta = 0.005$ on trials in which the US is absent. To simulate the effects of moderate doses of a cholinergic antagonist such as scopolamine, the hippocampal-region learning rate is decreased tenfold (i.e., $\beta = 0.005$ on trials in which the US is present and $\beta = 0.0005$ on trials in which the US is absent). To simulate the effects of high doses of a cholinergic agonist such as physostigmine, the hippocampal-region learning rate is increased (e.g., $\beta = 1.0$ on trials in which the US is present and $\beta = 0.1$ on trials in which the US is absent). No other parameters in the model are assumed to be altered by administration of these cholinergic drugs.

11 Emergent Themes

This book has focused on computational models of the hippocampal region and its interaction with other brain structures during simple forms of learning. In this final chapter, we highlight the most important themes that have emerged, and we stress their implication for future computational modeling.

11.1 HIPPOCAMPAL FUNCTION CAN BEST BE UNDERSTOOD IN TERMS OF HOW THE HIPPOCAMPUS INTERACTS AND COOPERATES WITH THE FUNCTIONING OF OTHER BRAIN SYSTEMS.

The hippocampus interacts with other brain regions that are its partners in learning and memory, including the entorhinal cortex, the basal forebrain, the cerebellum, and the primary sensory and motor cortices. In this partnership, the hippocampus acts as an information processor, taking input from some brain regions, operating on it, and sending the output to other brain regions.

Borrowing methods from computer science and cognitive science, theoreticians have attempted to specify how the hippocampus carries out its processing role and how its output is used by its partners. Various theories have grown out of this approach, including models that suggest a hippocampal role in learning stimulus-stimulus relationships, in incorporating contextual information during ongoing learning, in forming cue configurations, and so forth (see chapter 6 for a review). In particular, computational models have demonstrated that these information-processing accounts of hippocampal-region function can explain why certain kinds of learning behaviors are selectively disrupted or altered after hippocampal region damage, while others appear to be unaffected. The challenge now is to return to the laboratory to determine the extent to which these computational models stand up to rigorous empirical testing and to modify them accordingly.

11.2   PARTIAL VERSUS COMPLETE LESIONS MAY DIFFER
IN MORE THAN JUST DEGREE.

New selective techniques for experimental brain lesions are demonstrating that very subtle differences in the extent of damage can lead to broad differences in resulting behavior. For example, chapter 9 discussed how "hippocampal" damage can have very different implications depending on whether the lesion is selective to the hippocampus or extends to include nearby structures such as the entorhinal cortex. These recent results overturned a great deal of prior work which presumed that damage to any structure within the hippocampal region would produce similar results. In particular, many behavioral impairments resulting from damage to the hippocampal region turned out to depend not on the hippocampus at all, but rather on other nearby structures.[1] Several computational models (including those discussed in chapter 9) have made specific predictions about the effects of selective lesions on various tasks, and it is now up to researchers to empirically confirm or disconfirm those predictions.

Another area in which computational modeling may be helpful is in understanding the different implications of complete versus partial hippocampal lesion. Most amnesic individuals who are studied in research laboratories have more or less total loss of hippocampal tissue with resulting severe anterograde amnesia. But there are many people who have only partial loss of hippocampal tissue, resulting in intermediate memory impairments.

For example, some individuals with intractable epilepsy do not respond to drug treatment, and the seizures become so frequent and severe as to be life threatening. One option is surgical removal of the brain tissue where the seizures originate—often the anterior temporal lobes, including the amygdala and the anterior 2–3 cm of the hippocampus on one side of the brain.[2] Approximately 68% of patients undergoing this surgery become seizure-free, while another 23% report worthwhile reduction in seizures.[3]

These patients often also experience some memory loss following surgery, presumably due to partial loss of one hippocampus.[4] However, individuals with medial temporal lobe epilepsy generally report memory impairments even before surgery, and this is at least partially due to sclerosis (scarring) in the hippocampus as a result of repeated seizures.[5]

It should be possible to develop computational models that address partial hippocampal damage—for example, through removal of some percentage of hippocampal neurons—and predict the resulting constellation of behavioral impairments. This is a topic that has received relatively less study in the computational modeling community but that could have important clinical implications.

11.3   DISRUPTING A BRAIN SYSTEM HAS DIFFERENT EFFECTS THAN REMOVING IT.

Chapter 10 described data showing that eyeblink conditioning is not disrupted when the hippocampus is lesioned but is disrupted when the hippocampus is dysfunctional.[6] Such dysfunction can result from the lesion of modulatory structures such as medial septum or from the introduction of drugs such as scopolamine that disrupt modulatory inputs. Hippocampal dysfunction can also result from electrical stimulation or even the presence of scar tissue. Moreover, many so-called hippocampal lesions are, in fact, lesions to the fimbria/fornix that disrupt subcortical inputs to the hippocampus. In some cases, the effect of fimbria/fornix lesions appears similar to the effect of direct lesions to the hippocampus. But it is not clear whether this pattern will hold true over a wider range of behavioral tasks or whether fimbria/fornix lesions result in impairments that are more similar to the disruptions that occur from cholinergic antagonists such as scopolamine.

Here, computational modeling provides some important insight. For example, our scopolamine model in chapter 10 suggests that there are distinct and qualitative differences between hippocampal lesion and disruption due to changes in cholinergic inputs to the hippocampus. Although both may result in similar declarative memory deficits in humans, studies of simple learning paradigms such as classical conditioning illuminate subtle but important differences between lesion and disruption. The computational model provides a way to predict, *a priori*, which kinds of learning will be impaired or spared following lesion or disruption.

These distinctions and differences also have clinical implications. Memory rehabilitation techniques that work well in an individual with hippocampal lesion (such as following medial temporal damage) may be less effective in individuals with hippocampal disruption (such as following basal forebrain damage) and vice versa. Understanding the pattern of impaired and spared memory abilities in each population may help clinicians to develop therapies that are tailored to an individual's etiology and abilities.

11.4   STUDIES OF THE SIMPLEST FORMS OF ANIMAL LEARNING MAY BOOTSTRAP US TOWARD UNDERSTANDING MORE COMPLEX ASPECTS OF LEARNING AND MEMORY IN HUMANS.

Much of the modeling that is presented in this book begins by addressing data from studies of hippocampal function in animal learning and then builds on this animal research to seek a clearer understanding of the hippocampus in human learning and memory. Because comparative studies of animal and human learning have been so essential to the study of the neurobiology of learning, it is important to understand how complex forms of human learning relate to the more basic forms of learning that are seen in all animals.

"Typically, evolution works through endless variations on a limited repertory of themes," wrote the noted psychologist W. K. Estes. "Similar mechanisms for accomplishing the same functions appear at many stages and levels of both phylogeny and ontogeny, and, as a consequence, clues to understanding complex processes of human cognition sometimes come from studying simpler forms."[7]

For example, suppose one wants to study how people learn to categorize objects. A human has many different mechanisms for learning, ranging from simple classical conditioning all the way up to verbally mediated rules. This is far too much to attempt to study at once. Instead, a researcher may use a simpler model system, which abstracts out all but one kind of learning. One model system is rabbit eyeblink conditioning. It is generally assumed that rabbits do not have access to many higher-level forms of learning (such as verbally mediated rules) but are instead restricted to simpler forms of associative learning. The hope is that findings from studies of animal conditioning will scale up to more complex forms of learning in humans. Indeed, many of the basic principles of learning that are seen in conditioning are also manifested in higher-level forms of human cognition, such as learning complex categories and concepts.[8]

A related point was discussed in chapter 8, in which studies of cortical remapping in animals inspired a broader program for remediation of language-learning impairment in children. What is especially salient here is that the original animal work involved simple conditioning behaviors. On the surface, these learning behaviors have very little to do with the extraordinary complexities of human language acquisition, a subject that is still poorly understood. But by using these simple animal paradigms, researchers were able to grasp some of the fundamentals of how learning induces plasticity in the cortex. Apparently, the rules that govern this plasticity are independent of the particular learning paradigm or species being studied. Thus, researchers took insights gained by studying simpler learning processes and applied them to a far more complex phenomenon: language learning.

11.5   KEEP IT SIMPLE. KEEP IT USEFUL. KEEP IT TESTABLE.

Keep It Simple

A model's value to science is often inversely related to its complexity. The point of a model is to reduce the complexity of the real world and focus on a reduced set of phenomena. To accomplish this, the modeler must resist the urge to make the model as complex and "realistic" as possible. When models become so intricate as to be comprehensible only to other modelers, they lose their ability to function as effective tools for guiding empirical research. Whenever possible, we believe that a modeler should try to build new models on top of old ones, adding a minimum of new assumptions to capture a maximal amount of new data. The alternative is to add new parameters and complexity each time a new piece of data needs to be accounted for. Such a model quickly spirals out of control, becoming too complicated to be useful. Rather, the goal of modeling, as described by W. K. Estes, should be to "find out whether [one can] arrive at a small number of concepts and principles that, applied in varying combinations, could help illuminate a wide variety of psychological phenomena."[9] In other words, a good model is one that exemplifies the principle of parsimony, proposing the simplest possible hypothesis to explain the data at hand.

Keep It Useful

A model that is simple but realistic still has one more challenge: It must be useful. Models are tools and different models are useful for different purposes. A frequent trap for modelers and those who evaluate them is to judge a model's "utility" against a checklist of phenomena, such as determining which model accounts for the "most" behavioral data or incorporates the "most" anatomical detail. These comparisons must be made with caution. Anatomical detail is a good thing in a model of anatomical substrates, but it can needlessly complicate a model of higher-level behaviors. Similarly, a model that can correctly account for only a few pieces of behavioral data may be useful—if those data are particularly puzzling or important. A related trap is to assume that all models are necessarily in competition and that only one can be shown to be "correct." Rather, it is quite possible for two or more models to capture different aspects of anatomy and physiology and different kinds of behaviors. In many cases, different models can complement each other in much the same way that an architect may use several line drawings of the same building, ranging from close-ups of the wiring to broad views of the façade. Each describes a different aspect of the same subject, and each is useful for a different purpose.

Keep It Testable

Unlike the architect's diagrams, models must be more than mere illustrations. It is not enough for the model to show behaviors that are similar to those already observed in the laboratory. The model must generate strong, testable predictions. If animals or humans fail to behave in the way the model does, the model is discredited and must be revised or abandoned. Moreover, even if animal and human studies generate data that are in every way concordant with the model's predictions, this does not prove that the brain operates in the same way. Rather, it only shows that the assumptions embedded in the model are one possible way that the brain could work; there could be many other models that embed other assumptions and that generate the same data. However, as more and more data accumulate, we may become more and more convinced that a given model is the most plausible way to understand brain function. Thus, it is incumbent on the researchers who propose a model to note how their model can be tested and which model predictions, if disproven, would require the model to be abandoned.

CONCLUSION

We have tried to convey in this book how and why computational models have advanced our understanding of the neural bases of learning and memory. We feel strongly that it should be possible to understand these models and appreciate their value to science without delving into mathematical details. We have tried to communicate the fundamentals of neural-network modeling of hippocampal function to the broader scientific community, by focusing on the underlying principles rather than on the mathematical nuts and bolts.

In covering a range of models from a variety of researchers, we have tried to convey how it is possible for different models to capture different aspects of anatomy and physiology and different kinds of behaviors. In many cases, these models complement each other, the assumptions of one model being derived from the implications of another.

Many questions about hippocampal function in learning still remain unanswered. We believe that good models should raise as many new questions as answer old ones. Some of these open questions are empirical, and we have suggested, at several places in the book, what we think are some of the more pressing empirical issues that need to be resolved by further behavioral and neurobiological studies in animals and humans. Other open questions and unresolved issues that the models raise are of a more theoretical nature and suggest new modeling directions for the future. Although we have aimed this book primarily at nonmodelers, we hope that we may have excited a few of our readers to go on to become modelers themselves or to incorporate computational modeling into their own research programs through collaboration with modelers.

Glossary

The purpose of the glossary is to provide a quick reference for the reader who encounters a word in the text that was defined earlier in the book. Accordingly, the words listed below are defined in the (occasionally idiosyncratic) way in which they are used in the text. In some cases, these are more specialized definitions than might appear in a textbook or general-purpose dictionary. For more complete explanations, the reader is referred to the body of the text.

A1: See **Primary Auditory Cortex.**

Ablation: Surgical removal of a (brain) structure; may involve collateral damage to overlying structures.

Acetylcholine (abbreviated **ACh**): A brain chemical that acts as a neurotransmitter in the body, carrying signals to muscles, and a neuromodulator in the brain, mediating the responsiveness of neurons to other inputs.

Ach: See **Acetylcholine.**

ACoA: See **Anterior Communicating Artery.**

ACoA Syndrome: A cluster of symptoms that may follow aneurysm of the anterior communicating artery, including anterograde amnesia, personality changes, and confabulation; the precise symptoms depend on the severity of the aneurysm and on which brain structures are vascularized by the ACoA in that individual.

Acquired Equivalence: A conditioning paradigm in which two superficially dissimilar stimuli (e.g., A and B), having been associated with the same reinforcer, tend also to be associated with each other, so subsequent learning about A tends to generalize to B.

Acquisition: In conditioning, a paradigm that consists of learning a single CS-US association.

Activation Level: The overall probability that a neuron or node will become active or fire on the basis of the sum of its inputs. May also be interpreted as the strength of a node's response to its inputs.

Activation Rule: The rule by which the weighted inputs to a node are converted into node activation levels.

Active: The state in which a node or neuron passes a message on to other nodes or neurons.

AD: See **Alzheimer's Disease.**

Afferent: Of input to a neuron.

Afferent Neuron: A neuron that sends information to another neuron.

Aggregate Error: The difference between the actual US and the aggregate prediction of the US; usually equivalent to (US-CR).

Aggregate Prediction of the US: In the Rescorla-Wagner model, the prediction of US arrival based on all available CSs; used to generate a CR and to compute error for error-correction learning.

Agonist: A drug that facilitates neuronal transmission involving a specific kind of neurotransmitter—for example, by increasing the amount of neurotransmitter produced presynaptically, increasing the effectiveness of postsynaptic receptors, or delaying the removal of excess neurotransmitter from the synapse.

Allocortex: A simple form of cortex with only two cell layers, found in reptiles and birds and in some areas of mammalian cortex.

Alzheimer's Disease (abbreviated **AD**):   A progressive, degenerative, neurological illness that results in abnormal neuronal elements called plaques and tangles and that leads to memory loss, cognitive dysfunction, and eventually death.

Amnesia: Severe memory loss; see **Anterograde Amnesia** and **Retrograde Amnesia.**

Amnesic: Of or having to do with amnesia; also refers to an individual with anterograde amnesia.

Amygdala: A subcortical structure that is involved in emotional learning.

Aneurysm: A neurological condition in which the walls of a blood vessel are weakened and may balloon out under pressure and even burst; in this case, structures that depend on that blood vessel to supply oxygen and nutrients are deprived and may die.

Animal Model: Use of a particular animal preparation to capture some aspects of a phenomenon that is observed in humans.

Anoxia: Loss of oxygen supply to the brain, possibly leading to neuronal death.

Antagonist: A drug that impedes neuronal transmission involving a specific kind of neurotransmitter—for example, by decreasing the amount of neurotransmitter produced presynaptically or by blocking postsynaptic receptors.

Anterior: Toward the front.

Anterior Communicating Artery (abbreviated **ACoA**):   A blood vessel that supplies oxygen and nutrients to an area that may include the basal forebrain and frontal cortex; a frequent site of aneurysm in humans.

Anterograde Amnesia: A kind of memory dysfunction in which acquisition of new memories is impaired while older memories may survive intact. Certain kinds of nondeclarative memory may also be spared.

Architecture: The physical structure of a neural network, including nodes and how they are connected (but not the strengths of those connections or the pattern of node activations).

Aricept: See **Donepezil.**

Aspiration: Surgical removal of a (brain) structure by suction; may involve collateral damage to overlying structures.

Association: A link between two neurons, nodes, or concepts such that when one is activated, the other may be activated as well.

Association Cortex: Areas of cortex not necessarily limited to processing a single modality; specifically, those areas of cortex that are involved in integrating information, planning, and decision making.

Associational Weights: In a multilayer neural network, the upper layer of weights that connects internal-layer nodes to output-layer nodes, thus specifying how the representation of the current input should be associated with an output.

Associative Learning: Learning about relationships (associations) between stimuli.

Associative LTP: A possible mechanism for associative learning in the brain, whereby simultaneous activity in two neurons leads to a strengthening of the synapse between them.

Associative Weights: The efficacy of one node to cause activation in another node. Often defined as a number that may be modified through learning: If the number is positive, then activity in the first node tends to increase activity in the receiving node; if it is negative, then activity in the first node tends to depress activity in the receiving node.

Asymptote: The maximum possible value of a variable; appears as a leveling-off point in a graph of that variable.

Atrophy: Abnormal shrinkage.

Autoassociative Network (or **Autoassociator**):   A class of neural network, characterized by a high level of connectivity between nodes, that can store arbitrary input patterns and recall them later on the basis of partial cues.

Autoencoder Network (or **Autoencoder**):   A variant of an autoassociator that includes an internal layer of nodes; outputs may be trained to reconstruct the input pattern according to an error-correction learning rule.

Axon: The output process of a neuron.

Backprojection: Projections from a brain area back to other regions that originally provided input to that area.

Backpropagation: See **Error Backpropagation Learning Algorithm.**

Basal Forebrain: A group of structures lying near the bottom and front of the brain, including medial septum and nucleus basalis.

Best Frequency: The auditory frequency (pitch) that maximally activates a particular pyramidal neuron in primary auditory cortex.

β: See **Learning Rate.**

Bias: A parameter that is sometimes used in neural networks that specifies a node's innate activation level before any other input is received.

Bilateral: Referring to both sides (hemispheres) of the brain, as in bilateral lesion.

Blocking: A conditioning paradigm in which prior learning that one CS A predicts the US blocks or reduces the amount of learning about a second CS B during subsequent AB-US training.

CA: See **Cornu Ammonis.**

CA1:   A subfield of the hippocampus.

CA3:   A subfield of the hippocampus, noted for its high degree of internal recurrency.

Category Learning: Learning that individual stimuli belong in particular categories, according to some predefined rule.

Cell Synchronization: Firing of various neurons simultaneously or in a distinct rhythm with respect to one another.

Cerebellar: Of the **Cerebellum.**

Cerebellar Model: A model of cerebellum, proposed by R. Thompson, that assumes that the cerebellum is capable of error-correction learning by making use of an error signal provided by the inferior olive.

Cerebellum: A structure at the rear of the brain that is involved in coordination and fine control of movement.

Cerebral Cortex: A thin gray sheet of tissue forming the surface of the brain, where memories are stored. Different regions of cortex are involved in processing different kinds of information.

Cholinergic: Of acetylcholine.

Chunking: A hypothesized mechanism whereby a set of co-occurring stimuli come to be treated as a unary whole or configuration that can accrue associations with the US.

Classical Conditioning: Learning that a previously neutral stimulus (the conditioned stimulus or CS) predicts a response-evoking stimulus (the unconditioned stimulus or US). With repeated CS-US pairing, the subject comes to give an anticipatory response (the conditioned response or CR) to the CS alone.

Climbing Fibers: A pathway from inferior olive to cerebellum that may carry error information to guide error-correction learning in the cerebellum.

Coarse Coding: A form of representation in which each external event (stimulus or stimulus feature) is encoded as a pattern of activity over many nodes or components of a model.

Cognex: See **Tacrine.**

Cognitive Map: A mental model of the environment that an animal can use to navigate, hypothesized by Tolman and later implicit in many models of hippocampal function.

Columnar Architecture: A general organizing principle of cortex in which neurons directly above and below each other in the cortical sheet tend to be interconnected and activated by similar inputs, hence acting as a functional column.

Combinatorial Explosion: The dilemma that results when every possible configuration of inputs is coded explicitly with a single input node (as in the configural cue network): The representation of every configuration of 2 inputs requires 3 nodes, the representation of every configuration of 4 inputs requires 14 nodes, the representation of every configuration of 8 inputs requires 105 nodes, and so on.

Competitive Network: A class of unsupervised network in which nodes are divided into clusters and nodes within a cluster compete to respond to the input. Nodes that win the competition undergo weight changes to make them more likely to win the competition and respond to similar inputs in future.

Component Representation: A form of representation in which each external event (stimulus or stimulus feature) is encoded within one node or component of a model.

Component Stimulus: One of the individual stimuli comprising a compound stimulus.

Compound Stimulus: A complex stimulus consisting of two or more stimuli, always presented together.

Compression: In a network, an increase in the overlap between the representations of two stimuli, which will increase generalization between those stimuli.

Computational Model: A model that is formalized as a computer program and that can generate data to compare against the behavior of the physical system being modeled.

Conditioned Inhibition: A conditioning paradigm in which one CS A predicts the US unless it is paired with a second CS B.

Conditioned Response (abbreviated **CR**): A response that is learned as a result of classical conditioning.

Conditioned Stimulus (abbreviated **CS**): A previously neutral stimulus that comes to evoke a response as a result of classical conditioning.

Conditioning: Learning that one stimulus predicts a second, salient stimulus. Learning is typically measured in terms of a specific response. See **Classical Conditioning** and **Instrumental Conditioning.**

Configural Cue Network: A neural network model of configural learning, proposed by M. Gluck and G. Bower, that assumes that there is one input node representing each CS and each combination of CSs.

Configuration, or Configural Learning: Learning in which a compound stimulus may have different associations or different meaning than the component stimuli that compose it.

Connectionism: The study of the behavior of model neural networks.

Connectionist: Having to do with neural networks or connectionism.

Consolidation Period: Period during which newly formed memories still depend on hippocampus and will be disrupted by hippocampal damage.

Context: The background, usually continuous, stimuli that are present during an experiment (such as the sights, sounds, and texture of the conditioning apparatus).

Context Shift Effect: In conditioning, the finding that a response to a CS trained in one experimental context may be weakened if that CS is presented in a novel context.

Contextual Effects: In conditioning, paradigms that show sensitivity to the context in which training occurs. (See, e.g., **Context Shift Effect.**)

Contextual Sensitivity: The degree to which responses that are learned in one context may be altered or weakened in another context.

Control or Control Group: A subject or group of subjects whose behavior is assumed to be normal, for comparison with a subject or group of experiments whose behavior is manipulated by the experimenter. An *experimental control group* receives the same training but without the critical manipulation. (For example, if an experiment tests the effects of exposure to a CS, the control group might receive equivalent time in the experimental chamber but without presentation of the CS.) A *surgical control group* receives the same surgery but without damage to the critical structure. (For example, if an experiment tests the effects of hippocampal aspiration, the control group might receive the same surgery—anesthesia, incision, etc.—but without removal of the hippocampus.)

Cornea: The transparent coat of the eyeball covering the iris and pupil.

Corneal: Of the cornea.

Cornu Ammonis: An early name for the hippocampus, which survives today in the name of hippocampal subfields, including CA1 and CA3.

Cortex: See **Cerebral Cortex.** (There are cortical areas within the cerebellum as well.)

Cortical: Of the cortex.

Cortical Map: Representation of sensory input (or other information) in a roughly topographic fashion across a cortical surface.

Cortical Remapping: Changing the cortical map.

Cortico-Cerebellar Network: Within Gluck & Myers's cortico-hippocampal model, a network that incorporates some aspects of stimulus representation in cortex and mapping from representation to behavioral response in cerebellum.

Cortico-Hippocampal Model: Neural network model proposed by M. Gluck and C. Myers that assumes that the hippocampal region forms new stimulus representations that compress (make more similar) the representations of redundant stimuli while differentiating (making less similar) the representations of stimuli that predict different future events. These new representations are adopted by the cortex, which is the site of long-term storage, and mapped to behavioral responses.

CR: See **Conditioned Response.**

Credit Assignment: The problem of knowing how to train a network when many different weights may have contributed to the output error.

Criterion: In conditioning, the performance standard that must be mastered before the subject is said to have learned the task (e.g., 80% correct responding over the last ten trials).

Critical Period: The period extending through the first few weeks or months of life during which cortical maps are especially plastic.

CS: See **Conditioned Stimulus.**

CS-CS Learning: Learning associations between two stimuli (CSs) in the absence of (or independently of) explicit reinforcement.

CS-US Learning: Learning an association between a stimulus (CS) and a reinforcer (US); usually, learning that the CS predicts the US and should evoke an anticipatory response (CR).

Cue: An event (particularly a sensory event or stimulus) that is predictive of whether another event will occur.

$D(A, B)$:   A formal measure of the overlap in representation between two stimuli A and B, computed as the difference in responding to each stimulus summed across all internal-layer nodes in a network. For example, if there are three internal-layer nodes (N1, N2, and N3), then $D(A, B)$ is the difference between N1's responses to A and B *plus* the difference between N2's responses to A and B *plus* the difference between N3's responses to A and B.

Deafferent: Cut off from input; a neuron or brain region is completely or partially deafferented if its normal sources of input are disabled or destroyed.

Declarative Memory: Memory for individual facts or autobiographical events that is easily accessed by verbal recall.

Decrement: Decrease.

Deep Layers: In cortex, the cell layers closest to the interior of the brain.

Delay Conditioning: A conditioning paradigm in which CS onset occurs before US onset and CS and US terminate together.

Delayed Nonmatch to Sample (abbreviated **DNMS**):   A recognition task in which a sample object is presented, there is a short delay, and then the sample object and a novel object are presented; the subject must choose the novel object.

Delta Rule: Another name for the **Widrow-Hoff Learning Rule.**

Dendrites: The input processes of a neuron.

Dentate Gyrus: A structure that receives input from entorhinal cortex and produces output that input to hippocampal field CA3.

Desired Output: In a neural network, the value that a node should output to minimize error; often defined with respect to a teaching input.

Differentiation: In a network, a decrease in the overlap between the representations of two stimuli, which will decrease generalization between those stimuli.

Discrimination: In conditioning, a paradigm in which one stimulus (A+) predicts the US but a second stimulus (B−) does not.

Discrimination Reversal: See **Reversal.**

Distributed Representation: A form of representation in which each external event (stimulus or stimulus feature) is encoded as a pattern of activity over many nodes or components of a model.

DNMS: See **Delayed Nonmatch to Sample.**

Donepezil: A drug (brand name: Aricept) that acts as a cholinergic agonist by interfering with the processes that clean extra ACh out of the synapse. Currently marketed as a drug to relieve the symptoms of Alzheimer's disease.

Dysfunction: Impaired or abnormal function.

Easy-Hard Transfer: In conditioning, a paradigm in which learning a difficult discrimination is facilitated by prior learning on a simpler discrimination along the same stimulus continuum. For example, learning to discriminate two similarly bright gray squares might be facilitated by prior training to discriminate a very bright gray versus a very dark gray.

EC Lesion: Lesion that is limited to the entorhinal cortex (and possibly subiculum) but sparing hippocampus and dentate gyrus; note, however, that EC lesion disables the primary pathway by which information enters and exits the hippocampus, so EC lesion may functionally disable the hippocampus as well.

Electroencephalogram (abbreviated **EEG**):   A recording of the electrical activity of the brain.

Electrophysiology: Relating to the electrical activity in neurons.

Empirical: Relating to data collected from animal or human experiments (as distinct from data produced by model simulations).

Engram: Physical trace of a memory in the brain—for example, altered neuronal connectivity.

Entorhinal Cortex: A structure within the hippocampal region that provides the primary pathway by which sensory information enters and leaves the hippocampal region.

Entorhinal Model: A model of entorhinal cortex, proposed by C. Myers, M. Gluck, and R. Granger, that assumes that the entorhinal cortex is capable of compressing the representations of co-occurring stimuli.

Episodic Memory: A subdivision of declarative memory that includes memory for specific (often autobiographical) events.

Error: In a neural network, the difference between the desired node output and the actual node output, sometimes calculated across many output nodes.

Error Backpropagation Learning Algorithm: An algorithm for error-correction learning in multilayer networks: The upper layer of weights is trained according to the Widrow-Hoff rule to reduce the error between actual and desired outputs; error is then propagated backward to the lower layer of weights, proportional to their activation (and hence proportional to their contribution to the responses of upper-layer nodes).

Error-Correction Learning: Learning that tries to reduce the difference (error) between the actual network output and a desired or target output.

Errorless Learning: A conditioning paradigm in which subjects are prevented from making any errors during learning; typically, learning begins with a trivially easy version of the problem, and difficulty is slowly increased until the subjects can execute the desired task perfectly.

Etiology: The underlying cause of a brain abnormality (e.g., type of disease or injury).

Event-Specific Amnesia: A form of amnesia in which memory loss is restricted to a particular period of time, such as the duration of a violent crime or other trauma.

Excitatory Neurotransmitter: A neurotransmitter that increases the net activation of a post-synaptic neuron.

Exclusive-Or Task: An engineering version of the negative patterning task, which requires an output of 1.0 if either of two inputs is present but an output of 0.0 if both inputs are present.

Exemplar Model: A network in which one internal-layer node is constructed to represent each configuration of inputs which is actually encountered; proposed as a model of human category learning by researchers such as R. Nosofsky.

Exposure: In conditioning, presentation of one or more CSs without any US.

External Input: In a neural network, input that is provided to the network from outside the system.

External Output: In a neural network, output that is visible outside the network (and may be interpreted as a behavioral response).

Extinction: A conditioning paradigm in which prior CS-US pairing is followed by CS-alone presentation until the CS stops evoking a response.

Extra-Hippocampal: Relating to structures other than the hippocampus.

Extrinsic Input: Input to a brain region originating from outside that brain region.

Eyeblink Conditioning: A conditioning preparation in which a corneal airpuff or shock US evokes a reflexive eyeblink; the CS may be a tone or light, and the CR is an anticipatory eyeblink learned in response to the CS.

Facilitate: Affect positively.

Feature-Negative Discrimination: A conditioning paradigm in which one CS A predicts the US unless it is preceded by a second CS B.

Feature-Positive Discrimination: A conditioning paradigm in which one CS A predicts the US only when it is preceded by a second CS B.

Feedback: In a network, connections from one layer of nodes back to a previous layer of nodes; in a brain, connections from one brain area back to the neurons that provided the input to that brain area.

Feedforward: In a network, connections from one layer of nodes to a higher layer of nodes; in a brain, connections from one brain area to neurons in a brain area that represents a subsequent stage of processing.

Fibers of Passage: Fibers (e.g., axons) that pass through a brain structure or region and may sustain collateral damage if that structure or region is lesioned.

Figure Completion Task: A task in which subjects see progressively less fragmented drawings until they can identify the object; learning is demonstrated if, on subsequent trials, subjects can recognize the object on the basis of a more incomplete version.

Fimbria: The merger zone between hippocampus and fornix.

Fimbrial: Relating to the fimbria.

Fornix: A fiber tract connecting hippocampus with various subcortical structures, including medial septum.

Fugue: A kind of amnesia in which individuals forget their past and identity. Usually caused by psychological, not physical, trauma.

GABA (a Gamma-aminobutyric acid):   A inhibitory neurotransmitter in the brain.

GABAergic: Having to do with GABA.

Generalization: The degree to which learning about one stimulus transfers to another stimulus.

Generalization Gradient: A graph showing how a strong response trained to one stimulus generalizes to other stimuli as a function of similarity to the trained stimulus.

Granule Cells: The principal cells of the dentate gyrus (compare with most cortical regions, where the principal cells are pyramidal neurons).

H+EC Lesion: Lesion that includes the hippocampus and entorhinal cortex (and possibly dentate gyrus and subiculum); assumed to be functionally equivalent to a HR lesion.

Hasselmo's Model: A model of hippocampus, proposed by M. Hasselmo and colleagues, that assumes that septohippocampal inputs modulate hippocampal learning.

Hebbian Learning: Learning which proceeds according to Hebb's rule; forms the basis for much learning in self-organizing networks.

Hebb's Rule: The learning principle formalized by D. Hebb: When two nodes or neurons are repeatedly coactive, the weight between them is strengthened.

Hemisphere: One of the two left-right halves of the brain. Many structures, including hippocampus and cortex, have an analogous component in each hemisphere, though the particular functions in each hemisphere may vary slightly.

Herpes Encephalitis: A condition in which the herpes virus enters the brain and attacks neurons there.

HF: See **Hippocampal Formation.**

Hidden Node, Hidden Node Layer: Nodes in a neural network that receive inputs from other nodes and send output to other nodes (i.e., without receiving external inputs or generating external outputs).

Hierarchical Clustering: Grouping inputs according to progressively finer-grained categories (e.g., animal, mammal, dog, terrier).

Hippocampal: Of the hippocampus.

Hippocampal Formation: A subset of hippocampal-region structures, often defined as including the hippocampus and dentate gyrus but not entorhinal cortex.

Hippocampal Region: Used to refer to a collection of brain structures that are implicated in learning and memory, including hippocampus, dentate gyrus, subiculum, entorhinal cortex, and sometimes nearby perirhinal cortex, parahippocampal cortex, and fimbria/fornix.

Hippocampi: Plural of hippocampus.

Hippocampus: A brain structure, lying in each of the medial temporal lobes in humans, that plays a crucial structure in acquisition of new memories.

H Lesion: Lesion limited to the hippocampus (and possibly dentate gyrus and subiculum) but sparing entorhinal cortex.

HL: Hippocampal lesion; specifically, a lesion limited to the hippocampus but sparing nearby structures and fibers of passage.

Homunculus: Pictorial representation of a human form with various components exaggerated or shrunken to reflect the amount of cortical representation that component receives within a given region of cortex.

HR: See **Hippocampal Region.**

HR Lesion: Hippocampal-region lesion; specifically, a lesion that includes the hippocampus and all other structures in the hippocampal region.

Hypoxia: Reduction of oxygen supply to the brain, possibly leading to neuronal death.

Ibotenic Acid: A neurotoxin that, when injected into the brain, destroys neurons near the injection site but spares nearby fibers of passage.

IgG-Saporin: See **Saporin.**

Impair: Affect negatively.

Increment: Increase.

Inferior Olive: A brain structure that receives inputs regarding the conditioned response (CR) and the US and that may provide an error signal (US-CR) to the cerebellum, guiding error-correction learning there.

Information-Processing Theory: A theory that focuses on how different brain structures process information rather than on what specific tasks might be disrupted when these various structures are lesioned or disabled.

Informational Value of a Stimulus: The usefulness of a stimulus in predicting subsequent salient events (such as a US), relative to other available stimuli.

Inhibitory Interneuron: See **Interneuron.**

Inhibitory Neurotransmitter: A neurotransmitter that reduces the net activation of a postsynaptic neuron.

Initialize: In neural network models, the resetting of all connection weights to original values (either 0.0 or small random values) without changing the network architecture, learning rule, or training procedure.

Input Node: A node in a neural network that receives input from outside the network rather than from other nodes in the network.

Input Pattern: A series of external inputs provided to a network for storage or processing.

Instrumental Conditioning: A form of conditioning in which reinforcement is contingent on the response (e.g., if a rat presses a lever, a food reward is available; if the lever is not pressed, nothing happens). Often called *operant conditioning*. Contrast with classical conditioning, in which reinforcement (the US) arrives independent of whether a response (CR) is executed.

Intact: Not having been lesioned, damaged, or otherwise disrupted.

Interference: In a neural network, the phenomenon whereby newly stored patterns can overwrite or merge with previously stored patterns.

Intermediate-Term Memory: Memory that may last minutes to hours but that may be lost thereafter.

Internal Node, Internal-Node Layer: Nodes in a neural network that receive inputs from other nodes and send output to other nodes (i.e., without receiving external inputs nor generating external outputs).

Internal Recurrency: Connections from neurons in one brain region back to other neurons of the same class in the same region, as opposed to connections that travel on to other brain areas.

Interneuron: A type of neuron that typically projects only to other neurons within a local area and has an inhibitory effect on them.

Intrinsic Input: Input to a brain region originating within that brain region (e.g., recurrent collaterals).

Isocortex: A form of cortex with six cell layers, found only in mammals.

Kainic Acid: A neurotoxin that, when injected into the brain, destroys neurons near the injection site but may also destroy nearby fibers of passage; produces a less selective lesion than ibotenic acid.

Kohonen Network: See **Self-Organizing Feature Map.**

Language-Learning Impairment (abbreviated **LLI**):   A condition, associated with dyslexia, in which children show specific impairments in language processing without other intellectual deficits.

Latent Inhibition: A conditioning paradigm in which prior unreinforced exposure to one stimulus retards subsequent learning to associate that stimulus with the US.

Latent Learning: Learning that occurs in the absence of any explicit US.

Learned Irrelevance: A conditioning paradigm in which prior exposure to the CS and US, uncorrelated with each other, retards subsequent learning that the CS predicts the US.

Learning Curve: A graph showing how responding changes as a function of training trials.

Learning Rate (sometimes abbreviated β):   A parameter in a learning rule that specifies how large weight changes should be.

Learning Rule: A formal procedure for modifying a system to adapt responding based on experience; in neural networks, a rule for modifying weights between nodes.

Least-Mean-Squared Learning Rule (abbreviated **LMS**): Another name for the Widrow-Hoff Learning Rule.

Lesion: As a verb: To damage, destroy, or remove a portion of brain tissue in the course of experiment for the purpose of observing how behavior is modified. As a noun: A localized region of damage to the brain.

LLI: See **Language-Learning Impairment**.

LMS: See **Least-Mean-Squared Learning Rule.**

Local Representation: A form of representation in which each external event (stimulus or stimulus feature) is encoded within one node or component of a model.

Long-Term Memory: Memory that may last weeks or years.

Long-Term Potentiation (abbreviated **LTP**): A neuronal mechanism by which the synapse between two neurons may be strengthened depending on how the neurons' activity is correlated; a candidate mechanism for learning in the brain.

LTP: See **Long-Term Potentiation.**

M1: See **Primary Motor Cortex.**

Magnetic Resonance Imaging (abbreviated **MRI**): A technique for obtaining a detailed picture of the brain by recording molecular fluctuations in a magnetic field.

Medial Septum: A structure within the basal forebrain that projects acetylcholine and GABA to hippocampus.

Medial Temporal Lobe: The part of the human brain lying on the inside of the temporal lobe; corresponds roughly to the hippocampal region in animals.

Mere Exposure Effect: The finding that learning can occur following exposure to the CS in the absence of any explicit US.

Metrifonate: A drug that acts as a cholinergic agonist by interfering with the processes that clean extra ACh out of the synapse and thus increasing the opportunity for ACh to activate the postsynaptic neuron.

Microdialysis: A technique for measuring fluctuations in levels of neurotransmitters or other chemicals within a limited region of brain.

Millisecond (abbreviated **msec**): One-thousandth of a second.

Mirror Drawing: A task that involves learning to draw while observing hand movements reversed through a mirror. With practice, subjects show improvement in accuracy and speed.

Mispair: In the paired associate task, a nonrewarded pair that consists of one item from each of two rewarded pairs.

Modality: Of a particular kind of sensory stimulus (e.g., vision, audition).

Model: A simplified version of a physical system that captures some aspects of the physical system but eliminates others.

Momentum: A parameter sometimes used in neural networks that specifies that the weight change on the current trial should include some portion of the weight change on the previous trial; this helps to keep the weight moving in a consistent direction (positive or negative) over a series of trials and may speed learning in the network.

Mossy Fibers: Fibers arising in dentate gyrus and terminating in hippocampus.

MRI: See **Magnetic Resonance Imaging.**

msec: See **Millisecond.**

Multilayer Network: A neural network with at least one internal layer of nodes between the input and output node layers.

Multimodal: Involving more than one sensory modality.

Muscarinic Receptor: A subclass of cholinergic receptor that is also activated by the cholinergic agonist muscarine.

Negative Patterning: A conditioning paradigm in which either of two CSs predicts the US but the compound of both CSs predicts no US.

Neocortex: A form of cortex with six cell layers, found only in mammals. In mammals (particularly humans), most cerebral cortex is neocortex.

Network: A collection of interacting units, especially a neural network.

Neural Network: A group of interacting units (nodes) with adjustable connections (weights) between them; may be used as a model of similar processing between neurons (or groups of neurons) in the brain.

Neuroanatomy: The study of the anatomy of the brain with particular attention to connections between neurons or groups of neurons.

Neurology: The study of the nervous system, especially neurons.

Neuromodulator: A brain chemical that affects how neurons process incoming information.

Neuron: An information-processing cell in the brain or nervous system, which typically receives inputs from synapses on its dendrites, integrates information so received, and may become active, sending information on via its axons to other neurons.

Neuronal: Of neurons.

Neurophysiology: The study of the physiology of neurons, often with emphasis on electrical or chemical changes in neurons.

Neuropsychology: The study of the biological and neuronal basis of behavior, especially how brain injury or abnormality affects behavior.

Neuroradiography: Techniques for producing pictures of the structure or activity of the nervous system, especially the brain.

Neuroscience: The study of the brain and nervous system with particular attention to how neurons interact and function.

Neurotoxin: A chemical that, when injected into the brain, destroys neurons near the injection site.

Neurotransmitter: A brain chemical released by one neuron that may activate the receptor of another neuron and cause activation there; neurotransmitters thus carry messages between neurons.

Nicotinic Receptor: A subclass of cholinergic receptor that is also activated by the cholinergic agonist nicotine.

Node: A processing unit in a neural network that receives inputs, integrates them, and may become active and produce output; may be related to a neuron.

Nonmonotonic Development of the Stimulus Generalization Gradient: In conditioning, the finding of a broad generalization gradient early in training that is sharpened as training progresses.

Nonpairs: In the paired associate task, stimulus pairs consisting of one element from a rewarded pair and one element that is never part of a rewarded pair.

Novelty: In a network, the degree of difference between a current input pattern and all previously stored patterns; in an autoassociator or autoencoder, novelty can be estimated as the degree to which the output pattern differs from the input pattern (for a familiar, well-stored pattern, input and output patterns should be identical).

Nucleus Basalis: A structure within the basal forebrain that projects acetylcholine to cortex and amygdala.

Occasion Setting: A phenomenon in which a stimulus (called an *occasion-setter*) can mediate the association between a CS and US without itself entering into association with the US.

Olfaction: The sense of smell.

Olfactory: Of smell.

Olfactory Bulb: A region of the brain that receives inputs from olfactory receptor cells and projects to the olfactory cortex.

One-Layer Network: A neural network in which input nodes are connected to output nodes via a single layer of associative weights.

Output Node: A node in a neural network that sends output to an external target rather than to another node in the network.

Output Pattern: The pattern of activations produced by the output layer of a network.

Output Rule: The rule specifying how a node's activation level should be converted into a node output.

Overgeneralization: A tendency to generalize from one stimulus to other stimuli that are not sufficiently similar to warrant the same response.

Overtraining Reversal Effect: In conditioning, the finding that learning to reverse a discrimination can be facilitated if the original discrimination is overtrained, that is, trained for many more trials than are needed to acquire the desired responses.

Paired Associate Learning: A learning task that involves learning to associate arbitrary pairs of stimuli; certain pairs of stimuli are rewarded, but recombinations of these stimuli are not.

Paleocortex: A simple form of cortex with only two cell layers, found in reptiles and birds and in some areas of mammalian cortex.

Paradigm: The logical structure underlying an experiment independent of the particular stimuli used, the particular species tested, etc. For example, latent inhibition is a paradigm in which prior exposure to a stimulus is followed by learning to respond to that stimulus.

Paragraph Delayed Recall: A neuropsychological test of memory; the experimenter reads a short story and the subject is asked to repeat it after a delay of 5–15 minutes. Points are given for each item of the story that the subject correctly recalls.

Parahippocampal Cortex: An area of cortex lying near the entorhinal cortex and sometimes classed as part of the parahippocampal region.

Parahippocampal Region: The cortical areas lying near the hippocampus, including entorhinal cortex, perirhinal cortex and parahippocampal cortex.

Parallel Distributed Processing (abbreviated **PDP**):   A synonym for connectionism.

Parallel Fibers: A pathway by which sensory information reaches neurons in the cerebellum.

Parameter: A variable in an experiment or in a network that may be altered according to current needs (e.g., the number of CS exposures or the number of internal-layer nodes).

Pattern Completion: The ability of network (especially an autoassociative network) to take a partial or noisy version of a stored pattern as input and produce output that is the original stored version.

Pattern Recognition: The ability of a network (especially an autoassociative network) to take an arbitrary input and produce output that is the most similar stored pattern, thus "recognizing" the input as a distorted version of the stored pattern.

Pavlovian Conditioning: See **Classical Conditioning.**

PDP: See **Parallel Distributed Processing.**

Perceptron: An early name for a class of neural networks.

Perceptual Learning: A task in which subjects see progressively less fragmented drawings until they can identify the object; on subsequent trials, subjects can recognize the object on the basis of a more incomplete version.

Perforant Path: The fiber pathway from entorhinal cortex to hippocampus, which passes through (perforates) the intervening dentate gyrus.

Periallocortex: Cortex that is intermediate in structure between two-layer allocortex and six-layer neocortex, including the entorhinal cortex.

Perirhinal Cortex: An area of cortex lying near the entorhinal cortex and sometimes classed as part of the parahippocampal region.

Phasic: Of short duration, as a CS.

Phone: Any speech sound.

Phoneme: The smallest meaningful unit of speech in a language.

Physostigmine: A drug that acts as a cholinergic agonist by interfering with the processes that clean extra ACh out of the synapse and thus increasing the opportunity for ACh to activate the postsynaptic neuron.

Physostigmine Model: A variant of the cortico-hippocampal model in which the learning rate in the hippocampal region is inflated to simulate the effects of the cholinergic agonist physostigmine.

Piriform Cortex: See **Primary Olfactory Cortex.**

Piriform Model: A model of piriform (olfactory) cortex, proposed by R. Granger and colleagues, that assumes that the piriform cortex is capable of performing hierarchical clustering of odor inputs.

Place Cells: Neurons in the hippocampus that become active when the animal is in a particular region of space.

Plaques: In Alzheimer's disease, dense deposits outside and around neurons.

Plasticity: The ability of synapses to change so that firing in one neuron is more likely to affect activation of another neuron.

Polymodal: Involving more than one sensory modality.

Postrhinal Cortex: An area in the parahippocampal region of rats corresponding to the parahippocampal cortex in primates.

Postsynaptic Neuron: A neuron lying on the receiving end of a synapse.

Predictive Autoencoder: A variant on the autoencoder that includes additional output nodes to encode the expected reinforcement (or classification), given the current inputs.

Preparation: A particular learning system (e.g., rabbit eyeblink conditioning) that is used to refer both to the species and the response being learned.

PRER Lesion: Lesion of the parahippocampal region, including entorhinal cortex.

Presynaptic Neuron: A neuron that releases neurotransmitter into a synapse.

Primary Auditory Cortex (abbreviated **A1**):   The area of cortex where the first cortical processing of auditory input occurs; located in the temporal lobes in humans.

Primary Motor Cortex (abbreviated **M1**):   The area of cortex where simple motor movement commands are generated and projected to muscles.

Primary Olfactory Cortex (also called **Piriform Cortex**):   The area of cortex where the first cortical processing of odor input occurs.

Primary Sensory Cortex: The areas of cortex where the first cortical processing of sensory input occurs.

Primary Somatosensory Cortex (abbreviated **S1**):   The area of cortex where the first cortical processing of somatosensory (touch) input occurs; located near the top of the brain in humans.

Primary Visual Cortex (abbreviated **V1**):   The area of cortex where the first cortical processing of visual input occurs; located in the rear of the brain in humans.

Priming: An effect in which prior exposure to a stimulus affects the speed at which that same stimulus is subsequently recognized or processed.

Principal Components Analysis: A statistical technique for extracting the features of a data set that contain the most information and compressing or ignoring other, redundant features.

Principal Neurons: The neurons in a given brain region that are largely responsible for collecting input (especially from other brain regions), processing it, and passing it on to other brain regions. In most areas of cortex and in hippocampus, pyramidal neurons are the principal neurons; in dentate gyrus, granule cells are the principal neurons. Compare with interneurons, which collect and distribute information over local areas.

Procedural Memory: The class of memories that are incrementally acquired over many trials and may not be subject to conscious recollection (e.g., skills).

Projection: A connection from one brain region to another, typically formed by the axons of pyramidal neurons in the originating region synapsing on the dendrites of pyramidal neurons in the target region.

Psychogenic Amnesia: A kind of amnesia in which individuals may forget their past and identity. Usually due to psychological, not physical, trauma, psychogenic amnesia often resolves with time.

Punishment: An event or object that a subject seeks to avoid during the course of an experiment (e.g., shock).

Pyramidal Neuron: A kind of neuron that is generally involved in collecting input from widely divergent sources, processing information, and passing it on to other neurons in other brain areas. Compare with interneuron, which collects and distributes information over a local area.

Receptor: A region on the surface of a neuron that can be activated by a particular neurotransmitter, leading to a sequence of chemical and electrical changes within the neuron.

Recoding: Synonymous with rerepresentation.

Recurrent Collaterals: Connections from a neuron to its neighbors, as opposed to output processes that leave the brain region or contact other cell types.

Redundancy: The degree to which two stimuli or events reliably co-occur and are equally predictive of future reinforcement; high redundancy means that the stimuli always co-occur and can profitably be represented as two aspects of a single compound stimulus.

Reflex: A response to an external stimulus that is innate to an animal (or human) and does not have to be learned, such as a leg flexion in response to a foot shock or an eyeblink in response to a corneal airpuff; the stimulus that evokes such a reflexive response can serve as the unconditioned stimulus (US) in a classical conditioning experiment.

Reinforcement: An event that can serve to modify behavior, such as a reward or punishment.

Reinforcement Modulation Theories: Theories of learning that emphasize that the ability of the reinforcement (e.g., US) to drive learning depends on how unexpected it is, given all the information (e.g., CSs) present.

Representation: A scheme for relating events in the external world inside a neural network (or brain).

Representational Distortion: Altering various aspects of a representation, especially to emphasize "important" aspects while deemphasizing "less important" aspects.

Representational Weights: In a multilayer neural network, the lower layer of weights that connects input nodes to internal-layer nodes, thus specifying what representation an input pattern should evoke across the internal layer.

Rerepresentation: Forming a new representation, especially one that is more appropriate to the task at hand.

Rescorla-Wagner Model: A model of conditioning that embeds the Widrow-Hoff learning rule and assumes that CSs compete with one another for associative strength according to their informational value.

Retrograde Amnesia: A form of amnesia in which older memories are lost.

Reversal: In conditioning, a paradigm in which discrimination learning (e.g., A+, B−) is followed by learning opposite responses to the same stimuli (e.g., B+, A−).

Reward: An event or object that a subject seeks to obtain during the course of the experiment (e.g., food).

Runaway Excitation: In neural networks, a phenomenon in which activation of a subset of nodes results in activation of all the nodes to which they connect.

Runaway Synaptic Modification: In neural networks, synaptic modification that occurs during runaway excitation. If storage occurs while all nodes are active, then future activation of any one node may be enough to activate every node in the network.

S1: See **Primary Somatosensory Cortex.**

Salience: Effectiveness of a stimulus in eliciting attention or other processing resources.

Saporin: A neurotoxin that selectively destroys neurons that contain acetylcholine without damaging other kinds of neurons in the same area or damaging fibers of passage.

Schmajuk-DiCarlo Model (S-D Model): A neural network model of hippocampal-region function, proposed by N. Schmajuk and J. DiCarlo, that assumes that the hippocampal region is essential for implementing some aspects of the Rescorla-Wagner model (specifically, the ability to predict the US on the basis of all available cues) and also for forming new stimulus configurations in cortex. Simple learning to predict the US on the basis of individual CSs is assumed to occur in the cerebellum and can survive hippocampal-region damage.

Scopolamine: A drug that acts as a cholinergic antagonist, blocking cholinergic receptors and thus reducing opportunities for ACh to activate the postsynaptic neuron.

Scopolamine Model: A variant of the cortico-hippocampal model in which the learning rate in the hippocampal region is lowered to simulate the effects of the cholinergic antagonist scopolamine.

S-D Model: See **Schmajuk-DiCarlo Model.**

Self-Organizing Feature Map: A network that forms a topographic representation (map) of the input across its nodes.

Self-Organizing Network: A network that is capable of unsupervised learning.

Semantic Memory: A subdivision of declarative memory that includes memory for facts, such as vocabulary items or general knowledge about the world.

Sensory Cortex: An area of cortex devoted to processing (unimodal or polymodal) sensory cortex; compared with association cortex that is devoted to processing more abstract information such as goals and plans.

Sensory Modality: See **Modality.**

Sensory Modulation Theories: Theories of learning that emphasize the ability of CSs to enter into new associations, based on how much they add to the overall ability to predict reinforcement.

Sensory Preconditioning: A conditioning paradigm in which prior exposure to a compound of two stimuli (A and B) increases the amount that subsequent training about A will transfer to B.

Septal: Of the septum.

Septohippocampal Projection: The projection from medial septum to hippocampus, consisting of cholinergic and GABAergic fibers.

Septum: A collective term for the lateral septum and medial septum.

Sham Control: In an animal lesion experiment, a sham control is given the same surgical procedure but without the lesion. This allows the experimenter to deduce that any abnormalities in the lesioned animals are truly due to the absence of the lesioned structure and not simply to the surgical procedure itself.

Short-Term Memory: Short-duration (seconds to minutes) memory, typically lost if attention is diverted.

Sigmoidal: S-shaped. A sigmoidal activation function means that a node output is close to zero for a range of low activation values, climbs in a near-linear fashion for intermediate activation values, and then stabilizes close to 1.0 for a range of high activation values.

Simulation Run: One experiment with a single neural network, from initialization through learning. Typically, results with neural network models record the averaged performance of a number of independently initialized simulation runs.

Simultaneous Odor Discrimination: Task in which a rat is presented with two odors coming simultaneously from two odor ports and must poke its nose into the port delivering the correct odor.

Single-Layer Network: A neural network in which input nodes connect directly to output nodes via a single layer of associative weights.

Sit Control: In an experiment involving exposure to one or more stimuli, a sit control is a subject that is given equivalent time in the experimental chamber but without any exposure to the stimuli.

Somatosensory: Of the sense of touch.

Source Amnesia: A form of amnesia in which an individual may remember a piece of information but not the spatial or temporal context in which that information was learned.

Specificity: The ability to map similar stimuli to different responses, suppressing the tendency to generalize between them.

Spectrogram: See **Speech Spectrogram.**

Speech Spectrogram: A figure plotting the different sound frequencies in a speech event as a function of time.

Stimulus (plural: **Stimuli**): An event (especially a sensory event) that is processed by neurons in the brain (or nodes in a neural network).

Stimulus Configuration: See **Configuration.**

Stimulus Generalization Gradient: See **Generalization Gradient.**

Stimulus Interval Effects: In conditioning, a class of phenomena in which the timing of stimuli is particularly important, such as trace conditioning.

Stimulus-Meaning Learning: Learning an association between a stimulus and a salient future event or outcome (e.g., a reinforcer).

Stimulus Representation: See **Representation.**

Stimulus Selection: The process by which individual stimuli are tuned in or tuned out of attention or processing.

Stimulus-Stimulus Learning: Learning associations between two stimuli in the absence of (or independently of) explicit reinforcement.

Stop Consonants: Consonants such as /t/, /p/, and /b/ that involve a brief period of silence in the corresponding spectrogram.

Storage: In a network, the process by which a pattern is encoded by changing associative weights between nodes; in a brain, the process whereby information is encoded by altering synaptic connections between neurons.

Stratum Lacunosum-Moleculare: The layer of the hippocampus where extra-hippocampal inputs synapse onto the dendrites of pyramidal cells.

Stratum Pyramidale: The layer of the hippocampus containing pyramidal cell bodies.

Stratum Radiatum: The layer of the hippocampus where recurrent collaterals from other areas of hippocampus synapse onto the dendrites of pyramidal cells.

Stroke: A neurological condition that occurs when blood flow is interrupted, through either occlusion (blockage) or rupture of a blood vessel; structures downstream that depend on the blood vessel to supply oxygen and nutrients will be deprived and may die.

Subcortical: Having to do with the structures lying beneath the cerebral cortex in the brain.

Subiculum: A structure within the hippocampal region that lies between hippocampus and entorhinal cortex and may provide an output pathway from hippocampal region to subcortical structures such as amygdala.

Substrate: The brain regions, cells, or processes that underlie a particular behavior or function.

Successive Odor Discrimination: A task in which a rat is presented with one odor coming from an odor port; if the odor has been designated as rewarded, the rat should poke its nose into the odor port to obtain this reward; if the odor has been designated as nonrewarded, then the rat should remove its nose from the port area to initiate the next trial and the next odor.

Superficial Layers: In cortex, the cell layers closest to the surface.

Supervised Learning: Learning in which an external system (sometimes called a teaching input) monitors the response and generates an error measure, which can be used to guide learning. Error-correction learning (e.g., error backpropagation and the Widrow-Hoff rule) is a form of supervised learning.

Synapse: A small gap between neurons; a presynaptic neuron releases neurotransmitter into the synapse, where it may activate receptors in the postsynaptic neuron.

Synaptic Strength: The efficacy of a connection between two neurons.

Systemic Administration: Delivering a drug to the entire brain (as via injection into the blood or ventricles), as opposed to local administration by injection directly into a particular brain region.

Tacrine: A drug (brand name Cognex) that acts as a cholinergic agonist by interfering with the processes that clean extra ACh out of the synapse. Originally marketed as a drug to relieve the symptoms of Alzheimer's disease, Tacrine is no longer prescribed, owing to severe side effects, including liver failure.

Tangles: In Alzheimer's disease, twisted strands of fiber that accumulate inside neurons.

Taxonomy: System for classification.

Teaching Input: A special input to a neural network that defines the desired output for one or more nodes.

Temporal Lobes: The region of the brain in each hemisphere lying under the temples and ears.

Thalamus: A brain region that serves as a way station for all sensory information (except olfaction) to reach primary sensory cortex.

Theta Rhythm: A phenomenon in which large numbers of neurons begin to fire in synchronous bursts, approximately 4–8 times a second; associated with exploratory or learning behaviors.

Threshold: A parameter that is sometimes used in neural networks specifying the minimal level of node activation required before the node can become active.

Tonic: Prolonged, as a contextual stimulus.

Topographic: A form of representation in which physically similar inputs evoke activity in nodes (or neurons) that are adjacent in the network (or brain).

Trace Conditioning: A conditioning paradigm in which the CS occurs before the US but stops before the US arrives, leaving a short interval during which a memory, or "trace," of the CS must be maintained.

Transduce: To change energy from one form to another—for example, from chemical stimuli (odors) into electrical impulses (neuronal activity).

Transition: In speech, the change from one phoneme to another.

Trauma: Injury; especially a physical injury resulting in long-lasting behavioral effects.

Trial: In conditioning, the sequence of events consisting of CS presentation, CR generation, and US arrival or nonarrival. In neural network models, trials may also include intermixed presentation of the context alone, without any CS or US, to simulate the time the subject spends in the conditioning apparatus between presentations of CSs.

Unconditioned Response (abbreviated **UR**):   A reflexive response to an unconditioned stimulus—for example, a protective eyeblink in response to a corneal airpuff or a leg flexion in response to a foot shock.

Unconditioned Stimulus (abbreviated **US**):   A stimulus that evokes a reflexive response—for example, a corneal airpuff that evokes a protective eyeblink or a foot shock that evokes a leg flexion pulling the foot away.

Unilateral: Of or involving a single side (hemisphere) of the brain, as in a unilateral lesion; compare with **Bilateral.**

Unimodal: Involving a single sensory modality.

Unreinforced Learning: See **Latent Learning.**

Unsupervised Learning: Learning in which there is no external system to evaluate performance; instead, the system may develop its own strategy for representing information. Variants are autoassociative networks and competitive networks.

UR: See **Unconditioned Response.**

US: See **Unconditioned Stimulus.**

V1:   See **Primary Visual Cortex.**

Water Maze: A task in which an animal (typically a rat) is placed in a circular pool filled with opaque liquid and learns to escape to a hidden platform somewhere in the pool.

Weight: In a neural network, a number specifying the strength or efficacy of a connection between two nodes. A positive number specifies an excitatory connection; a negative number specifies an inhibitory connection.

Widrow-Hoff Rule: A neural network learning rule that specifies that the connection between two nodes should be changed proportionally to the error between the desired output and the actual output; applies only to networks with a single layer of weights and a well-defined desired output.

Working Memory: The form of memory that contains information relevant to the task at hand (e.g., task rules, goals, recent responses).

XOR Task: See **Exclusive-Or Task.**

Notes

CHAPTER 2

1. Julius Arantius, 1587, cited in W. Seifert, 1983, p. 625.

2. Scoville & Milner, 1957.

3. Milner, Corkin, & Teuber, 1968, p. 217.

4. Zola-Morgan, Squire, & Amaral, 1986.

5. See Zola-Morgan & Squire, 1993, for a full discussion of different conditions leading to anterograde amnesia.

6. See, e.g., Parkin et al., 1988, for a description of psychogenic amnesia.

7. See Kapur, 1993, for a review of such cases.

8. This study is reviewed in Squire & Zola-Morgan, 1988.

9. Milner, 1962.

10. Gabrieli et al., 1993.

11. See, e.g., Cohen, 1984; Haist, Musen, & Squire, 1991.

12. Mishkin & Delacour, 1975.

13. Mishkin, 1978; Zola-Morgan & Squire, 1986.

14. Freed, Corkin, & Cohen, 1987; Squire, Zola-Morgan, & Chen, 1988.

15. Zola-Morgan & Squire, 1993.

16. See, e.g., Mumby, Pinel, & Wood, 1990; Wible, Eichenbaum, & Otto, 1990; Winocur, 1990; Rothblat & Kromer, 1991; Otto & Eichenbaum, 1992.

17. Otto & Eichenbaum, 1992.

18. See, e.g., O'Keefe, 1979.

19. Wilson & McNaughton, 1993.

20. O'Keefe, 1979; Nadel & Willner, 1980.

21. Morris et al., 1982.

22. Morris et al., 1982.

23. Morris et al., 1982.

24. Wiener, Paul, & Eichenbaum, 1988.

25. See Gormezano, Kehoe, & Marshall, 1983, for review.

26. See, e.g., Schmajuk, Lam, & Christiansen, 1994.

27. See, e.g., Solomon et al., 1989.

28. Clark & Zola, 1998.

29. Kandel, 1976.

30. Schmaltz & Theios, 1972; Solomon & Moore, 1975; Solomon, 1977; Akase, Alkon, & Disterhoft, 1989.

31. Schmaltz & Theios, 1972.

32. Weiskrantz & Warrington, 1979; Daum, Channon, & Canavan, 1989; Woodruff-Pak, 1993; Gabrieli et al., 1995.

33. Berger et al., 1983.

34. Moyer, Deyo, & Disterhoft, 1990.

35. Moyer, Deyo, & Disterhoft, 1990.

36. Solomon et al., 1986; Moyer, Deyo, & Disterhoft, 1990. Note that other studies have shown no impairment in trace conditioning in hippocampal-lesioned animals (e.g., Port, Romano, & Patterson, 1986; James, Hardiman, & Yeo, 1987). The exact reason for these discrepancies is not yet clear but may reflect subtle differences in lesion extent between the studies or other paradigmatic differences such as the use of an airpuff US versus a shock US.

37. Thompson, 1972.

38. Port & Patterson, 1984.

39. See, e.g., Hirsh, 1974; Rudy & Sutherland, 1989; Eichenbaum, 1997.

40. Thompson et al., 1980, p. 262.

CHAPTER 3

1. Miller, Barnet, & Grahame, 1995.

2. See Maran & Baudry, 1995, for a review.

3. McCulloch & Pitts, 1943.

4. See, e.g., Deller, Proakis, & Hansen, 1993; Owens, 1993; Pitton, Wang, & Juang, 1996.

5. Widrow & Hoff, 1960.

6. McCulloch & Pitts, 1943; Rosenblatt, 1958; Widrow & Hoff, 1960; Rumelhart, Hinton, & Williams, 1986; Gluck & Bower, 1988a; Widrow & Winter, 1988; Minsky & Papert, 1998.

7. Stephen Grossberg and colleagues have been among the forefront in studying the plasticity-stability trade-off; see, e.g., Grossberg, 1980; Carpenter & Grossberg, 1991; Grossberg & Merrill, 1996.

8. See Widrow & Winter, 1988, for review.

9. Widrow, Winter, & Baxter (1988): recognizing rotated patterns; Widrow & Winter (1988): time-series prediction; Widrow, Gupta, & Maitra (1973): playing blackjack; Nguyen & Widrow (1989): truck backer-upper.

10. Widrow & Winter, 1988.

11. Rescorla & Wagner, 1972.

12. Pavlov, 1927.

13. Kamin, 1968.

14. Marchant & Moore, 1973; Solomon, 1977.

15. Solomon, 1977. Similar results obtain whether phase 3 consists of testing responses to the light CS alone (extinction testing) or of training a new response to the light CS.

16. Kamin, 1969.

17. Trabasso & Bower, 1964.

18. See, e.g., Rudy, 1974; Martin & Levey, 1991.

19. Rescorla & Wagner, 1972.

20. Sutton & Barto, 1981.

21. See, e.g., Walkenbach & Haddad, 1980; Miller, Barnet, & Grahame, 1995.

22. Frey & Sears, 1978; Gluck & Bower, 1988b; Siegel & Allan, 1996.

23. See, e.g., Bliss & Lømo, 1973; Barrionuevo & Brown, 1983; Levy & Steward, 1983; Lynch, 1986.

24. Hebb, 1949, p. 62.

25. W. James, 1890, p. 226.

26. Thompson, 1986.

27. Sears & Steinmetz, 1991.

28. Marr, 1969; Albus, 1971; Yeo, Hardiman, & Glickstein, 1985.

29. Gluck, Myers, & Thompson, 1994.

30. See Thompson, 1986.

31. Gluck, Myers, & Thompson, 1994.

32. Kim, Krupa, & Thompson, 1998.

33. Gluck, Myers, & Thompson, 1994.

34. See, e.g., Bolles & Fanselow, 1980; Fanselow, 1998.

35. See, e.g., Vriesen & Moscovitch, 1990; Schultz, Dayan, & Montague, 1997.

36. See, e.g., Lubow, 1973, 1997.

37. Latent inhibition is disrupted by hippocampal-region damage; see, e.g., Solomon & Moore, 1975; Kaye & Pearce, 1987; Shohamy, Allen, & Gluck, 1999. Sensory preconditioning is disrupted by hippocampal-region damage: Port & Patterson, 1984.

CHAPTER 4

1. Guttman & Kalish, 1956.

2. Shepard, 1987.

3. Shepard, 1987.

4. See, e.g., Ballard, Hinton, & Sejnowski, 1983; Georgopoulos et al., 1983.

5. One early, influential mathematical description of distributed representations was developed in the late 1950s by W. K. Estes and colleagues and was termed stimulus sampling theory (Atkinson & Estes, 1963; Neimark & Estes, 1967).

6. See, e.g., Hebb, 1949; Lashley, 1950.

7. For example, distributed representations in the visual system: Ballard, Hinton, & Sejnowski, 1983; in sensory and motor cortex: Georgopoulos et al., 1983, 1986.

8. Rescorla, 1976.

9. Rescorla, 1976.

10. Kehoe, 1988.

11. Gluck & Bower, 1988a, 1988b; Gluck, Bower, & Hee, 1989.

12. See, e.g., Gluck & Bower, 1988a, 1988b; Gluck, Bower, & Hee, 1989.

13. Gluck & Bower, 1988b; Gluck, Bower, & Hee, 1989.

14. See Nosofsky, 1984, 1988.

15. See, e.g., Nosofsky, 1984, 1988.

16. The backpropagation algorithm was discovered independently by Werbos (1974); Parker (1985); Le Cun (1986); and Rumelhart, Hinton, & Williams (1986). The last version is the most commonly cited version.

17. Minsky & Papert, 1969.

18. See, e.g., Rumelhart, Hinton, & Williams, 1986.

19. Funahashi, 1989; Hornik, Stinchcombe, & White, 1989.

20. Detecting forged signatures: Mighell, Wilkinson, & Goodman, 1989; pronouncing typewritten text: Sejnowski & Rosenberg, 1986; detecting faults in mechanical equipment: Robinson, Bodruzzaman, & Malkani, 1994; Japkowicz, Myers, & Gluck, 1995; interpreting sonar returns: Gorman & Sejnowski, 1988; diagnosing diseases: Falk et al., 1998.

21. See, e.g., Barto & Jordan, 1987; Durbin & Rumelhart, 1989; Hinton, 1989; Hanson, 1990; Mazzoni, Andersen, & Jordan, 1991.

22. See Crick & Asanuma, 1986, and Crick, 1989, for a review of such biological implausibilities associated with the backpropagation algorithm.

23. Parker, 1985; Stork, 1989; Schmajuk & DiCarlo, 1990.

24. Fitzsimonds, Song, & Poo, 1997.

CHAPTER 5

1. Hull, 1952.

2. Rescorla & Wagner, 1972.

3. See, e.g., Tolman, 1932.

4. Tolman & Honzick, 1930.

5. Hebb, 1949, p. 62.

6. Bliss & Lømo, 1973; Kelso, Ganong, & Brown, 1986.

7. See, e.g., Roman, Staubli, & Lynch, 1987; Gabriel et al., 1991; LeDoux, 1993.

8. Levy, Brassel, & Moore, 1983.

9. Anderson, 1977; Hinton, 1989.

10. See, e.g., Anderson, 1977.

11. See Tank & Hopfield, 1987, for a review.

12. Treves & Rolls, 1994.

13. Bliss & Lømo, 1973.

14. Marr, 1971.

15. See Willshaw & Buckingham, 1990, for a review.

16. See, e.g., McNaughton & Morris, 1987; McNaughton & Nadel, 1990; O'Reilly & McClelland, 1994; Hasselmo, Schnell, & Barkai, 1995; Recce & Harris, 1996; Rolls, 1996; Treves, Skaggs, & Barnes, 1996; Treves & Rolls, 1992.

17. Treves & Rolls, 1994.

18. Rolls, 1989.

19. Marr, 1971.

20. See, e.g., Lynch & Granger, 1992; Alvarez & Squire, 1994; Levy, 1994; McClelland, McNaughton, & O'Reilly, 1994; Treves & Rolls, 1994; Murre, 1996.

21. See, e.g., Wickelgren, 1979; Mishkin, 1982; Teyler & DiScenna, 1986; Buzsáki, 1996.

22. Ackley, Hinton, & Sejnowski, 1985; Elman & Zipser, 1987; Baldi & Hornik, 1989.

23. Hinton, 1989; Harnad, Hanson, & Lubin, 1994.

24. Japkowicz, 1999.

CHAPTER 6

1. Gluck & Myers, 1993.

2. Solso, 1991, pp. 287–290.

3. Gluck & Myers, 1993.

4. Levy, 1989, 1990.

5. Humans: Weiskrantz & Warrington, 1979; Daum, Channon, & Canavan, 1989; Woodruff-Pak, 1993; Gabrieli et al., 1995; rabbits: Schmaltz & Theios, 1972; Solomon & Moore, 1975; rats: Christiansen & Schmajuk, 1992; Schmajuk, Lam, & Christiansen, 1994.

6. See, e.g., Berger & Orr, 1983.

7. Odor discrimination in rats: Otto et al., 1991; object discrimination in monkeys: Zola-Morgan & Squire, 1986; Ridley et al., 1995; texture discrimination in rats: Whishaw & Tomie, 1991; frequency discrimination in rats: Marston, Everitt, & Robbins, 1993. In other paradigms, researchers have sometimes found that discrimination is indeed disrupted by hippocampal damage. For example, in one study in which rats were trained that one CS+ predicted a shock US while another CS− did not, normal but not hippocampal-lesioned rats learned to respond more to the CS+ than to the CS− (Micco & Schwartz, 1997).

8. See, e.g., Berger & Orr, 1983; Buchanan & Powell, 1980.

9. Gluck & Myers, 1993.

10. Fimbrial lesion abolishes sensory preconditioning in rabbit eyeblink conditioning: Port & Patterson, 1984; Port, Beggs, & Patterson, 1987.

11. Myers & Gluck, 1994.

12. See, e.g., Mackintosh, 1973.

13. Allen et al., 1998.

14. Model of instrumental conditioning: Myers & Gluck, 1996; model of category learning: Gluck, Oliver, & Myers, 1996.

15. See Bouton, 1991, and Bouton & Swartzentruber, 1991, for a review of why extinction represents more than simple unlearning of a CS-US association.

16. See, e.g., Bouton & Swartzentruber, 1991.

17. Berger & Orr, 1983.

18. Bouton & Swartzentruber, 1991.

19. Solomon, Van der Schaaf, Thompson, & Weisz, 1986; Moyer, Deyo, & Disterhoft, 1990.

20. Zackheim, Myers, & Gluck, 1998.

21. Moyer, Deyo, & Disterhoft, 1990; James, Hardiman, & Yeo, 1987.

22. Moyer, Deyo, & Disterhoft, 1990.

23. See, e.g., Levy, 1996; Wallenstein & Hasselmo, 1997.

24. Berger et al., 1983.

25. Miller & Steinmetz, 1997.

26. Berger & Thompson, 1978.

27. Cahusec et al., 1993.

28. Cahusec et al., 1993.

29. Deadwyler, West, & Lynch, 1979.

30. Bostock, Muller, & Kubie, 1991.

31. See, e.g., Schmajuk & Moore, 1988; Schmajuk & DiCarlo, 1991, 1992; Schmajuk, Gray, & Lam, 1996.

32. Schmajuk & DiCarlo, 1992.

33. Thompson, 1986.

34. The interested reader is referred to Schmajuk & DiCarlo, 1992, for a detailed mathematical explanation of the S-D model. See also Schmajuk & Moore, 1985.

35. Schmajuk & DiCarlo, 1992.

36. Schmajuk & DiCarlo, 1992; Schmajuk & Buhusi, 1997.

37. Buhusi & Schmajuk, 1996; Schmajuk, Gray, & Lam, 1996.

38. Schmajuk & Blair, 1993; Schmajuk, 1994.

39. Thompson, 1986.

40. Solomon, 1977.

41. Schmajuk & DiCarlo, 1992.

42. Following hippocampal damage, blocking may be impaired (Solomon, 1977; Rickert et al., 1978) or spared (Rickert et al., 1981; Garrud et al., 1984; Baxter, Holland, & Gallagher, 1997).

43. See Rudy & Sutherland, 1995, for a review.

44. See, e.g., Gallagher & Holland, 1992; Eichenbaum & Bunsey, 1995; Bussey et al., 1998; Han, Gallagher, & Holland, 1998.

45. See, e.g., Wickelgren, 1979; Sutherland & Rudy, 1989.

46. See, e.g., Rudy & Sutherland, 1989.

47. See, e.g., Whishaw & Tomie, 1991; Gallagher & Holland, 1992; Jarrard 1993.

48. Gallagher & Holland, 1992; Eichenbaum & Bunsey, 1995; Bussey et al., 1998; Han, Gallagher, & Holland, 1998.

49. Wiedemann, Georgilas, & Kehoe, 1999.

50. James Kehoe, personal communication.

51. Hirsh, 1974; Nadel & Willner, 1980; Winocur, Rawlins, & Gray, 1987; Penick & Solomon, 1991.

52. Haist, Musen, & Squire, 1991; Weiskrantz & Warrington, 1979.

53. Reducing attention to stimuli that are not significant: Grastyan et al., 1959; not correlated with reinforcement: Douglas & Pribam, 1966; Douglas, 1972; Kimble, 1968; or irrelevant with respect to predicting reinforcement: Moore, 1979; Solomon, 1979.

54. See, e.g., Mackintosh, 1975; Pearce and Hall, 1980.

55. See, e.g., Olton, 1983.

56. See, e.g., Olton, 1983; Rawlins, 1985; Buzsáki, 1989.

57. See, e.g., West et al., 1982; McNaughton & Barnes, 1990.

58. See, e.g., Wallenstein, Eichenbaum, & Hasselmo, 1998.

59. Eichenbaum, Otto, & Cohen, 1994.

60. Bunsey & Eichenbaum, 1993.

61. Gluck & Myers, 1995.

62. Wallenstein, Eichenbaum, & Hasselmo, 1998.

63. O'Keefe & Nadel, 1978; Nadel & Willner, 1980; Nadel, 1992.

64. See, e.g., Burgess & O'Keefe, 1996; Muller & Stead, 1996; Recce & Harris, 1996; Sharp, Blair, & Brown, 1996; Touretzky & Redish, 1996; Redish & Touretzky, 1997; Samsonovich & McNaughton, 1997; Redish, 1999.

65. See, e.g., Nadel, 1991.

66. O'Keefe, 1990.

67. See, e.g., Eichenbaum, Stewart, & Morris, 1990; Taube, 1991; Gluck & Myers, 1993.

68. Kubie & Ranck, 1983.

69. See, e.g., Eichenbaum et al., 1988; Eichenbaum, Mathews, & Cohen, 1989.

70. Eichenbaum & Buckingham, 1990; Eichenbaum, Cohen, et al., 1992.

71. Eichenbaum, Mathews, & Cohen, 1989.

72. See, e.g., Daum, Channon, & Gray, 1992; Gabrieli et al., 1995.

73. Mirror tracing: Gabrieli et al., 1993; cognitive skill learning: Knowlton, Ramus, & Squire, 1992.

74. Knowlton, Squire & Gluck, 1994; Reed et al., 1999.

75. Schacter, 1985.

76. See, e.g., Daum, Channon, & Canavan, 1989; Daum et al., 1991; Myers, Hopkins et al., 2000.

77. Myers, Oliver et al., 2000.

78. Myers, Oliver et al., 2000.

79. Myers, McGlinchey-Berroth et al., 2000.

CHAPTER 7

1. See, e.g., Pavlov, 1927; Hull, 1943; Konorski, 1967.

2. Hirsh, 1974.

3. O'Keefe & Nadel, 1978.

4. Good & Honey, 1991.

5. Nadel & Willner, 1980; Balsam & Tomie, 1985.

6. See, e.g., Good & Honey, 1991; Penick & Solomon, 1991; Kim & Fanselow, 1992; cf. Bouton & Swartzentruber, 1986.

7. Penick & Solomon, 1991.

8. Hsaio & Isaacson, 1971.

9. Hsaio & Isaacson, 1971.

10. Hirsh, 1974.

11. Rescorla & Wagner, 1972.

12. Good & Honey, 1991.

13. Good & Honey, 1991.

14. See, e.g., Mackintosh, 1975; Moore & Stickney, 1980.

15. See, e.g., Schmajuk, Thieme, & Blair, 1993; Brown & Sharp, 1995; Recce & Harris, 1996.

16. See, e.g., Burgess, O'Keefe, & Recce, 1993; Schmajuk et al., 1993.

17. Granger et al., 1996; Levy, 1996; Wallenstein & Hasselmo, 1997.

18. Myers & Gluck, 1994.

19. Honey & Good, 1993.

20. Myers & Gluck, 1994.

21. See, e.g., Antelman & Brown, 1972; Honey, Willis, & Hall, 1990; Good & Honey, 1991; Penick & Solomon, 1991; Kim & Fanselow, 1992; cf. Bouton & Swartzentruber, 1986.

22. Myers & Gluck, 1994.

23. Myers & Gluck, 1994.

24. See, e.g., Antelman & Brown, 1972; Penick & Solomon, 1991.

25. Lubow & Gewirtz (1995) give a full review of latent inhibition and attention.

26. Myers & Gluck, 1994.

27. Ackil et al., 1969; Solomon & Moore, 1975; McFarland, Kostas, & Drew, 1978; Kaye & Pearce, 1987; Han, Gallagher, & Holland, 1995.

28. Myers & Gluck, 1994.

29. Lubow, Rifkin, & Alek, 1976; Channell & Hall, 1983; Hall & Minor, 1984; Hall & Channell, 1985; Hall & Honey, 1989; Bouton & Brooks, 1993; Honey & Good, 1993; Zalstein-Orda & Lubow, 1994; Otto, Cousens, & Rajewski, 1997; Rosas & Bouton, 1997.

30. Myers & Gluck, 1994.

31. Context-alone trials can reduce latent inhibition: McIntosh & Tarpy, 1977; Westbrook, Bond, & Feyer, 1981; Kraemer & Roberts, 1984; Rosas & Bouton, 1997; see also Killcross et al., 1998a, 1998b. A conflicting study, finding no effect of context-alone trials: Hall & Minor, 1984.

32. Zalstein-Orda & Lubow, 1994.

33. Reiss & Wagner, 1972.

34. See Weiner & Feldon, 1997, for a full discussion of the role of nucleus accumbens in the attentional component of latent inhibition.

35. See Weiner, 1990, for discussion.

36. See, e.g., Holland, 1992.

37. In this case, although occasion setters B and C do not enter into direct associations with the US, there are circumstances in which they may become associated with A; see Holland, 1997.

38. Han, Gallagher, & Holland, 1998.

39. Jarrard & Davidson, 1991.

40. See, e.g., Hirsh, 1974.

41. Myers & Gluck, 1994; see also Eichenbaum, Stewart, & Morris, 1990; Taube, 1991.

42. See, e.g., Bouton & King, 1983; Bouton, 1984.

43. See, e.g., Bouton & King, 1983.

44. Bouton, 1991.

45. e.g., Bouton & Nelson, 1998.

46. See, e.g., Schmaltz & Theios, 1972; Wilson, Brooks, & Bouton, 1995.

47. See, e.g., Bouton & Peck, 1989; Bouton & Brooks, 1993.

48. Winocur & Olds, 1978; Hall & Honey, 1990.

49. Good & Honey, 1991; Bouton, 1993.

50. Winocur & Gilbert, 1984.

51. See, e.g., Winocur et al., 1987.

52. See, e.g., Winocur et al., 1987; Selden et al., 1991.

53. Myers & Gluck, 1994.

54. See, e.g., Bouton & King, 1983.

55. Hall & Honey, 1990.

56. Bouton & King, 1983.

57. Penick & Solomon, 1991.

58. See, e.g., Eichenbaum et al., 1988; Eichenbaum, Cohen et al., 1992.

59. Schacter, 1985.

60. Schacter, Harbluk, & McLachlan, 1984.

61. See also Schnider et al., 1996.

62. See, e.g., Oscar-Behrman & Zola-Morgan, 1980; Myers, Hopkins, et al., 2000. See also Daum et al., 1991.

63. Brooks & Baddeley, 1976.

64. Terrace, 1963, 1966.

65. Terrace, 1963.

66. See, e.g., Terrace, 1974.

67. Wilson et al., 1994.

68. Wilson et al., 1994.

69. Wilson et al., 1994.

CHAPTER 8

1. Gluck & Myers, 1993.

2. Guigon et al., 1994.

3. Wiesel, 1982.

4. See, e.g., Rasmusson, 1982; Merzenich et al., 1983; Wall & Cusick, 1984.

5. S. Clark et al., 1986; Wang et al., 1995.

6. Jenkins et al., 1990.

7. Jenkins et al., 1990.

8. Nudo et al., 1996.

9. See, e.g., Sutton et al., 1994; Goodall et al., 1997.

10. Researchers studying competitive networks include Marr, 1970; von der Malsburg, 1973; Fukushima, 1975; Grossberg, 1976; Kohonen, 1984; Rumelhart & Zipser, 1985; and Sutton et al., 1994.

11. Kohonen, 1988; Kohonen & Hari, 1999.

12. See, e.g., Rosenblatt, 1958; Marr, 1970; von der Malsburg, 1973; Fukushima, 1975; Grossberg, 1976; Kohonen, 1984; Rumelhart & Zipser, 1985.

13. Kohonen and colleagues have compiled a database of references to over 3000 applications of self-organizing feature maps that can be accessed via the Internet (http://www.icsi. berkeley.edu/~jagota/NCS/vol1.html). Another site listing extensive references to computational models of cortical maps is at http://www.cnl.salk.edu/~wiskott/Bibliographies/ CorticalMaps.html. Accessed June 21, 2000.

14. See, e.g., Kohonen, 1988; Kohonen & Hari, 1999.

15. See, e.g., Suzuki, 1996.

16. See, e.g., Anton, Lynch & Granger, 1991; Barkai et al., 1994.

17. Ambros-Ingerson, Granger, & Lynch, 1990; Granger et al., 1990.

18. Myers, Gluck, & Granger, 1995.

19. Eichenbaum et al., 1988.

20. Eichenbaum et al., 1988.

21. Staubli, Le, & Lynch, 1995.

22. Eichenbaum et al., 1988.

23. Eichenbaum, Otto, & Cohen, 1992.

24. Santibanez & Pinto Hamuy, 1957.

25. For example, simultaneous visual discrimination is sometimes impaired: Mishkin & Pribam, 1954; Pinto Hamuy et al., 1957; Zola-Morgan & Squire, 1985; Zola-Morgan, Squire, & Amaral, 1989a; sometimes spared: Ridley et al., 1995.

26. See, e.g., Staubli et al., 1987.

27. Gluck & Myers, 1996.

28. Swanson, 1979.

29. Otto et al., 1991.

30. Jarrard et al., 1984; Zola-Morgan, Squire, & Amaral, 1989b.

31. See, e.g., Hasselmo & Schnell, 1994; Myers et al., 1996.

32. Eichenbaum et al., 1988.

33. Myers & Gluck, 1996.

34. Eichenbaum, Mathews, & Cohen, 1989, p. 1214.

35. Eichenbaum, Mathews, & Cohen, 1989.

36. Myers & Gluck, 1996.

37. Myers & Gluck, 1996.

38. See, e.g., Szenthagothai, 1975; Lytton & Sejnowski, 1991; Steriade, McCormick, & Sejnowski, 1993; Guigon et al., 1994; Buonomano & Merzenich, 1995.

39. Bakin & Weinberger, 1990; Weinberger, 1993.

40. Weinberger, 1997.

41. Weinberger, Javid, & Lepan, 1993.

42. Bakin & Weinberger, 1990; Gao & Sugo, 1998; Kilgard & Merzenich, 1998.

43. See, e.g., Gao & Sugo, 1998.

44. Weinberger, 1997.

45. Bakin & Weinberger, 1996; Kilgard & Merzenich, 1998.

46. Baskerville, Schweitzer, & Herron, 1997; Sachdev et al., 1998.

47. Tallal, Miller, & Fitch, 1993.

48. Tallal et al., 1996.

49. Ambros-Ingerson, Granger, & Lynch, 1990.

CHAPTER 9

1. See, e.g., Mountcastle, 1979.

2. Amaral & Witter, 1989.

3. Zola-Morgan, Squire, & Ramus, 1994.

4. Jarrard, 1989; Jarrard & Davidson, 1991.

5. Price, 1973; van Hoesen & Pandya, 1975; Gluck & Granger, 1993; Woodhams et al., 1993.

6. Myers, Gluck, & Granger, 1995; see also Granger et al., 1996.

7. Myers, Gluck, & Granger, 1995.

8. Broad hippocampal-region damage may abolish latent inhibition (e.g., Ackil et al., 1969; Solomon & Moore, 1975; McFarland, Kostas, & Drew, 1978; Kaye & Pearce, 1987; Schmajuk, Lam, & Christiansen, 1994), but lesion limited to hippocampus (and sparing entorhinal cortex) may spare or even enhance latent inhibition (Jarrard, 1989; Clark, Feldon, & Rawlins, 1992; Honey & Good, 1993; Reilly, Harley, & Revusky, 1993; Purves, Bonardi, & Hall, 1995).

9. Yee, Feldon, & Rawlins, 1995; Shohamy, Allen, & Gluck, 1999.

10. Myers et al., 1995.

11. Mackintosh, 1973.

12. See also Bonardi & Hall, 1996.

13. Allen, Chelius, & Gluck, 1998.

14. Thompson, 1972.

15. Myers, Gluck, & Granger, 1995.

16. Lawrence, 1952; Mackintosh & Little, 1970; Marsh, 1969; Singer, Zental, & Riley, 1969; Haberlandt, 1971.

17. Gluck & Myers, 1993.

18. Gluck & Myers, 1993.

19. Myers, Gluck, & Granger, 1995.

20. See, e.g., Penick & Solomon, 1991.

21. Myers, Gluck, & Granger, 1995.

22. Honey & Good, 1993.

23. Myers, Gluck, & Granger, 1995.

24. Honey & Good, 1993.

25. Gluck & Myers, 1993.

26. See, e.g., Honey & Hall, 1989, 1991; Bonardi et al., 1993.

27. See especially Rolls, 1989, 1996, and Levy, 1985, 1990.

28. Rolls, 1989; Levy, 1990; McNaughton & Nadel, 1990.

29. Segal & Olds, 1973.

30. Segal & Olds, 1973.

31. Deadwyler, West, & Lynch, 1979.

32. Segal & Olds, 1973; Deadwyler, West, & Lynch, 1979.

33. Schmajuk & DiCarlo, 1992.

34. Schmajuk & Blair, 1993; Schmajuk, 1994; Buhusi & Schmajuk, 1996.

35. Buhusi & Schmajuk, 1996.

36. See Jarrard & Davidson, 1991, and Davidson, McKernan, & Jarrard, 1993, for a more complete comparison of different lesion techniques.

37. Buhusi, Gray, & Schmajuk, 1998.

38. Rolls, 1989, 1996.

39. See Rolls, 1996.

40. Rolls, 1989.

41. Young et al., 1997.

42. Eichenbaum, Otto, & Cohen, 1994.

43. Bunsey & Eichenbaum, 1993; Eichenbaum & Bunsey, 1995.

44. Bunsey & Eichenbaum, 1993.

45. See Eichenbaum & Bunsey, 1995.

46. Bunsey & Eichenbaum, 1993; Eichenbaum & Bunsey, 1995.

47. Gluck, Myers, & Goebel, 1994; Eichenbaum & Bunsey, 1995; Gluck & Myers, 1995.

48. Flicker, Ferris, & Reisberg, 1991; Masur et al., 1994.

49. de Leon et al., 1997.

50. Convit et al., 1993, 1995; de Leon et al., 1993a; Killiany et al., 1993.

51. de Leon et al., 1989.

52. Golomb et al., 1993.

53. Myers, Kluger, et al., 1998, in prep.

54. Myers, Kluger, et al., in prep.

55. Jones, 1993; Woodhams et al., 1993; Gómez-Isla et al., 1996.

CHAPTER 10

1. See Hasselmo, 1995, for a review.

2. See Hasselmo, 1995, for a review.

3. Vanderwolf, Leung, & Stewart, 1985; Lee et al., 1994.

4. Berry & Thompson, 1979; Feasey-Truger, Li, & Bruggencate, 1992; Everitt & Robbins, 1997.

5. See, e.g., Downs et al., 1972; Blozovski, Cudennec, & Garrigou, 1977.

6. See Spencer & Lal, 1983, for a review of scopolamine and its medical effects.

7. See Kopelman & Corn, 1988.

8. Solomon et al., 1983; Jarrard et al., 1984; Gluck & Myers, 1993.

9. See, e.g., Schmaltz & Theios, 1972.

10. Solomon et al., 1983, 1993; Bahro et al., 1995; Kaneko & Thompson, 1997.

11. Berry & Thompson, 1979.

12. Hasselmo & Bower, 1993; Hasselmo & Schnell, 1994; Hasselmo, Schnell, & Barkai, 1995.

13. Hasselmo, Schnell, & Barkai, 1995.

14. Hasselmo & Schnell, 1994.

15. See Hasselmo, 1995, for a review.

16. Meyer, 1996.

17. Harvey, Gormezano, & Cool-Hauser, 1983.

18. Ghoneim & Mewaldt, 1977; Peterson, 1977.

19. Hasselmo, Wyble, & Wallenstein, 1996.

20. Myers et al., 1996.

21. See also Lopes da Silva et al., 1985.

22. Solomon et al., 1983.

23. Myers et al., 1996; Myers, Ermita, et al., 1998.

24. Ogura & Aigner, 1993.

25. Kronforst-Collins et al., 1997.

26. See, e.g., Bartus, 1979; Dumery, Derer, & Blozovski, 1988; Miyamoto et al., 1989; Markowska, Olton, & Givens, 1995; see also Ennaceur & Meliani, 1992.

27. See, e.g., Jacobs, 1988.

28. Myers et al., 1996.

29. Chatterjee et al., 1993; see also Miyamoto et al., 1989.

30. Bartus, 1979; Kronforst-Collins et al., 1997.

31. Davis et al., 1978; Smith, Coogan, & Hart, 1986; Wetherell, 1992.

32. Myers, Ermita, et al., 1998.

33. Moore, Goodell, & Solomon, 1976.

34. Baxter, Holland, & Gallagher, 1997; see also Weiss, Freedman, & McGregor, 1974.

35. Harvey, Gormezano, & Cool-Hauser, 1983.

36. Myers, Ermita, et al., 1998.

37. Solomon et al., 1983.

38. Myers, Ermita, et al., 1998.

39. Solomon & Gottfried, 1981; Powell, Hernandez, & Buchanan, 1985.

40. Powell, Hernandez, & Buchanan, 1985.

41. Solomon & Gottfried, 1981.

42. Krnjevic & Ropert, 1982.

43. See also Woodruff-Pak et al., 1994a, 1994b.

44. Alonso & Kohler, 1982.

45. Lamour, Dutar, & Jobert, 1984.

46. Hasselmo & Schnell, 1994; Hasselmo, Schnell & Barkai, 1995.

47. The interested reader is referred to Hasselmo & Schnell, 1994, and Hasselmo, Schnell, & Barkai, 1995, for further details of the CA1 model.

48. Similar suggestions have been made by Gray, 1985, and Levy, 1989.

49. Wilson & Rolls, 1990.

50. Myers et al., 1996; Myers, Ermita, et al., 1998.

51. Rokers, Myers, & Gluck, 2000/in press.

52. Rokers, Myers, & Gluck, 2000/in press.

53. Jacobs, 1988; Gluck, Glauthier, & Sutton, 1992.

54. Montague, Dayan, & Sejnowski, 1996; Schultz, Dayan, & Montague, 1997; see also Pennartz, 1996.

55. Hasselmo et al., 1997.

56. Freund & Antal, 1988; Brazhnik et al., 1993.

57. Buzsáki, 1989; Buzsáki, Chen, & Gage, 1990.

58. See, e.g., Hasselmo, Wyble, & Wallenstein, 1996; Wallenstein & Hasselmo, 1997.

59. See Hasselmo, 1995, for a review.

60. Weinberger, 1997.

61. Bakin & Weinberger, 1996; Juliano, 1998; Kilgard & Merzenich, 1998.

62. Baskerville, Schweitzer, & Herron, 1997; Juliano, 1998; Sachdev et al., 1998.

63. See, e.g., Morris et al., 1992; Chatterjee et al., 1993.

64. Alexander & Freedman, 1984; Irle et al., 1992; DeLuca & Diamond, 1995.

65. Myers, DeLuca, et al., in preparation.

66. Weiskrantz & Warrington, 1979; Woodruff-Pak, 1993; Gabrieli et al., 1995.

67. Whitehouse et al., 1982; Kesner, 1988.

68. de Leon et al., 1993b.

69. Sunderland et al., 1985; Christensen et al., 1992.

70. Beatty, Butters, & Janowsky, 1986; Flicker, Serby, & Ferris, 1992; Flicker, Ferris, & Serby, 1992.

71. Tacrine: Knapp et al., 1994; Manning, 1994; Wagstaff & McTavish, 1994; physostigmine: Davis & Mohs, 1982; Thal et al., 1983; Sevush, Guterman, & Villalon, 1991; donepezil: Rogers, Friedhoff, & the Donepezil Study Group, 1996; Warren, Hier, & Pavel, 1998.

72. Bartus et al., 1985.

CHAPTER 11

1. See Zola-Morgan & Squire, 1993, for a review of how DNMS—once thought to depend on the hippocampus—is now known to depend more on nearby medial temporal structures.

2. Sperling et al., 1996.

3. Engel, 1993.

4. Oliver, 1988.

5. Miller, Munoz, & Finmore, 1993; Hermann et al., 1997.

6. See, e.g., Salafia et al., 1977; Solomon et al., 1983; Jarrard et al., 1984.

7. Estes, 1982.

8. Gluck & Bower, 1988a.

9. Estes, 1982.

References

Ackil, J., Mellgren, R., Halgren, C., & Frommer, G. (1969). Effects of CS preexposures on avoidance learning in rats with hippocampal lesions. *Journal of Comparative and Physiological Psychology, 69*(4), 739–747.

Ackley, D., Hinton, G., & Sejnowski, T. (1985). A learning algorithm for Boltzmann machines. *Cognitive Science, 9*, 147–169.

Akase, E., Alkon, D. L., & Disterhoft, J. F. (1989). Hippocampal lesions impair memory of short-delay conditioned eyeblink in rabbits. *Behavioral Neuroscience, 103*(5), 935–943.

Albus, J. (1971). A theory of cerebellar function. *Mathematical Bioscience, 10*, 25–61.

Alexander, M., & Freedman, M. (1984). Amnesia after anterior communicating artery rupture. *Neurology, 34*, 752–757.

Allen, M., Chelius, L., & Gluck, M. (1998). Selective entorhinal cortical lesions disrupt the learned irrelevance pre-exposure effect in the classically conditioned rabbit eyeblink response paradigm. *Society for Neuroscience Abstracts, 24*, 442.

Alonso, A., & Kohler, C. (1982). Evidence for separate projections of hippocampal pyramidal and non-pyramidal neurons to different parts of the septum in the rat brain. *Neuroscience Letters, 31*(3), 209–214.

Alvarez, P., & Squire, L. (1994). Memory consolidation and the medial temporal lobe: A simple network model. *Proceedings of the National Academy of Sciences, 91*, 7041–7045.

Amaral, D. G., & Witter, M. P. (1989). The three-dimensional organization of the hippocampal formation: A review of anatomical data. *Neuroscience, 31*(3), 571–591.

Ambros-Ingerson, J., Granger, R., & Lynch, G. (1990). Simulation of paleocortex performs hierarchical clustering. *Science, 247*, 1344–1348.

Anderson, J. (1977). Neural models with cognitive implications. In D. LaBerge & S. Samuels (Eds.), *Basic Processes in Reading: Perception and Comprehension* (pp. 27–90). Hillsdale, NJ: Lawrence Erlbaum Associates.

Antelman, S., & Brown, T. (1972). Hippocampal lesions and shuttlebox avoidance behavior: A fear hypothesis. *Physiology and Behavior, 9*, 15–20.

Anton, P., Lynch, G., & Granger, R. (1991). Computation of frequency-to-spatial transform by olfactory bulb glomeruli. *Biological Cybernetics, 65*, 407–414.

Atkinson, R., & Estes, W. (1963). Stimulus sampling theory. In R. Luce, R. Bush, & E. Galanter (Eds.), *Handbook of Mathematical Psychology*, vol. 2, New York: Wiley.

Bahro, M., Schreurs, B., Sunderland, T., & Molchan, S. (1995). The effects of scopolamine, lorazepam, and glycopyrrolate on classical conditioning of the human eyeblink response. *Psychopharmacology, 122*(4), 395–400.

Bakin, J. S., & Weinberger, N. M. (1990). Classical conditioning induces CS-specific receptive field plasticity in the auditory cortex of the guinea pig. *Brain Research, 536,* 271–286.

Bakin, J., & Weinberger, N. (1996). Induction of a physiological memory in the cerebral cortex by stimulation of the nucleus basalis. *Proceedings of the National Academy of Sciences USA, 93,* 11219–11224.

Baldi, P., & Hornik, K. (1989). Neural networks and principal component analysis: Learning from examples without local minima. *Neural Networks, 2,* 53–58.

Ballard, D., Hinton, G., & Sejnowski, T. (1983). Parallel visual computation. *Nature, 306*(5938), 21–26.

Balsam, P., & Tomie, A. (1985). *Context and Conditioning.* Hillsdale, NJ: Lawrence Erlbaum Associates.

Barkai, E., Bergman, R., Horwitz, G., & Hasselmo, M. (1994). Modulation of associative memory function in a biophysical simulation of rat piriform cortex. *Journal of Neurophysiology, 72*(2), 659–677.

Barrionuevo, G., & Brown, T. H. (1983). Associative long-term potentiation in hippocampal slices. *Proceedings of the National Academy of Sciences USA, 80,* 7347–7351.

Barto, A., & Jordan, M. (1987). Gradient following without backpropagation in layered nets. In *Proceedings of the IEEE First International Conference on Neural Networks* (vol. 2, pp. 629–636).

Bartus, R. (1979). Physostigmine and recent memory: Effects in young and aged nonhuman primates. *Science, 206,* 1087–1089.

Bartus, R., Dean, R., Pontecorvo, M., & Flicker, C. (1985). The cholinergic hypothesis: A historical overview, current perspective, and future directions. *Annals of the New York Academy of Sciences, 444,* 332–358.

Baskerville, K., Schweitzer, J., & Herron, P. (1997). Effects of cholinergic depletion on experience-dependent plasticity in the cortex of the rat. *Neuroscience, 80*(4), 1159–1169.

Baxter, M., Holland, P., & Gallagher, M. (1997). Disruption of decrements in conditioned stimulus processing by selective removal of hippocampal cholinergic input. *Journal of Neuroscience, 17*(13), 5230–5236.

Bear, M., Connors, B., & Paradiso, M. (1996). *Neuroscience: Exploring the Brain.* Philadelphia: Williams & Wilkins.

Beatty, W., Butters, N., & Janowsky, D. (1986). Patterns of memory failure after scopolamine treatment: Implications for cholinergic hypotheses of dementia. *Behavioral and Neural Biology, 45*(2), 196–211.

Berger, T., & Orr, W. (1983). Hippocampectomy selectively disrupts discrimination reversal learning of the rabbit nictitating membrane response. *Behavioral Brain Research, 8,* 49–68.

Berger, T., Rinaldi, P., Weisz, D., & Thompson, R. (1983). Single-unit analysis of different hippocampal cell types during classical conditioning of the rabbit nictitating membrane response. *Journal of Neurophysiology, 50,* 1197–1219.

Berger, T., & Thompson, R. (1978). Neuronal plasticity in the limbic system during classical conditioning of the rabbit nictitating membrane response. I: The hippocampus. *Brain Research, 145*(2), 323–346.

Berry, S., & Thompson, R. (1979). Medial septal lesions retard classical conditioning of the nictitating membrane response in rabbits. *Science, 205*, 209–211.

Bliss, T., & Lømo, T. (1973). Long-lasting potentiation of synaptic transmission in the dentate area of the anaesthetized rabbit following stimulation of the perforant path. *Journal of Physiology, 232*, 331–356.

Bloom, F., Lazerson, A., Hofstadter, L. (1985). *Brain, Mind and Behavior,* New York: W. Freeman.

Blozovski, D., Cudennec, A., & Garrigou, D. (1977). Deficits in passive-avoidance learning following atropine in the developing rat. *Psychopharmacology, 54*(2), 139–143.

Bolles, R., & Fanselow, M. (1980). A perceptual-defensive-recuperative model of fear and pain. *Behavioral and Brain Sciences, 3*, 291–301.

Bonardi, C., & Hall, G. (1996). Learned irrelevance: No more than the sum of CS and US pre-exposure effects? *Journal of Experimental Psychology: Animal Behavior Processes, 22*(2), 183–191.

Bonardi, C., Rey, V., Richmond, M., & Hall, G. (1993). Acquired equivalence of cues in pigeon autoshaping: Effects of training with common consequences and common antecedents. *Animal Learning and Behavior, 21*(4), 369–376.

Bostock, E., Muller, R., & Kubie, J. (1991). Experience-dependent modifications of hippocampal place cell firing. *Hippocampus, 1*(2), 193–206.

Bouton, M. (1984). Differential control by context in the inflation and reinstatement paradigms. *Journal of Experimental Psychology: Animal Behavior Processes, 10*(1), 56–74.

Bouton, M. (1991). Context and retrieval in extinction and in other examples of interference in simple associative learning. In L. Dachowski & C. F. Flaherty (Eds.), *Current Topics in Animal Learning: Brain, Emotion and Cognition* (pp. 25–53). Hillsdale, NJ: Lawrence Erlbaum Associates.

Bouton, M. (1993). Context, time and memory retrieval in the interference paradigms of Pavlovian learning. *Psychological Bulletin, 114*(1), 80–99.

Bouton, M., & Brooks, D. (1993). Time and context effects on performance in a Pavlovian discrimination reversal. *Journal of Experimental Psychology: Animal Behavior Processes, 19*(2), 1–15.

Bouton, M., & King, D. (1983). Contextual control of the extinction of conditioned fear: Tests for the associative value of the context. *Journal of Experimental Psychology: Animal Behavior Processes, 9*(3), 248–265.

Bouton, M., & Nelson, J. (1998). The role of context in classical conditioning: Some implications for cognitive behavior therapy. In W. O'Donohue (Ed.), *Learning and Behavior Therapy* (pp. 59–84). New York: Allyn & Bacon.

Bouton, M., & Peck, C. (1989). Context effects on conditioning, extinction and reinstatement in an appetitive conditioning paradigm. *Animal Learning and Behavior, 17*, 188–198.

Bouton, M., & Swartzentruber, D. (1986). Analysis of the associative and occasion-setting properties of contexts participating in a Pavlovian discrimination. *Journal of Experimental Psychology: Animal Behavior Processes, 12*, 333–350.

Bouton, M., & Swartzentruber, D. (1991). Sources of relapse after extinction in pavlovian and instrumental learning. *Clinical Psychology Review, 11,* 123–140.

Brazhnik, E., Vinogradova, O., Stafekhina, V., & Kitchigina, V. (1993). Acetylcholine, theta-rhythm and activity of hippocampal neurons in the rabbit. IV: Sensory stimulation. *Neuroscience, 53*(4), 993–1007.

Brooks, D., & Baddeley, A. (1976). What can amnesic patients learn? *Neuropsychologia, 14,* 111–122.

Brown, M., & Sharp, P. (1995). Simulation of spatial learning in the Morris water maze by a neural network model of the hippocampal formation and nucleus accumbens. *Hippocampus, 5,* 171–188.

Buchanan, S., & Powell, D. (1980). Divergencies in Pavlovian conditioned heart rate and eye-blink responses produced by hippocampectomy in the rabbit (*Oryctolagus cuniculus*). *Behavioral and Neural Biology, 30,* 20–38.

Buhusi, C., Gray, J., & Schmajuk, N. (1998). Perplexing effects of hippocampal lesions on latent inhibition: A neural network solution. *Behavioral Neuroscience, 112*(2), 316–351.

Buhusi, C., & Schmajuk, N. (1996). Attention, configuration and hippocampal function. *Hippocampus, 6,* 621–642.

Bunsey, M., & Eichenbaum, H. (1993). Critical role of the parahippocampal region for paired association learning in rats. *Behavioral Neuroscience, 107,* 740–747.

Buonomano, D., & Merzenich, M. (1995). Temporal information transformed into a spatial code by a neural network with realistic properties. *Science, 267,* 1028–1030.

Burgess, N., & O'Keefe, J. (1996). Neuronal computations underlying the firing of place cells and their role in navigation. *Hippocampus, 6*(6), 749–762.

Burgess, N., O'Keefe, J., & Recce, M. (1993). Using hippocampal "place cells" for navigation, exploiting phase coding. In S. Hanson, J. Cowan, & C. Giles (Eds.), *Advances in Neural Information Processing Systems* (vol. 5, pp. 929–936). San Mateo, CA: Morgan Kaufman.

Bussey, T., Warburton, E. C., Aggleton, J., & Muir, J. (1998). Fornix lesions can facilitate acquisition of the transverse patterning task: A challenge for "configural" theories of hippocampal function. *Journal of Neuroscience, 18*(4), 1622–1631.

Buzsáki, G. (1989). Two-stage model of memory-trace formation: A role for "noisy" brain states. *Neuroscience, 31*(3), 551–570.

Buzsáki, G. (1996). The hippocampo-neocortical dialogue. *Cerebral Cortex, 6*(2), 81–92.

Buzsáki, G., Chen, L., & Gage, F. (1990). Spatial organization of physiological activity in the hippocampal region: Relevance to memory formation. *Progress in Brain Research, 83,* 257–268.

Cahusec, P., Rolls, E., Miyashita, Y., & Niki, H. (1993). Modification of the responses of hippocampal neurons in the monkey during the learning of a conditional spatial response task. *Hippocampus, 3*(1), 29–42.

Carlson, N. R. (1986). *The Physiology of Behavior* (3rd ed.). London: Allyn & Bacon.

Carlson, N. R. (1997). *Physiology of Behavior* (6th ed). New York: Allyn and Bacon.

Carpenter, G., & Grossberg, S. (Ed.). (1991). *Pattern Recognition by Self-Organizing Neural Networks.* Cambridge, MA: MIT Press.

Channell, S., & Hall, G. (1983). Contextual effects in latent inhibition with an appetitive conditioning procedure. *Animal Learning and Behavior, 11*(1), 67–74.

Chatterjee, A., Morris, M., Bowers, D., Williamson, D., Doty, L., & Heilman, K. (1993). Cholinergic treatment of an amnesic man with a basal forebrain lesion: Theoretical implications. *Journal of Neurology, Neurosurgery and Psychiatry, 56,* 1282–1289.

Christensen, H., Maltby, N., Jorm, A., Creasey, H., & Broe, G. (1992). Cholinergic 'blockade' as a model of the cognitive deficits in Alzheimer's disease. *Brain, 115*(Pt. 6), 1681–1699.

Christiansen, B., & Schmajuk, N. (1992). Hippocampectomy disrupts the topography of the rat eyeblink response during acquisition and extinction of classical conditioning. *Brain Research, 595*(2), 206–214.

Clark, A., Feldon, J., & Rawlins, J. (1992). Aspiration lesions of rat ventral hippocampus disinhibit responding in conditioned suppression or extinction, but spare latent inhibition and the partial reinforcement extinction effect. *Neuroscience, 48*(4), 821–829.

Clark, R., & Zola, S. (1998). Trace eyeblink classical conditioning in the monkey: A nonsurgical method and behavioral analysis. *Behavioral Neuroscience, 112*(5), 1062–1068.

Clark, S., Allard, T., Jenkins, W., & Merzenich, M. (1986). Cortical map reorganization following neurovascular island skin transfers on the hands of adult owl monkeys. *Society for Neuroscience Abstracts, 12,* 391.

Cohen, N. (1984). Preserved learning capacity in amnesia: Evidence for multiple learning systems. In L. Squire & N. Butters (Eds.), *Neuropsychology of Memory* (pp. 83–103). New York: Guilford Press.

Convit, A., de Leon, M., Golomb, J., George, A., Tarshish, C., Bobinski, M., Tsui, W., de Santi, S., Wegiel, J., & Wisniewski, H. (1993). Hippocampal atrophy in early Alzheimer's disease, anatomic specificity and validation. *Psychiatry Quarterly, 64,* 371–387.

Convit, A., de Leon, M., Tarshish, C., De Santi, S., Kluger, A., Rusinek, H., & George, A. (1995). Hippocampal volume losses in minimally impaired elderly. *The Lancet, 345,* 266.

Crick, F. (1989). The recent excitement about neural networks. *Nature, 337,* 129–132.

Crick, F., & Asanuma, C. (1986). Certain aspects of the anatomy and physiology of the cerebral cortex. In D. Rumelhart & J. McClelland (Ed.), *Parallel Distributed Processing: Explorations in the Microstructure of Cognition* (pp. 333–371). Cambridge, MA: MIT Press.

Daum, I., Channon, S., & Canavan, A. (1989). Classical conditioning in patients with severe memory problems. *Journal of Neurology, Neurosurgery and Psychiatry, 52,* 47–51.

Daum, I., Channon, S., & Gray, J. (1992). Classical conditioning after temporal lobe lesions in man: Sparing of simple discrimination and extinction. *Behavioral Brain Research, 52,* 159–165.

Daum, I., Schugens, M., Channon, S., Polkey, C., & Gray, J. (1991). T-maze discrimination and reversal learning after unilateral temporal or frontal lobe lesions in man. *Cortex, 27*(4), 613–622.

Davidson, T., McKernan, M., & Jarrard, L. (1993). Hippocampal lesions do not impair negative patterning: A challenge to configural association theory. *Behavioral Neuroscience, 107*(2), 227–234.

Davis, K., & Mohs, R. (1982). Enhancement of memory processes in Alzheimer's disease with multiple-dose intravenous physostigmine. *American Journal of Psychiatry, 139,* 1421–1424.

Davis, K., Mohs, R., Tinklenberg, J., Pfefferbaum, A., Hollister, L., & Kopell, B. (1978). Physostigmine: Improvement of long-term memory processes in normal humans. *Science, 201,* 272–274.

de Leon, M., George, A., Golomb, J., Tarshish, C., Convit, A., Kluger, A., de Santi, S., McRae, T., Ferris, S., Reisberg, B., Ince, C., Rusinek, H., Bobinski, M., Quinn, B., Miller, D., & Wisniewski, H. (1997). Frequency of hippocampal formation atrophy in normal aging and Alzheimer's disease. *Neurobiology of Aging, 18*(1), 1–11.

de Leon, M., George, A., Stylopoulos, L., Smith, G., & Miller, D. (1989). Early marker for Alzheimer's disease: The atrophic hippocampus. *The Lancet,* 672–673.

de Leon, M., Golomb, J., George, A., Convit, A., Rusinek, H., Morys, J., Bobinski, M., de Santi, S., Tarshish, C., Narkiewicz, O., & Wisniewski, H. (1993b). Hippocampal formation atrophy: Prognostic significance for Alzheimer's Disease. In B. Corain, K. Iqbal, M. Nicolini, B. Winblad, H. Wisniewski, & P. Zatta (Eds.), *Alzheimer's Disease: Advances in Clinical and Brain Research* (pp. 35–46). New York: John Wiley & Sons.

de Leon, M., Golomb, J., George, A., Convit, A., Tarshish, C., McRae, T., de Santi, S., Smith, G., Ferris, S., Noz, M., & Rusinek, H. (1993a). The radiologic prediction of Alzheimer's Disease: The atrophic hippocampal formation. *American Journal of Neuroradiology, 14,* 897–906.

Deadwyler, S., West, M., & Lynch, G. (1979). Activity of dentate granule cells during learning: Differentiation of perforant path input. *Brain Research, 169,* 29–43.

Deller, J., Jr., Proakis, J., & Hansen, J. (1993). *Discrete-Time Processing of Speech Signals.* New York: Macmillan Press.

DeLuca, J., & Diamond, B. (1995). Aneurysm of the anterior communicating artery: A review of neuroanatomical and neurophysiological sequelae. *Journal of Clinical and Experimental Neuropsychology, 17*(1), 100–121.

Douglas, R. (1972). Pavlovian conditioning and the brain. In R. Boakes & M. Halliday (Eds.), *Inhibition and Learning.* London: Academic Press.

Douglas, R., & Pribam, K. (1966). Learning and limbic lesions. *Neuropsychologia, 4,* 192–222.

Downs, D., Cardozo, C., Schneiderman, N., Yehle, A., VanDercar, D., & Zwilling, G. (1972). Central effects of atropine upon aversive classical conditioning in rabbits. *Psychopharmacologia, 23,* 319–333.

Dumery, V., Derer, P., & Blozovski, D. (1988). Enhancement of passive avoidance learning through small doses of intra-amygdaloid physostigmine in the young rat: Its relation to the development of acetylcholinesterase. *Developmental Psychobiology, 21*(6), 553–565.

Durbin, R., & Rumelhart, D. E. (1989). Product units: A computationally powerful and biologically plausible extension to backpropagation. *Neural Computation, 1,* 133–142.

Eichenbaum, H. (1997). Declarative memory: Insights from cognitive neurobiology. *Annual Review of Psychology, 48,* 547–572.

Eichenbaum, H., & Buckingham, J. (1990). Studies on hippocampal processing: Experiment, theory and model. In M. Gabriel & J. Moore (Eds.), *Learning and Computational Neuroscience: Foundations of Adaptive Networks* (pp. 171–231). Cambridge, MA: MIT Press.

Eichenbaum, H., & Bunsey, M. (1995). On the binding of associations in memory: Clues from studies on the role of the hippocampal region in paired associate learning. *Current Directions in Psychological Science, 4*(1), 19–23.

Eichenbaum, H., Cohen, N. J., Otto, T., & Wible, C. (1992). Memory representation in the hippocampus: Functional domain and functional organization. In L. R. Squire, G. Lynch, N. M. Weinberger, & J. L. McGaugh (Eds.), *Memory Organization and Locus of Change* (pp. 163–204). Oxford: Oxford University Press.

Eichenbaum, H., Fagan, A., Mathews, P., & Cohen, N. J. (1988). Hippocampal system dysfunction and odor discrimination learning in rats: Impairment or facilitation depending on representational demands. *Behavioral Neuroscience, 102*(3), 331–339.

Eichenbaum, H., Mathews, P., & Cohen, N. J. (1989). Further studies of hippocampal representation during odor discrimination learning. *Behavioral Neuroscience, 103*(6), 1207–1216.

Eichenbaum, H., Otto, T., & Cohen, N. J. (1992). The hippocampus—What does it do? *Behavioral and Neural Biology, 57*, 2–36.

Eichenbaum, H., Otto, T., & Cohen, N. J. (1994). Two functional components of the hippocampal memory system. *Behavioral and Brain Sciences, 17*(3), 449–518.

Eichenbaum, H., Stewart, C., & Morris, R. G. M. (1990). Hippocampal representation in place learning. *Journal of Neuroscience, 10*(11), 3531–3542.

Elman, J., & Zipser, D. (1987). *Learning the hidden structure of speech* (Tech. Report No. 8701). San Diego: Institute for Cognitive Science, University of California.

Engel, J. (1993). Outcome with respect to epileptic seizures. In J. Engel (Ed.), *Surgical Treatment of the Epilepsies* (pp. 609–621). New York: Raven.

Ennaceur, A., & Meliani, K. (1992). Effects of physostigmine and scopolamine on rats' performances in object-recognition and radial-maze tests. *Psychopharmacology, 109*, 321–330.

Ermita, B., Allen, M., Gluck, M., Zaborszky, L. (1999). Effects of neurotoxic lesions of the medial septum on motor-reflex learning in the rabbit. *Abstracts of the Society for Neuroscience Annual Meeting (Miami, Florida)*, vol. 24, p. I-191.

Estes, W. K. (1982). *Models of Learning, Memory, and Choice.* New York: Praeger.

Everitt, B., & Robbins, T. (1997). Central cholinergic systems and cognition. *Annual Review of Psychology, 48*, 649–684.

Falk, C., Gilchrist, J., Pericak-Vance, M., & Speer, M. (1998). Using neural networks as an aid in the determination of disease status: Comparison of clinical diagnosis to neural-network predictions in a pedigree with autosomal dominant limb-girdle muscular dystrophy. *American Journal of Human Genetics, 62*, 941–949.

Fanselow, M. (1998). Pavlovian conditioning, negative feedback and blocking: Mechanisms that regulate association formation. *Neuron, 20*, 625–627.

Feasey-Truger, K., Li, B., & Bruggencate, G. (1992). Lesions of the medial septum which produce deficits in working/spatial memory do not impair long-term potentiation in the CA3 region of the rat in hippocampus in vivo. *Brain Research, 591*(2), 296–304.

Fitch, R., Miller, S., & Tallal, P. (1997). Neurobiology of speech perception. *Annual Review of Neuroscience, 20*, 331–353.

Fitzsimonds, R., Song, H.-J., & Poo, M.-M. (1997). Propagation of activity-dependent synaptic depression in simple neural networks. *Nature, 388*, 439–448.

Flicker, C., Ferris, S., & Reisberg, B. (1991). Mild cognitive impairment in the elderly: Predictors of dementia. *Neurology, 41,* 1006–1009.

Flicker, C., Ferris, S., & Serby, M. (1992). Hypersensitivity to scopolamine in the elderly. *Psychopharmacology, 107,* 437–441.

Flicker, C., Serby, M., & Ferris, S. (1990). Scopolamine effects on memory, language, visuospatial praxis and psychomotor speed. *Psychopharmacology, 100*(2), 243–250.

Freed, D., Corkin, S., & Cohen, N. (1987). Forgetting in HM: A second look. *Neuropsychologia, 25*(3), 461–471.

Freund, T., & Antal, M. (1988). GABA-containing neurons in the septum control inhibitory interneurons in the hippocampus. *Nature, 336,* 170–173.

Frey, P., & Sears, R. (1978). Models of conditioning incorporating the Rescorla-Wagner associative axiom, a dynamic attention process, and a catastrophe rule. *Psychological Review, 85,* 321–340.

Fukushima, K. (1975). Cognitron: A self-organizing multilayered neural network. *Biological Cybernetics, 20*(3/4), 121–136.

Funahashi, K.-I. (1989). On the approximate realization of continuous mappings by neural networks. *Neural Networks, 2,* 183–192.

Funnell, E. (1995). A case of forgotten knowledge. In R. Campbell & M. Conway (Eds.), *Broken Memories: Case Studies in Memory Impairments* (pp. 225–236). Cambridge, MA: Blackwell.

Gabriel, M., Vogt, B., Kubota, Y., Poremba, A., & Kang, E. (1991). Training-stage related neuronal plasticity in limbic thalamus and cingulate cortex during learning: a possible key to mnemonic retrieval. *Behavioural Brain Research, 46*(2), 175–185.

Gabrieli, J., Corkin, S., Mickel, S., & Crowden, J. (1993). Intact acquisition and long-term retention of mirror-tracing skill in Alzheimer's Disease and in global amnesia. *Behavioral Neuroscience, 107*(6), 899–910.

Gabrieli, J., McGlinchey-Berroth, R., Carrillo, M., Gluck, M., Cermack, L., & Disterhoft, J. (1995). Intact delay-eyeblink classical conditioning in amnesia. *Behavioral Neuroscience, 109*(5), 819–827.

Gaffan, D. (1997). Episodic and semantic memory and the role of the not-hippocampus. *Trends in Cognitive Sciences, 1*(7), 246–248.

Gallagher, M., & Holland, P. C. (1992). Preserved configural learning and spatial learning impairment in rats with hippocampal damage. *Hippocampus, 2*(1), 81–88.

Gao, E., & Sugo, N. (1998). Experience-dependent corticofugal adjustment of midbrain frequency map in bat auditory system. *Proceedings of the National Academy of Sciences USA, 95,* 12663–12670.

Garrud, P., Rawlins, J., Mackintosh, N., Goodall, G., Cotton, M., & Feldon, J. (1984). Successful overshadowing and blocking in hippocampectomized rats. *Behavioral Brain Research, 12,* 39–53.

Gazzaniga, M., Ivry, R., & Mangun, G. (1998). *Cognitive Neuroscience: The Biology of the Mind.* New York: Norton.

Georgopoulos, A., Kalaska, J., Caminiti, R., & Massey, J. (1983). Interruption of motor cortical discharge subserving aimed arm movements. *Experimental Brain Research, 49*(3), 327–340.

Georgopoulos, A., Schwartz, A., & Kettner, R. (1986). Neuronal population coding of movement direction. *Science, 233,* 1416–1419.

Ghoneim, M., & Mewaldt, S. (1977). Studies on human memory: The interactions of diazepam, scopolamine and physostigmine. *Psychopharmacology, 52,* 1–6.

Gluck, M., & Bower, G. (1988a). From conditioning to category learning: An adaptive network model. *Journal of Experimental Psychology: General, 117*(3), 225–244.

Gluck, M., & Bower, G. (1988b). Evaluating an adaptive network model of human learning. *Journal of Memory and Language, 27,* 166–195.

Gluck, M., Bower, G., & Hee, M. (1989). A configural-cue network model of animal and human associative learning. In *11th Annual Conference of Cognitive Science Society* (pp. 323–332). Ann Arbor, MI.

Gluck, M., Glauthier, P., & Sutton, R. (1992). Adaptation of cue-specific learning rates in network models of human category learning. In *Proceedings of the Fourteenth Annual Meeting of the Cognitive Science Society,* Bloomington, IL.

Gluck, M., & Granger, R. (1993). Computational models of the neural bases of learning and memory. *Annual Review of Neuroscience, 16,* 667–706.

Gluck, M., & Myers, C. (1993). Hippocampal mediation of stimulus representation: A computational theory. *Hippocampus, 3,* 491–516.

Gluck, M., & Myers, C. (1995). Representation and association in memory: A neurocomputational view of hippocampal function. *Current Directions in Psychological Science, 4*(1), 23–29.

Gluck, M., & Myers, C. (1996). Integrating behavioral and physiological models of hippocampal function. *Hippocampus, 6,* 643–653.

Gluck, M., Myers, C., & Goebel, J. (1994). A computational perspective on dissociating hippocampal and entorhinal function (Response to Eichenbaum, et al.). *Behavioral and Brain Sciences, 17,* 478–479.

Gluck, M., Myers, C., & Thompson, R. (1994). A computational model of the cerebellum and motor-reflex conditioning. In S. Zornetzer, J. Davis, C. Lau, & T. McKenna (Eds.), *An Introduction to Neural and Electronic Networks* (pp. 91–98). New York: Academic Press.

Gluck, M., Oliver, L., & Myers, C. (1996). Late-training amnesic deficits in probabilistic category learning: A neurocomputational analysis. *Learning and Memory, 3,* 326–340.

Gollin, E. (1960). Developmental studies of visual recognition of incomplete objects. *Perceptual and Motor Skills, 11,* 289–298.

Golomb, J., de Leon, M., Kluger, A., George, A., Tarshish, C., & Ferris, S. (1993). Hippocampal atrophy in normal aging: An association with recent memory impairment. *Archives of Neurology, 50*(9), 967–973.

Gómez-Isla, T., Price, J., McKeel, D., Morris, J., Growdon, J., & Hyman, B. (1996). Profound loss of layer II entorhinal cortex neurons occurs in very mild Alzheimer's Disease. *Journal of Neuroscience, 16*(14), 4491–4500.

Good, M., & Honey, R. (1991). Conditioning and contextual retrieval in hippocampal rats. *Behavioral Neuroscience, 105*(4), 499–509.

Goodall, S., Reggia, J., Chen, Y., Ruppin, E., & Whitney, C. (1997). A computational model of acute focal cortical lesions. *Stroke, 28*(1), 101–109.

Gorman, R. P., & Sejnowski, T. (1988). Analysis of hidden units in a layered network trained to classify sonar targets. *Neural Networks, 1*(1), 75–89.

Gormezano, I., Kehoe, E. J., & Marshall, B. S. (1983). Twenty years of classical conditioning research with the rabbit. *Progress in Psychobiology and Physiological Psychology, 10,* 197–275.

Granger, R., Ambros-Ingerson, J., Staubli, U., & Lynch, G. (1990). Memorial operation of multiple, interacting simulated brain structures. In M. A. Gluck & D. E. Rumelhart (Eds.), *Neuroscience and Connectionist Theory* (pp. 95–129). Hillsdale, NJ: Lawrence Erlbaum Associates.

Granger, R., Wiebe, S., Taketani, M., & Lynch, G. (1996). Distinct memory circuits comprising the hippocampal region. *Hippocampus, 6,* 567–578.

Grastyan, E., Lissak, K., Madarasz, I., & Donhoffer, H. (1959). Hippocampal electrical activity during the development of conditioned reflexes. *Electroencephalography and Clinical Neurophysiology, 11,* 409–430.

Gray, J. A. (1985). Memory buffer and comparator can share the same circuitry. *Behavioral and Brain Sciences, 8*(3), 501.

Grossberg, S. (1976). Adaptive pattern classification and recoding: Part I. *Biological Cybernetics, 23,* 121–134.

Grossberg, S. (1980). How does a brain build a cognitive code? *Psychological Review, 89,* 529–572.

Grossberg, S., & Merrill, J. (1996). The hippocampus and cerebellum in adaptively timed learning, recognition and movement. *Journal of Cognitive Neuroscience, 8*(3), 257–277.

Guigon, E., Grandguillaume, P., Otto, I., Boutkhil, L., & Burnod, Y. (1994). Neural network models of cortical functions based on the computational properties of the cerebral cortex. *Journal of Physiology (Paris), 88,* 291–308.

Guttman, N., & Kalish, H. (1956). Discriminability and stimulus generalization. *Journal of Experimental Psychology, 51,* 79–88.

Haberlandt, K. (1971). Transfer along a continuum in classical conditioning. *Learning and Motivation, 2,* 164–172.

Haist, F., Musen, G., & Squire, L. R. (1991). Intact priming of words and non-words in amnesia. *Psychobiology, 19*(4), 275–285.

Hall, G., & Channell, S. (1985). Differential effects of contextual change on latent inhibition and on the habituation of an orienting response. *Journal of Experimental Psychology: Animal Behavior Processes, 11*(3), 470–481.

Hall, G., & Honey, R. (1989). Contextual effects in conditioning, latent inhibition, and habituation: Associative and retrieval functions of contextual cues. *Journal of Experimental Psychology: Animal Behavior Processes, 15*(3), 232–241.

Hall, G., & Honey, R. (1990). Context-specific conditioning in the conditioned-emotional-response procedure. *Journal of Experimental Psychology: Animal Behavior Processes, 16*(3), 271–278.

Hall, G., & Minor, H. (1984). A search for context-stimulus associations in latent inhibition. *Quarterly Journal of Experimental Psychology, 36B,* 145–169.

Han, J.-S., Gallagher, M., & Holland, P. (1995). Hippocampal lesions disrupt decrements but not increments in conditioned stimulus processing. *Journal of Neuroscience, 15*(11), 7323–7329.

Han, J.-S., Gallagher, M., & Holland, P. (1998). Hippocampal lesions enhance configural learning by reducing proactive interference. *Hippocampus, 8,* 138–146.

Hanson, S. (1990). A stochastic version of the delta rule. *Physica D, 42,* 265–272.

Harnad, S., Hanson, S., & Lubin, J. (1994). Learned categorical perception in neural nets: Implications for symbol grounding. In V. Honavar & L. Uhr (Eds.), *Symbol Processors and Connectionist Network Models in Artificial Intelligence and Cognitive Modeling: Steps Toward Principled Integration* (pp. 191–206). New York: Academic Press.

Harvey, J., Gormezano, I., & Cool-Hauser, V. (1983). Effects of scopolamine and methylscopolamine on classical conditioning of the rabbit nictitating membrane response. *Journal of Pharmacology and Experimental Therapeutics, 225*(1), 42–49.

Hasselmo, M. (1995). Neuromodulation and cortical function: Modeling the physiological basis of behavior. *Behavioural Brain Research, 67,* 1–27.

Hasselmo, M., & Bower, J. (1993). Acetylcholine and memory. *Trends in Neurosciences, 16*(6), 218–222.

Hasselmo, M., Linster, C., Patil, M., Ma, D., & Cekic, M. (1997). Noradrenergic suppression of synaptic transmission may influence cortical "signal-to-noise" ratio. *Journal of Neurophysiology, 77,* 3326–3339.

Hasselmo, M., & Schnell, E. (1994). Laminar selectivity of the cholinergic suppression of synaptic transmission in rat hippocampal region CA1: Computational modeling and brain slice physiology. *Journal of Neuroscience, 14*(6), 3898–3914.

Hasselmo, M., Schnell, E., & Barkai, E. (1995). Dyamics of learning and recall at excitatory recurrent synapses and cholinergic modulation in rat hippocampal region CA3. *Journal of Neuroscience, 15*(7), 5249–5262.

Hasselmo, M., Wyble, B., & Wallenstein, G. (1996). Encoding and retrieval of episodic memories: Role of cholinergic and GABAergic modulation in hippocampus. *Hippocampus, 6*(6), 693–708.

Hebb, D. (1949). *The Organization of Behavior.* New York: Wiley.

Hermann, B., Seidenberg, M., Schoenfeld, J., & Davies, K. (1997). Neuropsychological characteristics of the syndrome of mesial temporal lobe epilepsy. *Archives of Neurology, 54*(4), 369–376.

Hilgard, E., Atkinson, R., & Atkinson, R. (1975). *Introduction to Psychology* (6th ed.). New York: Harcourt, Brace, Jovanovich.

Hilgard, E., & Bower, G. (1975). *Theories of Learning* (4th ed.). Englewood Cliffs, NJ: Prentice Hall.

Hinton, G. (1989). Connectionist learning procedures. *Artificial Intelligence, 40,* 185–234.

Hinton, G. (1992). How neural networks learn from experience. *Scientific American,* September, 145–151.

Hirsh, R. (1974). The hippocampus and contextual retrieval of information from memory: A theory. *Behavioral Biology, 12,* 421–444.

Holland, P. (1992). Occasion setting in Pavlovian conditioning. In D. Medin (Ed.), *The Psychology of Learning and Motivation* (pp. 69–125). New York: Acadamic Press.

Holland, P. (1997). Brain mechanisms for changes in processing of conditioned stimuli in Pavlovian conditioning: Implications for behavior theory. *Animal Learning and Behavior, 25*(4), 373–399.

Honey, R., & Good, M. (1993). Selective hippocampal lesions abolish the contextual specificity of latent inhibition and conditioning. *Behavioral Neuroscience, 107*(1), 23–33.

Honey, R., & Hall, G. (1989). Acquired equivalence and distinctiveness of cues. *Journal of Experimental Psychology: Animal Behavior Processes, 15*(4), 338–346.

Honey, R., & Hall, G. (1991). Acquired equivalence and distinctiveness of cues using a sensory-preconditioning procedure. *Quarterly Journal of Experimental Psychology, 43B,* 121–135.

Honey, R., Willis, A., & Hall, G. (1990). Context specificity in pigeon autoshaping. *Learning and Motivation, 21,* 125–136.

Hornik, K., Stinchcombe, M., & White, H. (1989). Multilayer feedforward networks are universal approximators. *Neural Networks, 2,* 359–366.

Hsaio, S., & Isaacson, R. (1971). Learning of food and water positions by hippocampus damaged rats. *Physiology and Behavior, 6,* 81–83.

Hull, C. (1943). *Principles of Behavior.* New York: Appleton-Century-Crofts.

Hull, C. (1952). *A Behavior System: An Introduction to Behavior Theory Concerning the Individual Organism.* New Haven: Yale University Press.

Irle, E., Woura, B., Kunert, H., Hampl, J., & Kunze, S. (1992). Memory disturbances following anterior communicating artery rupture. *Annals of Neurology, 31*(5), 473–480.

Jacobs, R. A. (1988). Increased rates of convergence through learning rate adaptation. *Neural Networks, 1,* 295–307.

James, G., Hardiman, M., & Yeo, C. (1987). Hippocampal lesions and trace conditioning in the rabbit. *Behavioural Brain Research, 23*(2), 109–116.

James, W. (1890). *Psychology (Briefer Course).* New York: Holt.

Japkowicz, N. (1999) *Concept-learning in the absence of counter-examples: An Autoassociation-Based Approach to Classification.* Ph.D. Thesis, Rutgers University.

Japkowicz, N., Myers, C., & Gluck, M. (1995). A novelty detection approach to classification. In *Proceedings of the International Joint Conference on Artificial Intelligence,* Montreal: Morgan Kaufman Publishers.

Jarrard, L. (1989). On the use of ibotenic acid to lesion selectively different components of the hippocampal formation. *Journal of Neuroscience Methods, 29,* 251–259.

Jarrard, L. (1993). On the role of the hippocampus in learning and memory in the rat. *Behavioral and Neural Biology, 60,* 9–26.

Jarrard, L., & Davidson, T. (1991). On the hippocampus and learned conditional responding: Effects of aspiration versus ibotenate lesions. *Hippocampus, 1,* 107–117.

Jarrard, L., Okaichi, H., Steward, O., & Goldschmidt, R. (1984). On the role of hippocampal connections in the performance of place and cue tasks: Comparisons with damage to hippocampus. *Behavioral Neuroscience, 98*(6), 946–954.

Jenkins, W., Merzenich, M., Ochs, M., Allard, T., & Guic-Robles, E. (1990). Functional reorganization of primary somatosensory cortex in adult owl monkeys after behaviorally controlled tactile stimulation. *Journal of Neurophysiology, 63*(1), 82–104.

Jones, R. (1993). Entorhinal-hippocampal connections: A speculative view of their function. *Trends in Neurosciences, 16*(2), 58–64.

Juliano, S. (1998). Mapping the sensory mosaic. *Science, 279,* 1653–1714.

Kalat, J. (1995). *Biological Psychology* (5th ed). New York: Brooks/Cole.

Kamin, L. (1968). "Attention-like" processes in classical conditioning. In M. Jones (Ed.), *Miami Symposium on the Prediction of Behavior, 1967: Aversive stimulation* (pp. 9–32). Coral Gables, FL: University of Miami Press.

Kamin, L. (1969). Predictability, surprise, attention and conditoning. In B. Campbell & R. Church (Eds.), *Punishment and Aversive Behavior* (pp. 279–296). New York: Appleton-Century-Crofts.

Kandel, E. R. (1976). *Cellular Basis of Behavior.* San Francisco: W. H. Freeman & Co.

Kaneko, T., & Thompson, R. (1997). Disruption of trace conditioning of the nictitating membrane response in rabbits by central cholinergic blockade. *Psychopharmacology, 131,* 161–166.

Kapur, N. (1993). Focal retrograde amnesia in neurological disease: A critical review. *Cortex, 29,* 217–234.

Kaye, H., & Pearce, J. (1987). Hippocampal lesions attenuate latent inhibition and the decline of the orienting response in rats. *Quarterly Journal of Experimental Psychology, 39B,* 107–125.

Kehoe, E. J. (1988). A layered network model of associative learning. *Psychological Review, 95*(4), 411–433.

Kelso, S. R., Ganong, A. H., & Brown, T. H. (1986). Hebbian synapses in hippocampus. *Proceedings of the National Academy of Science USA, 83,* 5326–5330.

Kesner, R. (1988). Reevaluation of the contribution of the basal forebrain cholinergic system to memory. *Neurobiology of Aging, 9,* 609–616.

Kilgard, M., & Merzenich, M. (1998). Cortical map reorganization enabled by nucleus basalis activity. *Science, 279,* 1714–1718.

Killcross, A., Kiernan, M., Dwyer, D., & Westbrook, R. (1998a). Loss of latent inhibition of contextual conditioning following non-reinforced context exposure in rats. *Quarterly Journal of Experimental Psychology B, 51*(1), 75–90.

Killcross, A., Kiernan, M., Dwyer, D., & Westbrook, R. (1998b). Effects of retention interval on latent inhibition and perceptual learning. *Quarterly Journal of Experimental Psychology, 51*(1), 59–74.

Killiany, R., Moss, M., Albert, M., Sandoor, T., Tieman, J., & Jolesz, F. (1993). Temporal lobe regions on magnetic resonance imaging identify patients with early Alzheimer's disease. *Archives of Neurology, 50,* 949–954.

Kim, J. J., & Fanselow, M. S. (1992). Modality-specific retrograde amnesia of fear. *Science, 256,* 675–677.

Kim, J., Krupa, D., & Thompson, R. (1998). Inhibitory cerebello-olivary projections and blocking effect in classical conditioning. *Science, 279*, 570–573.

Kimble, D. P. (1968). Hippocampus and internal inhibition. *Psychological Bulleting, 70*(5), 285–295.

Knapp, M., Knopman, D., Solomon, P., Pendlebury, W., Davis, C., & Gracon, S. (1994). A 30–week randomized controlled trial of high-dose Tacrine in patients with Alzheimer's Disease. *Journal of the American Medical Association, 271*(13), 985–991.

Knowlton, B., Ramus, S., & Squire, L. (1992). Intact artificial grammar learning in amnesia: Dissociation of classification learning and explicit memory for specific instances. *Psychological Science, 3*(3), 172–179.

Knowlton, B., Squire, L., & Gluck, M. (1994). Probabilistic classification learning in amnesia. *Learning and Memory, 1*, 106–120.

Kohonen, T. (1984). *Self-Organization and Associative Memory*. New York: Springer-Verlag.

Kohonen, T. (1988). The "neural" phonetic typewriter. *IEEE Computer, 21*, 11–22.

Kohonen, T., & Hari, R. (1999). Where the abstract feature maps of the brain might come from. *Trends in the Neurosciences, 22*(3), 135–139.

Konorski, J. (1967). *Integrative activity of the brain: An interdisciplinary approach.* Chicago: University of Chicago Press.

Kopelman, M., & Corn, T. (1988). Cholinergic "blockade" as a model for cholinergic depletion: A comparison of the memory deficits with those of Alzheimer-type dementia and the alcoholic Korsakoff syndrome. *Brain, 111* (part 5), 1079–1110.

Kraemer, P., & Roberts, W. (1984). The influence of flavor preexposure and test interval on conditioned taste aversions in the rat. *Learning and Motivation, 15*, 259–278.

Krnjevic, K., & Ropert, N. (1982). Electrophysiological and pharmacological characteristics of facilitation of hippocampal populations spikes by stimulation of the medial septum. *Neuroscience, 7*(9), 2165–2183.

Kronforst-Collins, M., Moriearty, P., Ralph, M., Becker, R., Schmidt, B., Thompson, L., & Disterhoft, J. (1997). Metrifonate treatment enhances acquisition of eyeblink conditioning in aging rabbits. *Pharmacology, Biochemistry and Behavior, 56*(1), 103–110.

Kubie, J. L., & Ranck, J. B., Jr. (1983). Sensory-behavioral correlates in individual hippocampus neurons in three situations: Space and context. In W. Seifert (Ed.), *Neurobiology of the Hippocampus* (pp. 433–447). London: Academic Press.

Kuffler, S., Nicholls, J., & Martin, A. (1984). *From Neuron to Brain: A Cellular Approach to the Function of the Nervous System.* Sunderland, MA: Sinauer Associates.

Lamour, Y., Dutar, P., & Jobert, A. (1984). Septo-hippocampal and other medial septum-diagonal band neurons: Electrophysiological and pharmacological properties. *Brain Research, 309*(2), 227–239.

Lashley, K. (1950). In search of the engram. In *Physiological Mechanisms in Animal Behavior: Symposium of the Society for Experimental Biology.* New York: Academic Press.

Lawrence, D. H. (1952). The transfer of a discrimination along a continuum. *Journal of Comparative and Physiological Psychology, 45,* 511–516.

Le Cun, Y. (1986). Learning processes in an asymmetric threshold network. In E. Bienenstock, F. Fogelman Souli, & G. Weisbuch (Eds.), *Disordered Systems and Biological Organization.* Berlin: Springer-Verlag.

LeDoux, J. (1993). Emotional memory systems in the brain. *Behavioural Brain Research, 58,* 69–79.

Lee, M., Chrobak, J., Sik, A., Wiley, R., & Buzsáki, G. (1994). Hippocampal theta activity following selective lesion of the septal cholinergic system. *Neuroscience, 62*(4), 1033–1047.

Levy, W. (1985). An information/computation theory of hippocampal function. *Society for Neuroscience Abstracts, 11,* 493.

Levy, W. (1989). A computational approach to hippocampal function. In R. Hawkins & G. Bower (Eds.), *Psychology of Learning and Motivation* (pp. 243–304). London: Academic Press.

Levy, W. (1990). Hippocampal theories and the information/computation perspective. In L. Erinoff (Ed.), *NIDA Monographs: Neurobiology of Drug Abuse: Learning and Memory* (pp. 116–125). Rockville, MD: U.S. Department of Health and Human Services, National Institute on Drug Abuse.

Levy, W. (1994). Unification of hippocampal function via computational considerations. In *Proceedings of the World Congress on Neural Networks, 1994,* (vol. 4, pp. IV-661–IV-666). San Diego.

Levy, W. (1996). A sequence predicting CA3 is a flexible associator that learns and uses context to solve hippocampal-like tasks. *Hippocampus, 6,* 579–590.

Levy, W., Brassel, S. E., & Moore, S. D. (1983). Partial quantification of the associative synaptic learning rule of the dentate gyrus. *Neuroscience, 8*(4), 799–808.

Levy, W., & Steward, O. (1983). Temporal contiguity requirements for long-term potentiation/depression in the hippocampus. *Neuroscience, 8*(4), 791–797.

Lopes da Silva, F., Groenewegen, H., Holsheimer, J., Room, P., Witter, M., van Groen, T., & Wadman, W. (1985). The hippocampus as a set of partially overlapping segments with a topographically organized system of inputs and outputs: The entorhinal cortex as a sensory gate, the medial septum as a gain-setting system and the ventral striatum as a motor interface. In G. Buzsáki & C. Vanderwolf (Eds.), *Electrical Activity of the Archicortex* (pp. 83–106). Budapest: Akademiai Kiado.

Lubow, R. (1973). Latent Inhibition. *Psychological Bulletin, 79,* 398–407.

Lubow, R. (1997). Latent inhibition as a measure of learned inattention: Some problems and solutions. *Behavioural Brain Research, 88,* 75–83.

Lubow, R., & Gewirtz, J. (1995). Latent inhibition in humans: Data, theory and implications for schizophrenia. *Psychological Bulletin, 117*(1), 87–103.

Lubow, R., Rifkin, B., & Alek, M. (1976). The context effect: The relationship between stimulus pre-exposure and environmental pre-exposure determines subsequent learning. *Journal of Experimental Psychology: Animal Behavior Processes, 2*(1), 38–47.

Lynch, G. (1986). *Synapses, Circuits and the Beginnings of Memory.* London: MIT Press.

Lynch, G., & Granger, R. (1992). Variations in synaptic plasticity and types of memory in corticohippocampal networks. *Journal of Cognitive Neuroscience, 4*(3), 189–199.

Lytton, W., & Sejnowski, T. (1991). Simulations of cortical pyramidal neurons synchronized by inhibitory interneurons. *Journal of Neurophysiology, 66*(3), 1059–1079.

Mackintosh, N. (1973). Stimulus selection: Learning to ignore stimuli that predict no change in reinforcement. In R. Hinde & J. Stevenson-Hinde (Eds.), *Constraints on Learning: Limitations and Predispositions* (pp. 75–96). New York: Academic Press.

Mackintosh, N. J. (1975). A theory of attention: Variations in the associability of stimuli with reinforcement. *Psychological Review, 82*(4), 276–298.

Mackintosh, N. J., & Little, L. (1970). An analysis of transfer along a continuum. *Canadian Journal of Psychology, 24*(5), 362–369.

Manning, F. (1994). Tacrine therapy for the dementia of Alzheimer's Disease. *American Family Physician, 50*(4), 819–826.

Maran, S., & Baudry, M. (1995). Properties and mechanisms of long-term synaptic plasticity in the mammalian brain: Relationships to learning and memory. *Neurobiology of Learning and Memory, 63*, 1–18.

Marchant, H., & Moore, J. (1973). Blocking of the rabbit's conditioned nictitating membrane response in Kamin's two-stage paradigm. *Journal of Experimental Psychology, 101*(1), 155–158.

Markowska, A., Olton, D., & Givens, B. (1995). Cholinergic manipulations in the medial septal area: Age-related effects on working memory and hippocampal electrophysiology. *Journal of Neuroscience, 15*(3, Pt. 1), 2063–2073.

Marr, D. (1969). A theory of cerebellar cortex. *Journal of Physiology, 202*(2), 437–470.

Marr, D. (1970). A theory for cerebral neocortex. *Proceedings of the Royal Society of London, B176*(43), 161–234.

Marr, D. (1971). Simple memory: A theory for archicortex. *Proceedings of the Royal Society, London, B262*(841), 23–81.

Marsh, G. (1969). An evaluation of three explanations for the transfer of discrimination effect. *Journal of Comparative and Physiological Psychology, 68*(2), 268–275.

Marston, H., Everitt, B., & Robbins, T. (1993). Comparative effects of excitotoxic lesions of the hippocampus and septum/diagonal band on conditional visual discrimination and spatial learning. *Neuropsychologia, 31*(10), 1099–1118.

Martin, I., & Levey, A. (1991). Blocking observed in human eyelid conditioning. *Quarterly Journal of Experimental Psychology B: Comparative and Physiological Psychology, 43*(3), 233–256.

Masur, D., Sliwinski, M., Lipton, R., Blau, A., & Crystal, H. (1994). Neuropsychological prediction of dementia and the absence of dementia in healthy elderly persons. *Neurology, 44*, 1427–1432.

Mazzoni, P., Andersen, R., & Jordan, M. (1991). A more biologically plausible learning rule for neural networks. *Proceedings of the National Academy of Sciences USA, 88*, 4433–4437.

McClelland, J., McNaughton, B., & O'Reilly, R. (1994). *Why we have complementary learning systems in the hippocampus and neocortex: Insights from the successes and failures of connectionist models of learning and memory* (Technical Report PDP.CNS.94.1). Pittsburgh: Carnegie Mellon University.

McCulloch, W., & Pitts, W. (1943). A logical calculus of the ideas immanent in nervous activity. *Bulletin of Mathematical Biophysics, 5,* 115–133.

McFarland, D., Kostas, J., & Drew, W. (1978). Dorsal hippocampal lesions: Effects of preconditioning CS exposure on flavor aversion. *Behavioral Biology, 22,* 398–404.

McIntosh, S., & Tarpy, R. (1977). Retention of latent inhibition in a taste-aversion paradigm. *Bulletin of the Psychonomic Society, 9,* 411–412.

McNaughton, B., & Barnes, C. (1990). From cooperative synaptic enhancement to associative memory: Bridging the abyss. *Seminars in the Neurosciences, 2,* 403–416.

McNaughton, B., & Morris, R. (1987). Hippocampal synaptic enhancement and information storage. *Trends in Neuroscience, 10*(10), 408–415.

McNaughton, B., & Nadel, L. (1990). Hebb-Marr networks and the neurobiological representation of action in space. In M. Gluck & D. Rumelhart (Eds.), *Neuroscience and Connectionist Theory* (pp. 1–63). Hillsdale, NJ: Lawrence Erlbaum Associates.

Merzenich, M., Kaas, J., Wall, J., Nelson, R., Sur, M., & Felleman, D. (1983). Topographic reorganization of somatosensory cortical areas 3b and 1 in adult monkeys following restricted deafferentation. *Neuroscience, 8,* 33–55.

Meyer, J. (1996). Hippocampal acetylcholine increases during eyeblink conditioning in the rabbit. *Physiology and Behavior, 60*(5), 1199–1203.

Micco, D., & Schwartz, M. (1997). Effects of hippocampal lesions upon the development of Pavlovian internal inhibition in rats. *Journal of Comparative and Physiological Psychology, 76*(3), 371–377.

Mighell, D., Wilkinson, T., & Goodman, J. (1989). Backpropagation and its application to handwritten signature verification. In D. Touretzky (Ed.), *Advances in Neural Information Processing Systems I* (pp. 340–347). San Mateo, CA: Morgan Kaufmann.

Miller, D., & Steinmetz, J. (1997). Hippocampal activity during classical discrimination-reversal eyeblink conditioning in rabbits. *Behavioral Neuroscience, 111*(1), 70–79.

Miller, L., Munoz, D., & Finmore, M. (1993). Hippocampal sclerosis and human memory. *Archives of Neurology, 50*(4), 391–394.

Miller, R., Barnet, R., & Grahame, N. (1995). Assessment of the Rescorla-Wagner Model. *Psychological Bulletin, 117*(3), 363–386.

Milner, B. (1962). Les troubles de la memoire accompagnant des lesions hippocampiques bilaterales. In P. Passouant (Ed.), *Physiologie de l'hippocampe.* Paris: Centre National de la Recherche Scientifique.

Milner, B., Corkin, S., & Teuber, J. (1968). Further analysis of the hippocampal amnesic syndrome: A 14–year follow-up study of HM. *Neuropsychologia, 6,* 215–234.

Minsky, M., & Papert, S. (1969). *Perceptrons.* Cambridge, MA: MIT Press.

Minsky, M., & Papert, S. (1998). *Perceptrons: Expanded Edition.* Cambridge, MA: MIT Press.

Mishkin, M. (1978). Memory in monkeys severely disrupted by combined but not by separate removal of amygdala and hippocampus. *Nature, 273,* 297–299.

Mishkin, M. (1982). A memory system in the monkey. *Philosophical Transactions of the Royal Society of London [Biology], 298,* 85–92.

Mishkin, M., & Delacour, J. (1975). An analysis of short-term visual memory in the monkey. *Journal of Experimental Psychology: Animal Behavior Processes, 1*(4), 326–334.

Mishkin, M., & Pribam, K. (1954). Visual discrimination performance following partial ablation of the temporal lobe. I: Ventral vs. lateral. *Journal of Comparative and Physiological Psychology, 47,* 14–20.

Mishkin, M., Vargha-Khadem, F., & Gadian, D. (1998). Amnesia and the organization of the hippocampal system. *Hippocampus, 8,* 212–216.

Miyamoto, M., Narumi, S., Nagaoka, A., & Coyle, J. (1989). Effects of continuous infusion of cholinergic drugs on memory impairment in rats with basal forebrain lesions. *Journal of Pharmacology and Experimental Therapy, 248*(2), 825–835.

Montague, P., Dayan, P., & Sejnowski, T. (1996). A framework for mesencephalic dopamine systems based on predictive Hebbian learning. *Journal of Neuroscience, 16*(5), 1936–1947.

Moore, J. (1979). Brain processes and conditioning. In A. Dickinson & R. Boakes (Eds.), *Mechanisms of Learning and Behavior* (pp. 111–142). Hillsdale, NJ: Lawrence Erlbaum Associates.

Moore, J., Goodell, N., & Solomon, P. (1976). Central cholinergic blockade by scopolamine and habituation, classical conditioning, and latent inhibition of the rabbit's nictitating membrane response. *Physiological Psychology, 4*(3), 395–399.

Moore, J., & Stickney, K. (1980). Formation of attentional-associative networks in real time: Role of the hippocampus and implications for conditioning. *Physiological Psychology, 8*(2), 207–217.

Morris, M., Bowers, D., Chatterjee, A., & Heilman, K. (1992). Amnesia following a discrete basal forebrain lesion. *Brain, 115,* 1827–1847.

Morris, R. (1983). An attempt to dissociate "spatial-mapping" and "working-memory" theories of hippocampal function. In W. Seifert (Ed.), *Neurobiology of the Hippocampus* (pp. 405–432). London: Academic Press.

Morris, R., Garrud, P., Rawlins, J., & O'Keefe, J. (1982). Place navigation impaired in rats with hippocampal lesions. *Nature, 297,* 681–683.

Mountcastle, V. (1979). An organizing principle for cerebral function: The unit module and the distributed system. In F. Schmitt & F. Worden (Eds.), *The Neurosciences: Fourth Study Program* (pp. 21–42). Cambridge, MA: MIT Press.

Moyer, J., Deyo, R., & Disterhoft, J. (1990). Hippocampectomy disrupts trace eye-blink conditioning in rabbits. *Behavioral Neuroscience, 104*(2), 243–252.

Muller, R., & Stead, M. (1996). Hippocampal place cells connected by Hebbian synapses can solve spatial problems. *Hippocampus, 6*(6), 709–719.

Mumby, D., Pinel, J., & Wood, E. (1990). Non-recurring-items delayed nonmatching-to-sample in rats: A new paradigm for testing nonspatial working memory. *Psychobiology, 18*(3), 321–326.

Murre, J. (1996). TraceLink: A model of amnesia and consolidation of memory. *Hippocampus, 6*(6), 675–684.

Myers, C., DeLuca, J., Schultheis, M., Schnirman, G., Ermita, B., Diamond, B., Warren, S., & Gluck, M. (in preparation). Impaired eyeblink classical conditioning in individuals with antero-grade amnesia resulting from anterior communicating artery aneurysm.

Myers, C., Ermita, B., Harris, K., Hasselmo, M., Solomon, P., & Gluck, M. (1996). A computational model of the effects of septohippocampal disruption on classical eyeblink conditioning. *Neurobiology of Learning and Memory, 66,* 51–66.

Myers, C., Ermita, B., Hasselmo, M., & Gluck, M. (1998). Further implications of a computational model of septohippocampal cholinergic modulation in eyeblink conditioning. *Psychobiology, 26*(1), 1–20.

Myers, C., & Gluck, M. (1994). Context, conditioning and hippocampal re-representation. *Behavioral Neuroscience, 108*(5), 835–847.

Myers, C., & Gluck, M. (1996). Cortico-hippocampal representations in simultaneous odor discrimination learning: A computational interpretation of Eichenbaum, Mathews & Cohen (1989). *Behavioral Neuroscience, 110*(4), 685–706.

Myers, C., Gluck, M., & Granger, R. (1995). Dissociation of hippocampal and entorhinal function in associative learning: A computational approach. *Psychobiology, 23*(2), 116–138.

Myers, C., Hopkins, R., Kesner, R., & Gluck, M. (2000). Localized hippocampal damage impairs acquisition, but not reversal, of a spatial discrimination in humans. *Psychobiology, 28*(3).

Myers, C., Kluger, A., Golomb, J., Ferris, S., de Leon, M., & Gluck, M. (1998). Predicting risk for Alzheimer's Dementia with a feature-irrelevant transfer task. *Abstracts of the Society for Neuroscience Annual Meeting (Los Angeles, CA),* 2116.

Myers, C., Kluger, A., Golomb, J., Ferris, S., de Leon, M., Schnirman, G., & Gluck, M. (in preparation). Hippocampal atrophy disrupts transfer generalization in non-demented elderly subjects.

Myers, C., McGlinchey-Berroth, R., Warren, S., Monti, L., Brawn, C., & Gluck, M. (2000). Latent learning in medial temporal amnesia: Evidence for disrupted representational but preserved attentional processes. *Neuropsychology, 14,* 3–15.

Myers, C., Oliver, L., Warren, S., & Gluck, M. (2000). Stimulus exposure effects in human associative learning. *Quarterly Journal of Experimental Psychology, 53B,* 173–187.

Nadel, L. (1991). The hippocampus and space revisited. *Hippocampus, 1*(3), 221–229.

Nadel, L. (1992). Multiple memory systems: What and why. *Journal of Cognitive Neuroscience, 4*(3), 179–188.

Nadel, L., & Willner, J. (1980). Context and conditioning: A place for space. *Physiological Psychology, 8*(2), 218–228.

Neimark, E., & Estes, W. (Eds.) (1967) *Stimulus Sampling Theory.* San Francisco: Holden-Day.

Nguyen, D., & Widrow, B. (1989). The truck backer-upper: An example of self-learning in neural networks. In *Proceedings of the International Joint Conference on Neural Networks IJCNN-90* (vol. II, pp. 357–363). Washington, DC.

Nosofsky, R. (1984). Choice, similarity, and the context theory of classification. *Journal of Experimental Psychology: Learning, Memory and Cognition, 10,* 104–114.

Nosofsky, R. (1988). Exemplar-based accounts of relations between classification, recognition and typicality. *Journal of Experimental Psychology: Learning, Memory and Cognition, 14*(4), 700–708.

Nudo, R., Milliken, G., Jenkins, W., & Merzenich, M. (1996). Use-dependent alterations of movement representations in primary motor cortex of adult squirrel monkeys. *Journal of Neuroscience, 16*(2), 785–807.

Ogura, H., & Aigner, T. (1993). MK-801 impairs recognition memory in Rhesus monkeys: Comparison with cholinergic drugs. *Journal of Pharmacology and Experimental Therapeutics, 266*, 60–64.

O'Keefe, J. (1979). A review of the hippocampal place cells. *Progress in Neurobiology, 13*, 419–439.

O'Keefe, J. (1983). Spatial memory within and without the hippocampal system. In W. Seifert (Ed.), *Neurobiology of the Hippocampus* (pp. 375–403). London: Academic Press.

O'Keefe, J. (1990). A computational theory of the hippocampal cognitive map. In J. Storm-Mathisen, J. Zimmer, & O. Ottersen (Eds.), *Progress in Brain Research* (vol. 83, pp. 301–312). New York: Elsevier Science.

O'Keefe, J., & Nadel, L. (1978). *The Hippocampus as a Cognitive Map.* Oxford: Clarendon University Press.

Oliver, A. (1988). Risk and benefit in the surgery of epilepsy: Complications and positive results on seizure and intellectual function. *Acta Neurologica Scandinavia, 78* (suppl. 117), 114–121.

Olton, D. (1983). Memory functions and the hippocampus. In W. Seifert (Ed.), *Neurobiology of the Hippocampus* (pp. 335–373). London: Academic Press.

O'Reilly, R., & McClelland, J. (1994). Hippocampal conjunctive encoding, storage, and recall: Avoiding a tradeoff. *Hippocampus, 4*, 661–682.

Oscar-Berman, M., & Zola-Morgan, S. (1980). Comparative neuropsychology and Korsakoff's syndrome. I: Spatial and visual reversal learning. *Neuropsychologia, 18*, 499–512.

Otto, T., Cousens, G., & Rajewski, K. (1997). Odor-guided fear conditioning in rats. 1: Acquisition, retention and latent inhibition. *Behavioral Neuroscience, 111*(6), 1257–1264.

Otto, T., & Eichenbaum, H. (1992). Complementary roles of the orbital prefrontal cortex and the perirhinal-entorhinal cortices in an odor-guided delayed-nonmatching-to-sample task. *Behavioral Neuroscience, 106*(5), 762–775.

Otto, T., Schottler, F., Staubli, U., Eichenbaum, H., & Lynch, G. (1991). Hippocampus and olfactory discrimination learning: Effects of entorhinal cortex lesions on olfactory learning and memory in a successive-cue, go-no-go task. *Behavioral Neuroscience, 105*(1), 111–119.

Owens, F. (1993). *Signal Processing of Speech.* New York: McGraw Hill.

Parker, D. (1985). *Learning Logic.* Cambridge, MA: MIT, Center for Computational Research in Economics and Management Science.

Parkin, A., Leng, N., & Stanhope, N. (1988). Memory impairment following ruptured aneurysm of the anterior communicating artery. *Brain and Cognition, 7*, 231–243.

Pavlov, I. (1927). *Conditioned Reflexes.* London: Oxford University Press.

Pearce, J., & Hall, G. (1980). A model for Pavlovian learning: Variations in the effectiveness of conditioned but not of unconditioned stimuli. *Psychological Review, 87*, 532–552.

Penick, S., & Solomon, P. (1991). Hippocampus, context and conditioning. *Behavioral Neuroscience, 105*(5), 611–617.

Pennartz, C. (1996). The ascending neuromodulatory systems in learning by reinforcement: Comparing computational conjectures with experimental findings. *Brain Research Reviews, 21,* 219–245.

Peterson, R. (1977). Scopolamine induced learning failures in man. *Psychopharmacologia, 52,* 283–289.

Pinto Hamuy, T., Santibanez, G., Gonzales, C., & Vicencio, E. (1957). Changes in behavior and visual discrimination preferences after selective ablations of the temporal cortex. *Journal of Comparative and Physiological Psychology, 50,* 379–385.

Pitton, J. W., Wang, K., & Juang, B.-H. (1996). Time-frequency analysis and auditory modeling for automatic speech recognition. *Proceedings of the IEEE, 84,* 1199–1214.

Port, R., Beggs, A., & Patterson, M. (1987). Hippocampal substrate of sensory associations. *Physiology and Behavior, 39,* 643–647.

Port, R., & Patterson, M. (1984). Fimbrial lesions and sensory preconditioning. *Behavioral Neuroscience, 98,* 584–589.

Port, R., Romano, A., & Patterson, M. (1986). Stimulus duration discrimination in the rabbit: Effects of hippocampectomy on discrimination and reversal learning. *Physiological Psychology, 4*(3, 4), 124–129.

Powell, D., Hernandez, L., & Buchanan, S. (1985). Intraseptal scopolamine has differential effects on Pavlovian eye blink and heart rate conditioning. *Behavioral Neuroscience, 99*(1), 75–87.

Price, J. (1973). An autoradiographic study of complementary laminar patterns of termination of afferent fiber to the olfactory cortex. *Journal of Comparative Neurology, 150,* 87–108.

Purves, D., Bonardi, C., & Hall, G. (1995). Enhancement of latent inhibition in rats with electrolytic lesions of the hippocampus. *Behavioral Neuroscience, 109*(2), 366–370.

Ramachandran, R., & Mammone, R. (Eds.). (1995). *Modern Methods of Speech Processing.* New York: Kluwer Academic Publishing.

Rasmusson, D. (1982). Reorganization of raccoon somatosensory cortex following removal of the fifth digit. *Journal of Comparative Neurology, 205,* 313–326.

Rawlins, J. (1985). Associations across time: The hippocampus as a temporary memory store. *Behavioral and Brain Sciences, 8,* 479–496.

Recce, M., & Harris, K. (1996). Memory for places: A navigational model in support of Marr's theory of hippocampal function. *Hippocampus, 6,* 735–748.

Redish, A. (1999). *Beyond the Cognitive Map: From Place Cells to Episodic Memory.* Cambridge, MA: MIT Press.

Redish, A., & Touretzky, D. (1997). Cognitive maps beyond the hippocampus. *Hippocampus, 7*(1), 15–35.

Reed, J., Squire, L., Patalano, A., Smith, E., & Jonides, J. (1999). Learning about categories that are defined by object-like stimuli despite impaired declarative memory. *Behavioral Neuroscience, 113,* 411–419.

Reed, R., & Marks, R. (1999). *Neural Smithing: Supervised Learning in Artificial Neural Networks.* Cambridge, MA: MIT Press.

Reilly, S., Harley, C., & Revusky, S. (1993). Ibotenate lesions of the hippocampus enhance latent inhibition in conditioned taste aversion and increase resistance to extinction in conditioned taste preference. *Behavioral Neuroscience, 107*(6), 996–1004.

Reiss, S., & Wagner, A. (1972). CS habituation produces a "latent inhibition effect" but no active "conditioned inhibition". *Learning and Motivation, 3,* 237–245.

Rescorla, R. (1976). Stimulus generalization: Some predictions from a model of Pavlovian conditioning. *Journal of Experimental Psychology: Animal Behavior Processes, 2*(1), 88–96.

Rescorla, R., & Wagner, A. (1972). A theory of Pavlovian conditioning: Variations in the effectiveness of reinforcement and non-reinforcement. In A. Black & W. Prokasy (Eds.), *Classical Conditioning II: Current Research and Theory* (pp. 64–99). New York: Appleton-Century-Crofts.

Rickert, E., Bennett, T., Lane, P., & French, J. (1978). Hippocampectomy and the attenuation of blocking. *Behavioral Biology, 22,* 147–160.

Rickert, E., Lorden, J., Dawson, R., & Smyly, E. (1981). Limbic lesions and the blocking effect. *Physiology and Behavior, 26,* 601–606.

Ridley, R., Timothy, C., Maclean, C., & Baker, H. (1995). Conditional learning and memory impairments following neurotoxic lesion of the CA1 field in hippocampus. *Neuroscience, 67*(2), 263–275.

Robinson, T., Bodruzzaman, M., & Malkani, M. (1994). Search for an improved time-frequency technique for neural network-based helicopter gearbox fault detection and classification. In *World Congress on Neural Networks* (vol. 2, pp. 238–243). San Diego.

Rogers, S., Friedhoff, L., & the Donepezil Study Group (1996). The efficacy and safety of donepezil in patients with Alzheimer's disease: Results of a US multicentre, randomized, double-blind, placebo-controlled trial. *Dementia, 7,* 293–303.

Rokers, B., Myers, C., & Gluck, M. (2000). A dynamic model of learning in the septo-hippocampal system. *Neurocomputing, 32–33,* 501–507.

Rolls, E. (1989). Functions of neuronal networks in the hippocampus and cerebral cortex in memory. In R. Cotterill (Ed.), *Models of Brain Function* (pp. 15–33). New York: Cambridge University Press.

Rolls, E. (1996). A theory of hippocampal function in memory. *Hippocampus, 6,* 601–620.

Roman, F., Staubli, U., & Lynch, G. (1987). Evidence for synaptic potentiation in a cortical network during learning. *Brain Research, 418,* 221–226.

Rosas, J., & Bouton, M. (1997). Additivity of the effects of retention interval and context change on latent inhibition: Toward resolution of the context forgetting paradox. *Journal of Experimental Psychology: Animal Behavior Processes, 23*(3), 283–294.

Rosenblatt, F. (1958). The perceptron: A probabilistic model for information storage and organization in the brain. *Psychology Review, 65,* 386–408.

Rothblat, L., & Kromer, L. (1991). Object recognition memory in the rat: The role of the hippocampus. *Behavioural Brain Research, 42,* 25–32.

Rudy, J. (1974). Stimulus selection in animal conditioning and paired-associate learning: Variation in associative processing. *Journal of Verbal Learning and Verbal Behavior, 13,* 282–296.

Rudy, J., & Sutherland, R. (1989). The hippocampal formation is necessary for rats to learn and remember configural discriminations. *Behavioural Brain Research, 34,* 97–109.

Rudy, J., & Sutherland, R. (1995). Configural association theory and the hippocampal formation: An appraisal and reconfiguration. *Hippocampus, 5,* 375–398.

Rumelhart, D., Hinton, G., & Williams, R. (1986). Learning internal representations by error propagation. In D. Rumelhart & J. McClelland (Eds.), *Parallel Distributed Processing: Explorations in the Microstructure of Cognition* (pp. 318–362). Cambridge, MA: MIT Press.

Rumelhart, D., & Zipser, D. (1985). Feature discovery by competitive learning. *Cognitive Science, 9,* 75–112.

Sachdev, R., Lu, S.-M., Wiley, R., & Ebner, F. (1998). Role of the basal forebrain cholinergic projection in somatosensory cortical plasticity. *Journal of Neurophysiology, 79,* 3216–3228.

Salafia, W., Romano, A., Tynan, T., & Host, K. (1977). Disruption of rabbit (*Oryctolagus cuniculus*) nictitating membrane conditioning by posttrial electrical stimulation of hippocampus. *Physiology and Behavior, 18,* 207–212.

Samsonovich, A., & McNaughton, B. (1997). Path integration and cognitive mapping in a continuous attractor network model. *Journal of Neuroscience, 17*(15), 5900–5920.

Santibanez, G., & Pinto Hamuy, T. (1957). Olfactory discrimination deficits in monkeys with temporal lobe ablations. *Journal of Comparative and Physiological Psychology, 50,* 472–474.

Schacter, D. (1985). Multiple forms of memory in humans and animals. In N. Weinberger, J. McGaugh, & G. Lynch (Eds.), *Memory Systems of the Brain: Animal and Human Cognitive Processes* (pp. 351–379). New York: Guildford Press.

Schacter, D., Harbluk, J., & McLachlan, D. (1984). Retrieval without recollection: An experimental analysis of source amnesia. *Journal of Verbal Learning and Verbal Behavior, 23,* 593–611.

Schmajuk, N. (1994). Stimulus configuration, classical conditioning, and spatial learning: Role of the hippocampus. In *World Congress on Neural Networks* (vol. 2, pp. II723–II728). San Diego: INNS Press.

Schmajuk, N., & Blair, H. (1993). Stimulus configuration, spatial learning and hippocampal function. *Behavioural Brain Research, 59,* 1–15.

Schmajuk, N., & Buhusi, C. (1997). Stimulus configuration, occasion setting and the hippocampus. *Behavioral Neuroscience, 111*(2), 235–258.

Schmajuk. N., & DiCarlo, J. (1990). *Backpropagation, classical conditioning and hippocampal function.* Chicago: Northwestern University.

Schmajuk, N., & DiCarlo, J. (1991). A neural network approach to hippocampal function in classical conditioning. *Behavioral Neuroscience, 105*(1), 82–110.

Schmajuk, N., & DiCarlo, J. (1992). Stimulus configuration, classical conditioning and hippocampal function. *Psychological Review, 99,* 268–305.

Schmajuk, N., Gray, J., & Lam, Y.-W. (1996). Latent inhibition: A neural network approach. *Journal of Experimental Psychology: Animal Behavior Processes, 22*(3), 321–349.

Schmajuk, N., Lam, Y.-W., & Christiansen, B. (1994). Latent inhibition of the rat eyeblink response: Effect of hippocampal aspiration lesions. *Physiology and Behavior, 55*(3), 597–601.

Schmajuk, N., & Moore, J. (1985). Real-time attentional models for classical conditioning. *Physiological Psychology, 13*(4), 278–290.

Schmajuk, N., & Moore, J. (1988). The hippocampus and the classically conditioned nictitating membrane response: A real-time attentional model. *Psychobiology, 16*(1), 20–35.

Schmajuk, N., Thieme, A., & Blair, H. (1993). Maps, routes, and the hippocampus: A neural network approach. *Hippocampus, 3*(3), 387–400.

Schmaltz, L., & Theios, J. (1972). Acquisition and extinction of a classically conditioned response in hippocampectomized rabbits (*Oryctolagus cuniculus*). *Journal of Comparative and Physiological Psychology, 79,* 328–333.

Schnider, A., Gutbrod, K., Hess, C., & Schroth, G. (1996). Memory without the context: Amnesia with confabulations after infarction of the right capsular genu. *Journal of Neurology, Neurosurgery and Psychiatry, 61*(2), 186–193.

Schultz, W., Dayan, P., & Montague, P. (1997). A neural substrate of prediction and reward. *Science, 275,* 1593–1599.

Scoville, W., & Milner, B. (1957). Loss of recent memory after bilateral hippocampal lesions. *Journal of Neurology, Neurosurgery and Psychiatry, 20,* 11–21.

Sears, L., & Steinmetz, J. (1991). Dorsal accessory olive activity diminishes during acquisition of the rabbit classically conditioned eyelid response. *Brain Research, 545*(1–2), 114–122.

Segal, M., & Olds, J. (1973). Activity of units in the hippocampal circuit of the rat during differential classical conditioning. *Journal of Comparative and Physiological Psychology, 82*(2), 195–204.

Seifert, W. (1983). In W. Seifert (Ed.), *Neurobiology of the Hippocampus* (p. 625). New York: Academic Press.

Sejnowski, T., & Rosenberg, C. (1986). *NETtalk: A parallel network that learns to read aloud* (JHU Technical Report No. JHU/EECS-86/01). Baltimore: Johns Hopkins University.

Selden, N., Everitt, B., Jarrard, L., & Robbins, T. (1991). Complementary roles for the amygdala and hippocampus in aversive conditioning to explicit and contextual cues. *Neuroscience, 42*(2), 335–350.

Sevush, S., Guterman, A., & Villalon, A. (1991). Improved verbal learning after outpatient oral physostigmine therapy in patients with dementia of the Alzheimer type. *Journal of Clinical Psychiatry, 52*(7), 300–303.

Sharp, P., Blair, H., & Brown, M. (1996). Neural network modeling of the hippocampal formation spatial signals and their possible role in navigation: A modular approach. *Hippocampus, 6*(6), 720–734.

Shepard, R. (1987). Towards a universal law of generalization for psychological science. *Science, 237,* 1317–1323.

Shohamy, D., Allen, M., & Gluck, M. (1999). Dissociating entorhinal and hippocampal function in latent inhibition of the classically conditioned eyeblink response. *Abstracts of the Society for Neuroscience Annual Meeting (Miami, FL), 25,* 40.14.

Siegel, S., & Allan, L. (1996). The widespread influence of the Rescorla-Wagner model. *Psychonomic Bulletin and Review, 3*(3), 314–321.

Singer, B., Zental, T., & Riley, D. (1969). Stimulus generalization and the easy-to-hard effect. *Journal of Comparative and Physiological Psychology, 69*(3), 528–535.

Smith, C., Coogan, J., & Hart, S. (1986). Effects of physostigmine on memory test performance in normal volunteers. *Psychopharmacology, 1986*(3), 364–366.

Solomon, P. (1977). Role of the hippocampus in blocking and conditioned inhibition of the rabbit's nictitating membrane. *Journal of Comparative and Physiological Psychology, 91*(2), 407–417.

Solomon, P. (1979). Temporal versus spatial information processing theories of hippocampal function. *Psychological Bulletin, 86,* 1272–1279.

Solomon, P., & Gottfried, K. (1981). The septohippocampal cholinergic system and classical conditioning of the rabbit's nictitating membrane response. *Journal of Comparative and Physiological Psychology, 95*(2), 322–330.

Solomon, P., Groccia-Ellison, M., Flynn, D., Mirak, J., Edwards, K., Dunehew, A., & Stanton, M. (1993). Disruption of human eyeblink conditioning after central cholinergic blockade with scopolamine. *Behavioral Neuroscience, 107*(2), 271–279.

Solomon, P., & Moore, J. (1975). Latent inhibition and stimulus generalization of the classically conditioned nictitating membrane response in rabbits (*Oryctolagus cuniculus*) following dorsal hippocampal ablation. *Journal of Comparative and Physiological Psychology, 89,* 1192–1203.

Solomon, P., Pomerleau, D., Bennett, L., James, J., & Morse, D. (1989). Acquisition of the classically conditioned eyeblink response in humans over the life span. *Psychology and Aging, 4*(1), 34–41.

Solomon, P., Solomon, S., Van der Schaaf, E., & Perry, H. (1983). Altered activity in the hippocampus is more detrimental to classical conditioning than removing the structure. *Science, 220,* 329–331.

Solomon, P., Van der Schaaf, E., Thompson, R., & Weisz, D. (1986). Hippocampus and trace conditioning of the rabbit's classically conditioned nictitating membrane response. *Behavioral Neuroscience, 100*(5), 729–744.

Solso, R. (1991). *Cognitive Psychology* (3rd ed.). Boston: Allyn & Bacon.

Spencer, D., & Lal, H. (1983). Effects of anticholinergic drugs on learning and memory. *Drug Development Research, 3,* 489–502.

Sperling, M., O'Connor, M., Saykin, A., & Plummer, C. (1996). Temporal lobectomy for refractory epilepsy. *Journal of the American Medical Association, 276,* 470–475.

Squire, L., & Knowlton, B. (1995). Memory, hippocampus and brain systems. In M. Gazzaniga (Ed.), *The Cognitive Neurosciences.* Cambridge, MA: MIT Press, pp. 825–837.

Squire, L., & Zola, S. (1998). Episodic memory, semantic memory and amnesia. *Hippocampus, 8,* 205–211.

Squire, L., & Zola-Morgan, S. (1988). Memory: Brain systems and behavior. *Trends in Neuroscience, 11*(4), 170–175.

Squire, L., Zola-Morgan, S., & Chen, K. (1988). Human amnesia and animal models of amnesia: Performance of amnesic patients on tests designed for the monkey. *Behavioral Neuroscience, 102*(2), 210–221.

Staubli, U., Fraser, D., Faraday, R., & Lynch, G. (1987). Olfaction and the "data" memory system in rats. *Behavioral Neuroscience, 101*(6), 757–765.

Staubli, U., Le, T., & Lynch, G. (1995). Variants of olfactory memory and their dependencies on the hippocampal formation. *Journal of Neuroscience, 15*(2), 1162–1171.

Steriade, M., McCormick, D., & Sejnowski, T. (1993). Thalamocortical oscillations in the sleeping and aroused brain. *Science, 262,* 679–685.

Stone, G. (1986). An analysis of the delta rule and the learning of statistical associations. In D. Rumelhart & J. McClelland, *Parallel Distributed Processing: Explorations in the Microstructure of Cognition* (vol. 1, pp. 444–459). Cambridge, MA: MIT Press.

Stork, D. (1989). Is backpropagation biologically plausible? In *Proceedings of the International Joint Conference on Neural Networks* (vol. II, pp. 241–246). Washington, D.C.

Sunderland, T., Tariot, P., Murphy, D., Weingartner, H., Mueller, E., & Cohen, R. (1985). Scopolamine changes in Alzheimer's disease. *Psychopharmacology, 87*(2), 247–249.

Sutherland, R., & Rudy, J. (1989). Configural association theory: The role of the hippocampal formation in learning, memory and amnesia. *Psychobiology, 17*(2), 129–144.

Sutton, G., Reggia, J., Armentrout, S., & D'Autrechy, C. L. (1994). Cortical map reorganization as a competitive process. *Neural Computation, 6,* 1–13.

Sutton, R., & Barto, A. (1981). Toward a modern theory of adaptive networks: Expectation and prediction. *Psychological Review, 88,* 135–170.

Suzuki, W. (1996). Neuroanatomy of the monkey entorhinal, perirhinal and parahippocampal cortices: Organization of cortical inputs and interconnections with amygdala and striatum. *Seminars in the Neurosciences, 8,* 3–12.

Swanson, L. (1979). The hippocampus: New anatomical insights. *Trends in Neurosciences, 2,* 9–12.

Szenthagothai, J. (1975). The "module-concept" in cerebral cortex architecture. *Brain Research, 95,* 475–496.

Tallal, P., Miller, S., Bedi, G., Byma, G., Wang, X., Nagarajan, S., Schreiner, C., Jenkins, W., & Merzenich, M. (1996). Language comprehension in language-learning impaired children improved with acoustically modified speech. *Science, 271,* 81–84.

Tallal, P., Miller, S., & Fitch, R. (1993). Neurobiological basis of speech: A case for the preeminence of temporal processing. *Annals of the New York Academy of Sciences, 682,* 27–47.

Tank, D., & Hopfield, J. (1987). Collective comptuation in neuronlike circuits. *Scientific American, 257*(6), 62–70.

Taube, J. (1991). Space, the final hippocampal frontier? *Hippocampus, 1*(3), 247–249.

Terrace, H. (1963). Discrimination learning with and without "errors." *Journal of Experimental Analysis of Behavior, 6*(1), 1–27.

Terrace, H. (1966). Discrimination learning and inhibition. *Science, 154,* 3757.

Terrace, H. (1974). On the nature of non-responding in discrimination learning with and without errors. *Journal of the Experimental Analysis of Behavior, 22,* 151–159.

Teyler, T., & DiScenna, P. (1986). The hippocampal memory indexing theory. *Behavioral Neuroscience, 100*(2), 147–154.

Thal, L., Fuld, P., Masur, D., & Sharpless, N. (1983). Oral physostigmine and lecithin improves memory in Alzheimer disease. *Annals of Neurology, 13,* 491–496.

Thompson, R. (1972). Sensory preconditioning. In R. Thompson & J. Voss (Eds.), *Topics in Learning and Performance* (pp. 105–129). New York: Academic Press.

Thompson, R. (1986). The neurobiology of learning and memory. *Science, 233,* 941–947.

Thompson, R., Berger, R., Berry, S., Hoehler, F., Kettner, R., & Weisz, D. (1980). Hippocampal substrate of classical conditioning. *Physiological Psychology, 8*(2), 262–279.

Tolman, E. (1932). *Purposive Behavior in Animals and Men.* New York: Appleton-Century-Croft. Reprint, University of California Press, 1949.

Tolman, E., & Honzik, C. (1930). Introduction and removal of reward, and maze performance in rats. *University of California Publications in Psychology, 4,* 257–275.

Touretzky, D., & Redish, A. (1996). Theory of rodent navigation based on interacting representations of space. *Hippocampus, 6*(3), 247–270.

Trabasso, T., & Bower, G. (1964). Concept identification. In R. Atkinson (Ed.), *Studies in Mathematical Psychology.* Stanford, CA: Stanford University Press.

Trabasso, T., & Bower, G. (1968). *Attention in Learning.* New York: Wiley.

Treves, A., & Rolls, E. (1992). Computational constraints suggest the need for two distinct input systems to the hippocampal CA3 network. *Hippocampus, 2*(2), 189–200.

Treves, A., & Rolls, E. (1994). Computational analysis of the role of the hippocampus in memory. *Hippocampus, 4*(3), 374–391.

Treves, A., Skaggs, W., & Barnes, C. (1996). How much of the hippocampus can be explained by functional constraints? *Hippocampus, 6*(6), 666–674.

Vanderwolf, C., Leung, L.-W., & Stewart, D. (1985). Two afferent pathways mediating hippocampal rhythmical slow-wave activity. In G. Buzsáki & C. Vanderwolf (Eds.), *Electrical Activity of the Archicortex* (pp. 47–66). Budapest: Akademiai Kiado.

van Hoesen, G., & Pandya, D. (1975). Some connections of the entorhinal (area 28) and perirhinal (area 35) cortices of the rhesus monkey. I: Temporal lobe afferents. *Brain Research, 95,* 1–24.

Vargha-Khadem, F., Gadian, D., Watkins, K., Connelly, A., Van Paesschen, W., & Mishkin, M. (1997). Differential effects of early hippocampal pathology on episodic and semantic memory. *Science, 277,* 376–332.

von der Malsburg, C. (1973). Self-organizing of orientation sensitive cells in the striate cortex. *Kybernetik, 14,* 85–100.

Vriesen, E., & Moscovitch, M. (1990). Memory for temporal order and conditional associative-learning in patients with Parkinson's Disease. *Neuropsychologia, 28*(12), 1283–1293.

Wagner, A., & Rescorla, R. (1972). Inhibition in Pavlovian conditioning: Application of a theory. In R. Boake & M. Halliday (Eds.), *Inhibition and Learning* (pp. 301–336). London: Academic Press.

Wagstaff, A., & McTavish, D. (1994). Tacrine: A review of its pharmacodynamic and pharmacokinetic properties, and therapeutic efficacy in Alzheimer's disease. *Drugs and Aging, 4*(6), 510–540.

Walkenbach, J., & Haddad, N. (1980). The Rescorla-Wagner theory of conditioning: A review of the literature. *The Psychological Record, 30*, 497–509.

Wall, J., & Cusick, C. (1984). Cutaneous responsiveness in primary somatosensory (S-I) hindpaw cortex before and after partial hindpaw deafferentation in adult rats. *Journal of Neuroscience, 4*, 1499–1515.

Wallenstein, G., Eichenbaum, H., & Hasselmo, M. (1998). The hippocampus as an associator of discontiguous events. *Trends in Neurosciences, 21*, 317–323.

Wallenstein, G., & Hasselmo, M. (1997). GABAergic modulation of hippocampal population activity: Sequence learning, place field development, and the phase precession effect. *Journal of Neurophysiology, 78*(1), 393–408.

Wang, X., Merzenich, M., Sameshima, K., & Jenkins, W. (1995). Remodelling of hand representation in adult cortex determined by timing of tactile stimulation. *Nature, 378*, 71–75.

Warren, S., Hier, D., & Pavel, D. (1998). Visual form of Alzheimer's disease and its response to anticholinersterase therapy. *Journal of Neuroimaging, 8*(4), 249–252.

Weinberger, N. (1993). Learning-induced changes of auditory receptive fields. *Current Opinion in Neurobiology, 3*, 570–577.

Weinberger, N. (1997). Learning-induced receptive field plasticity in the primary auditory cortex. *Seminars in Neuroscience, 9*, 59–67.

Weinberger, N., Javid, R., & Lepan, B. (1993). Long-term retention of learning-induced receptive field plasticity in auditory cortex. *Proceedings of the National Academy of Sciences USA, 90*, 2394–2398.

Weiner, I. (1990). Neural substrates of latent inhibition: The switching model. *Psychological Bulletin, 108*(3), 442–461.

Weiner, I., & Feldon, J. (1997). The switching model of latent inhibition: An update of neural substrates. *Behavioural Brain Research, 88*, 11–25.

Weiskrantz, L., & Warrington, E. (1979). Conditioning in amnesic patients. *Neuropsychologia, 17*, 187–194.

Weiss, K., Friedman, R., & McGregor, S. (1974). Effects of septal lesions on latent inhibition and habituation of the orienting response in rats. *Acta Neurobiologica Experimentalis, 34*, 491–504.

Werbos, P. (1974) *Beyond Regression: New Tools for Prediction and Analysis in the Behavioral Sciences.* Ph.D. Thesis, Harvard University.

West, M. (1990). Stereological studies of the hippocampus: A comparison of the hippocampal subdivisions of diverse species including hedgehogs, laboratory rodents, wild mice and men. *Progress in Brain Research, 83,* 13–36.

West, M., Christian, E., Robinson, J., & Deadwyler, S. (1982). Evoked potentials in the dentate gyrus reflect the retention of past sensory events. *Neuroscience Letters, 28,* 325–329.

Westbrook, R. F., Bond, N., & Feyer, A.-M. (1981). Short- and long-term decrements in toxicosis-induced odor-aversion learning: The role of duration of exposure to an odor. *Journal of Experimental Psychology: Animal Learning and Behavior, 7*(4), 362–381.

Wetherell, A. (1992). Effects of physostigmine on stimulus encoding in a memory-scanning task. *Psychopharmacology, 109,* 198–202.

Whishaw, I., & Tomie, J.-A. (1991). Acquisition and retention by hippocampal rats of simple, conditional and configural tasks using tactile and olfactory cues: Implications for hippocampal function. *Behavioral Neuroscience, 105*(6), 787–797.

Whitehouse, P., Price, D., Struble, R., Clark, A., Coyle, J., & DeLong, M. (1982). Alzheimer's disease and senile dementia: Loss of neurons in the basal forebrain. *Science, 215,* 1237–1239.

Wible, C., Eichenbaum, H., & Otto, T. (1990). A task designed to demonstrate a declarative memory representation of odor cues in rats. *Society for Neuroscience Abstracts, 16*(6), 605.

Wickelgren, W. (1979). Chunking and consolidation: A theoretical synthesis of semantic networks, configuring in conditioning, S-R versus cognitive learning, normal forgetting, the amnesic syndrome, and the hippocampal arousal system. *Psychological Review, 86*(1), 44–60.

Widrow, B., Gupta, N., & Maitra, S. (1973). Punish/reward: Learning with a critic in adaptive systems. *IEEE Transactions on Systems, Man and Cybernetics, SMC-3*(5), 455–465.

Widrow, B., & Hoff, M. (1960). Adaptive switching circuits. *Institute of Radio Engineers, Western Electronic Show and Convention Record, 4,* 96–104.

Widrow, B., & Winter, R. (1988). Neural nets for adaptive filtering and adaptive pattern recognition. *IEEE Computer,* March, 1988, 25–39.

Widrow, B., Winter, R., & Baxter, R. (1988). Layered neural nets for pattern recognition. *IEEE Transactions on Acoustics, Speech and Signal Processing, 36*(7), 1109–1118.

Wiedemann, G., Georgilas, A., & Kehoe, E. J. (1999). Temporal specificity in patterning of the rabbit nictitating membrane response. *Animal Learning and Behavior, 27*(1), 99–107.

Wiener, S., Paul, C., & Eichenbaum, H. (1988). Spatial and behavioral correlates of hippocampal neuronal activity. *Journal of Neuroscience, 9*(8), 2737–2763.

Wiesel, T. (1982). Postnatal development of the visual cortex and the influence of environment. *Nature, 299,* 583–591.

Willshaw, D., & Buckingham, J. (1990). An assessment of Marr's theory of the hippocampus as a temporary memory store. *Philosophical Transactions of the Royal Society of London, B329,* 205–215.

Wilson, A., Brooks, D., & Bouton, M. (1995). The role of the rat hippocampal system in several effects of context in extinction. *Behavioral Neuroscience, 109*(5), 828–836.

Wilson, B., Baddeley, A., Evans, J., & Shiel, A. (1994). Errorless learning in the rehabilitation of memory impaired people. *Neuropsychological Rehabilitation, 4*(3), 307–326.

Wilson, F., & Rolls, E. (1990). Learning and memory is reflected in the responses of reinforcement-related neurons in the primate basal forebrain. *Journal of Neuroscience, 10,* 1254–1267.

Wilson, M., & McNaughton, B. (1993). Dynamics of the hippocampal ensemble code for space. *Science, 261,* 1055–1058.

Winocur, G. (1990). Anterograde and retrograde amnesia in rats with dorsal hippocampal or dorsomedial thalamic lesions. *Behavioral Brain Research, 38,* 145–154.

Winocur, G., & Gilbert, M. (1984). The hippocampus, context and information processing. *Behavioral and Neural Biology, 40,* 27–43.

Winocur, G., & Olds, J. (1978). Effects of context manipulation on memory and reversal learning in rats with hippocampal lesions. *Journal of Comparative and Physiological Psychology, 92*(2), 312–321.

Winocur, G., Rawlins, J., & Gray, J. (1987). The hippocampus and conditioning to contextual cues. *Behavioral Neuroscience, 101*(5), 617–625.

Woodhams, P., Celio, M., Ulfig, N., & Witter, M. (1993). Morphological and functional correlates of borders in the entorhinal cortex and hippocampus. *Hippocampus, 3* (Special Issue on Entorhinal–Hippocampal Interaction, eds. R. Nitsch & T. Ohm), 303–311.

Woodruff-Pak, D. (1993). Eyeblink classical conditioning in HM: Delay and trace paradigms. *Behavioral Neuroscience, 107*(6), 911–925.

Woodruff-Pak, D., Li, Y., Kazmi, A., & Kem, W. (1994a). Nicotinic cholinergic system involvement in eyeblink classical conditioning in rabbits. *Behavioral Neuroscience, 108*(3), 486–493.

Woodruff-Pak, D., Li, Y., & Kem, W. (1994b). A nicotinic agonist (GTS-21), eyeblink classical conditioning, and nicotinic receptor binding in rabbit brain. *Brain Research, 645*(1–2), 309–317.

Yee, B., Feldon, J., & Rawlins, J. (1995). Latent inhibition in rats is abolished by NMDA-induced neuronal loss in the retrohippocampal region, but this lesion effect can be prevented by systemic haloperidol treatment. *Behavioral Neuroscience, 109*(2), 227–240.

Yeo, C., Hardiman, M., & Glickstein, M. (1985). Classical conditioning of the nictitating membrane response of the rabbit. I: Lesions of the cerebellar nuclei. *Experimental Brain Research, 60*(1), 87–98.

Young, B., Otto, T., Fox, G., & Eichenbaum, H. (1997). Memory representation within the parahippocampal region. *Journal of Neuroscience, 17*(13), 5183–5195.

Zackheim, J., Myers, C., & Gluck, M. (1998). A temporally sensitive recurrent network model of occasion setting. In N. Schmajuk & P. Holland (Eds.), *Occasion Setting: Associative Learning and Cognition in Animals* (pp. 319–342). Washington, DC: American Psychological Association.

Zalstein-Orda, N., & Lubow, R. (1994). Context control of negative transfer induced by preexposure to irrelevant stimuli: Latent inhibition in humans. *Learning and Motivation, 26,* 11–28.

Zigmond, M., Bloom, F., Landis, S., Roberts, J., & Squire, L. (1999a). *Fundamental Neuroscience.* New York: Academic Press.

Zigmond, M., Bloom, F., Landis, S., Roberts, J., & Squire, L. (1999b). *Fundamental Neuroscience Images, Version 1.0*. New York: Academic Press.

Zola-Morgan, S., & Squire, L. (1985). Medial temporal lesions in monkeys impair memory on a variety of tasks sensitive to human amnesia. *Behavioral Neuroscience, 99*(1), 22–34.

Zola-Morgan, S., & Squire, L. (1986). Memory impairment in monkeys following lesions limited to the hippocampus. *Behavioral Neuroscience, 100*(2), 155–160.

Zola-Morgan, S., & Squire, L. (1993). Neuroanatomy of memory. *Annual Review of Neuroscience, 16*, 547–563.

Zola-Morgan, S., Squire, L., & Amaral, D. (1986). Human amnesia and the medial temporal region: Enduring memory impairments following a bilateral lesion limited to field CA1 of the hippocampus. *Journal of Neuroscience, 6*(10), 2950–2967.

Zola-Morgan, S., Squire, L., & Amaral, D. (1989a). Lesions of the amygdala that spare adjacent cortical regions do not impair memory or exacerbate the impairment following lesions of the hippocampal formation. *Journal of Neuroscience, 9*(6), 1922–1936.

Zola-Morgan, S., Squire, L., & Amaral, D. (1989b). Lesions of the hippocampal formation but not lesions of the fornix or the mammillary nuclei produce long-lasting memory impairment in monkeys. *Journal of Neuroscience, 9*(3), 898–913.

Zola-Morgan, S., Squire, L., & Ramus, S. (1994). Severity of memory impairment in monkeys as a function of locus and extent of damage within the medial temporal lobe memory system. *Hippocampus, 4*(4), 483–495.

Author Index

Page references followed by letters *f* and *n* indicate figures and notes, respectively. Page references enclosed in square brackets indicate textual references to endnotes.

Gage, F., [336n57], 388n57

Gallagher, M., [171n42], 174, [174n44], [176n47], [176n48], [202n27], [207n38], 271, [325n34], 379n42, 379n44, 379n47, 379n48, 381n27, 388n34

Ganong, A. H., [114n6], 377n6

Gao, E., [251n42], [251n43], 384n42, 384n43

Garrigou, D., [309n5], 387n5

Garrud, P., [29n21], [29n22], [29n23], [171n42], 373n21, 373n22, 374n23, 379n42

Gazzaniga, M., 16f

George, A., 296f, [296n49], [296n50], [296n51], [297n52], [341n68], 386n49, 386n50, 386n51, 386n52, 389n68

Georgilas, A., [176n49], 379n49

Georgopoulos, A., [87n4], [87n7], 376n4, 376n7

Gewirtz, J., [202n25], 381n25

Ghoneim, M., [317n18], 387n18

Gilbert, M., [209n50], 382n50

Gilchrist, J., [109n20], 377n20

Givens, B., [322n26], 387n26

Glauthier, P., [334n53], 388n53

Glickstein, M., [72n28], 375n28

Gluck, M., [34n32], 35f, [52n6], 53, 66, [69n22], [72n29], [73n33], [74n33], [78n37], 97, [97n11], 99n, [99n12], [99n13], [109n20], [145n1], [148n3], 150, 152f, [152n5], [156n9], [157n11], 159f, [159n13], 160f, [160n14], [162n20], [179n61], [180n61], [180n67], [181n72], [182n73], [182n74], [182n76], [182n77], 183f, [183n78], [183n79], 184, 184f, 186, 198f, [198n18], [198n20], 199f, [199n22], [201n23], [202n26], 203f, [203n28], [203n30], 204f, [207n41], [210n53], 211f, [212n62], [215n1], [237n18], 239f, [241n27], [243n31], 244f, 246f, [247n33], 249f, [249n36], [249n37], 257, [266n5], [266n6], [268n7], [271n9], 272f, [272n10], 273f, [273n13], [273n15], [274n17], [275n18], [275n19], 276f, [278n21], [279n23], [280n25], [293n47], [297n53], 298f, 300f, [301n54], 303, 303f, [309n8], 310f, 319, [319n20], 320f, [320n23], 321f, [322n28], 323f, 325f, [325n32], 326f, [326n36], 327f, [328n38], 329f, [332n50], [332n51], [334n52], [334n53], 340f, [340n65], [340n66], 342, [348n8], 356, 357, 374n6, 374n32, 375n22, 375n29, 375n31, 376n11, 376n12, 376n13,

376n30, 376n33, 376n37, 378n1, 378n3, 378n5, 378n9, 378n11, 378n13, 378n14, 378n20, 380n61, 380n67, 380n72, 380n73, 380n74, 380n76, 380n77, 380n78, 380n79, 381n18, 381n20, 381n22, 381n23, 381n26, 381n28, 381n30, 382n41, 382n53, 383n1, 383n62, 384n18, 384n27, 384n31, 384n33, 384n36, 384n37, 385n5, 385n6, 385n7, 385n9, 385n10, 385n13, 385n15, 385n17, 385n18, 385n19, 385n21, 386n23, 386n25, 386n47, 386n53, 386n54, 387n8, 387n20, 387n23, 387n28, 388n32, 388n36, 388n38, 388n50, 388n51, 388n52, 388n53, 389n8, 389n65, 389n66

Goebel, J., [293n47], 386n47

Goldschmidt, R., [243n30], [309n8], [347n6], 384n30, 387n8, 389n6

Golomb, J., 296f, [296n49], [296n50], [297n52], [297n53], 298f, 300f, [301n54], [341n68], 386n49, 386n50, 386n52, 386n53, 386n54, 389n68

Gómez-Isla, T., [302n55], 386n55

Gonzales, C., [240n25], 384n25

Good, M., 190f, [190n4], [191n6], [193n12], [193n13], 198f, [198n19], [199n21], [203n29], [209n49], 271, [271n8], 276f, [278n22], [279n24], 381n4, 381n6, 381n12, 381n13, 381n19, 381n21, 382n29, 382n49, 385n8, 385n22, 386n24

Goodall, G., [171n42], 379n42

Goodall, S., [223n9], 383n9

Goodell, N., [325n33], 326f, 388n33

Goodman, J., [109n20], 376n20

Gorman, R. P., [109n20], 377n20

Gormezano, I., [33n25], 59f, 60f, [317n17], [326n35], 327f, 374n25, 387n17, 388n35

Gottfried, K., [328n39], [330n41], 388n39, 388n41

Gracon, S., [341n71], 389n71

Grahame, N., [43n1], [68n21], 374n1, 375n21

Grandguillaume, P., [218n2], [250n38], 383n2, 384n38

Granger, R., [124n20], [196n17], 234, [234n16], [234n17], 235f, 237, [237n18], 250, [257n49], [266n5], [266n6], [268n7], [272n10], [273n15], [275n19], 276f, [278n21], [279n23], 303, 357, 377n20, 381n17, 384n16, 384n17,

Subject Index

Page references followed by *t* and *f* refer to tables and figures, respectively.